Tracey Cox is Australia's foremost sex and relationships writer and has a degree in psychology. A former associate editor of *Cosmopolitan*, she contributes regularly to leading women's magazines.

HOT SEX

HOW TO DO IT

TRACEY COX

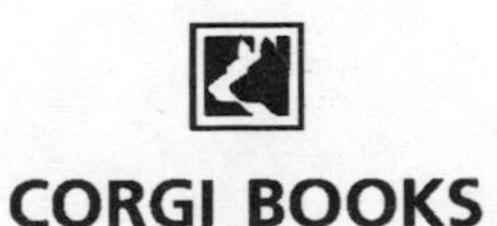

HOT SEX
A CORGI BOOK : 0 552 14707 9

First publication in Great Britain

PRINTING HISTORY
Corgi edition published 1999

3 5 7 9 10 8 6 4 2

Corgi Books are published by Transworld Publishers Ltd, 61–63 Uxbridge Road, London W5 5SA, in Australia by Transworld Publishers, c/o Random House Australia Pty Ltd, 20 Alfred Street, Milsons Point, NSW 2061, in New Zealand by Transworld Publishers, c/o Random House New Zealand, 18 Poland Road, Glenfield, Auckland and in South Africa by Transworld Publishers, c/o Random House (Pty) Ltd, Endulini, 5a Jubilee Road, Parktown 2193.

Edited by Jane Bowring
Text design by Cheryl Collins Design

Reproduced, printed and bound in Great Britain by Cox & Wyman Ltd, Reading, Berkshire.

In memory of James Rupert Murdoch 1988–1989

Contents

Acknowledgements

Many people have contributed to this book, both with information and moral support. At the risk of sounding like an Oscar winner, I really would like to thank my family (Shirley, Terry, Patrick, Maureen, Nigel, Deborah, Doug, Charles and Madeleine) and *all* my friends and work colleagues who supported and encouraged me when I needed it most.

Special thanks go to: Deborah Murdoch, my clever sister, for casting an experienced medical eye over the technical chapters and so generously sharing her expertise; Nigel Cox, my brother, for bravely providing an intimate male perspective without ever telling me to mind my own business; Ute Junker, for reading every word of the manuscript, ever so tactfully pointing out my errors and putting up with the anxiety attacks; Janet Muggivan, for her inspired publicity and marketing ideas and unwavering belief in both the project and me; Pat Ingram, the best editor in the business, who took me under her wing and taught me so much about journalism and life; Eric Fleming, Janet Hall and Grant Brecht, three of Australia's most respected psychologists, who've cheerfully given up so much of their time to teach me about sex and relationships; Shona Martyn, Jude McGee and Jane Bowring for having faith in the idea and guiding me through my introduction to book publishing with such good humour and style; Edith Weisberg, from Family Planning, who lent her formidable expertise to Chapter 6; Di Palmer, manager of Sydney's Club Femme, for making sense of all the weird and wonderful contraptions she sells in her erotica store; Amanda Dwyer, owner/operator of Salon Kitty's, who shared her sex secrets; Gerard Webster, a psychologist specialising in sexual abuse, who contributed immensely to several chapters in the book; Fiona Lecren, from Australian Birth Control, and Genevieve Graham, from the Child Protection Enforcement Agency, for advising on serious sex-related issues.

A huge thank you also to everyone who bared their souls anonymously and contributed real-life quotes and advice throughout the book; and the sex diary authors and the sex workers, Olivia and David, for their wonderfully frank guides in the foreplay chapter.

Thanks to the various magazines who allowed me to use some small sections from my previously published stories. Some of the information contained in this book originally appeared in:

Cosmopolitan: 'Blow Him Away', October 1996; 'The Top 10 Lies About Sex', February 1995; 'The 50 Most Intimate Things to Do With a Man', November 1994; 'The New Sex Rules', April 1995; *Australian Women's Forum:* 'Masturbation: At Your Fingertips', May 1996; 'The Sex Diaries', March 1995; *marie claire:* 'Complete Guide to Contraception', February 1996.

Publisher's Note

This book was originally published in Australia so a few changes have been made to the text in order to make the information as relevant and helpful as possible for readers in the UK.

Introduction

Anyone can be good in bed. Genital size doesn't matter. Looks don't matter. You don't have to have legs up to your chin, arms like Arnie, drive a sportscar or be rolling in it to be the best lover your partner's ever had. But you *do* need a good, working knowledge of your subject. And that's easier said than done.

Nearly everyone talks about sex. We're always boasting about how *fabulous* so-and-so is in bed and hinting at the real reason why we look so tired at work (nudge, nudge, wink, wink). But it's a rare person who'll confess details or talk specifics. Jane might well confide that Brad gives the best oral she's ever had but she doesn't launch into a lick-by-lick analysis of *why* – and I bet you don't ask for one.

That's why we buy sex books – to find out the nitty-gritty details about things we're too embarrassed to ask friends or lovers. Trouble is, few deliver what we really want to know. Sex manuals tend to gloss over the practical bread-and-butter stuff and, instead, talk in generalities – like how women need clitoral stimulation and men's bottoms are a veritable hot spot. Great advice but, if you haven't got the foggiest of what to do with it, useless.

This is where *Hot Sex* is different. Instead of assuming you know everything, I've assumed you know nothing and have dished up *all* the gory details in an easy-to-follow, step-by-step format. The only way I could have been more explicit and specific is to be there in the bedroom with you, guiding your hands and whatever else you're using (and, to tell the truth, I'd really rather not.)

That's not to say the book *only* deals with the basics. Experienced lovers will get heaps out of *Hot Sex* because there are enough advanced tips, tricks and techniques to keep even Madame Lash happy. But I *do* suggest everyone reads the introductory chapters. Very often it's the people who *think* they know what they're doing who need educating the most. Sex is a bit like typing. You can get by using two fingers, but you'll never be as good as someone who did the secretarial course and practised every night. Going back to the grass-roots level, even if it's just to check you're on the right track, isn't a bad idea for all of us. Don't let anyone tell you otherwise: sex skills can be learned and we can *all* improve on them.

I've written the book using everyday language for similar reasons. The correct, technical terms sound terribly authoritative but if *you* don't know that a wet dream is actually called a nocturnal emission, you wouldn't have a clue what I was talking about if I used this term. Sometimes, the words I use aren't even accurate. Most people say 'sperm' when they actually mean 'semen', for instance. But, hey, if that's what you call it, that's what I've called it a lot of the time because I want you to relate to what I'm saying.

I'm also guilty of making some broad generalisations about sex. Hopefully, there aren't too many but if you read something that you personally don't agree with, forgive me. If I covered every single individual preference, research finding, exception and extreme, I'd still be madly typing away at my computer!

Hot Sex is designed to be read cover to cover but it is equally useful if you dip into it for inspiration when the mood strikes. Because good sex is only possible if *both* the people having it are committed to making it great, I've included guides for him and her wherever possible. *Hot Sex* isn't ageist either. There's info on all the different stages of our sexual lives: everything from first-time masturbation and losing your virginity to having sex when you're pregnant and taking the monotony out of monogamy. Add hints on ditching those inhibitions, tips on building effective communication skills and heaps of relationship advice, and you really can't help but shred the sheets!

HOT SEX

Masturbation

The first, most important, skip-it-and-you're-doomed step to becoming a sexpert

Human beings are funny creatures. We'll chortle over whether to swallow or not swallow and turn that disastrous attempt at a new intercourse position into dinner party fodder, but when it comes to the most innocent, basic sexual act of all, we're about as likely to 'fess up as the guy in the corner suffering silently from an attack of piles. We might well be the most sexually uninhibited generation so far, but masturbation, particularly female masturbation, still has a dirty name.

Even my friends, used to me blurting out all sorts of bizarre sex statistics, aren't comfortable with it.

'What do you do to break the boredom of sitting behind a computer for hours on end?' a girlfriend asked me recently, during lunch with a group of friends.

'Drink coffee mostly,' I answered. 'Oh – and I masturbate. It's a little treat that breaks up the day and perks me up no end.'

There was a deathly silence. Knives and forks paused mid-air, someone choked on a mouthful of wine. *'Excuse me?'* my friend spluttered, redder than the beetroot on her plate.

'I said I take masturbation breaks,' I repeated lamely. And even *I* started to feel a tad embarrassed.

'You don't talk about it. The most you'll say to your mates is, "I went home and had a wank." But you always say it jokingly, so they don't really know if it's true. Not once has another guy ever turned to me and said, "How do you do it?" If he did, I'd probably think he was gay.'

Scott, 18, student

The fact is, although everybody does it (and if they don't, they should), few admit it and *no-one* discusses it freely. Masturbation remains one of the few sex subjects that can make the most liberated person blush. The same girl who'll cheerfully masturbate when she's between partners feels guilty if she continues when she's getting regular sex. Lots still view masturbation as something you do when 'you can't get any', fearing that if they're 'reduced' to masturbating, they're not sexually desirable enough to score 'the real thing'.

In reality, the more sexually active you are, the more likely you are to masturbate, regardless of whether you do or don't have a partner. Kinsey, the world's best known sex expert, found people who masturbated early in life led more vigorous sex lives than those who didn't, and continued having an active sex life long past when the average person stopped.

This is one area where men come up trumps. Most women masturbate about once a week, often not doing it regularly until their late teens. Most men masturbate at least twice as often, and started doing so around 12 or 13 years of age. Of the women who have discovered its joys, virtually all can masturbate to orgasm – 95 per cent of us, in fact (and some researchers put that figure even higher). On the opposite side, if you're a female who has never masturbated, statistics indicate it's quite likely you've never had an orgasm in your life. Pretty strong support for solo sex!

The truth is good girls *do* do it and if you never have and won't try, give up now on ever having a fulfilling sex life. Masturbation is a sure way (often the only way) to discover what turns you on sexually, and unless you know how to excite yourself, you've got zero chance of telling your partner how to. Few of us are lucky enough to start our sexual lives with a lover who's so patient and skilled he can teach us about our own body. Besides, masturbating is good for you. It releases tension, frees inhibitions, is gloriously liberating – and beats the hell out of counting sheep if you're having trouble dropping off!

Convinced but have no idea how it's done? It takes a brave person (and a few million drinks) to ask even your closest friend to tell you stroke-by-stroke how to do it. Luckily, you don't need to. In this chapter, you'll find no-nonsense, no-holds-barred, practical information on everything you ever wanted and needed to know about solo sex.

> 'The first time I masturbated, I was riddled with guilt. I'd heard horrible things about it: it was socially unacceptable, something you shouldn't do, it was dirty and messy. The general impression was only dirty old men wank. I now consider masturbating extremely healthy but while no-one now denies doing it, no-one really admits it either. My fantasies usually revolve around the person I'm with. I'll deliberately watch her face and her movements while we're making love, then replay them as I masturbate. I relive the sensations and try to copy the same technique she used on me to add reality. I love going down on her and most of my fantasies revolve around giving her oral sex. Sometimes, I'll catch myself moving my tongue as I'm masturbating, I'm so far into the fantasy.'
>
> Tim, 32, sales representative

A BIOLOGY LESSON THEY DIDN'T GIVE YOU AT SCHOOL

Sex is an acquired skill and you need to do your homework to become an expert. You'll never master the guitar without finding out where to put your fingers to play a note and sex is no different: you need to know some basic anatomy. Surprisingly few people take time out to discover how their body's sexual response system works. For men, this isn't too much of a problem. The penis is easy to study – all he has to do is look down and play around a little. Women's bits aren't in view and it's for that reason I've directed both of the following biological body tours to females. Out of the two of you, you probably know least about his and your own genitals. Combine this with some 'field research' – touching and testing the areas that are meant to feel good when stimulated – and you're well on the way to becoming a sexpert.

It's best if you work through the anatomy and masturbation exercises solo first, before repeating the exercise with your partner.

Learn how to give *yourself* maximum pleasure and you'll have more chance of successfully passing this knowledge on. Follow the directions faithfully and by the end of the chapter, you should both know your own and each other's hot spots. There's no exam. I'm not suggesting either of you learn the correct technical terms for every part of each other's genitals off by heart. 'Darling, do you like it when I touch you there?' is just as effective (if not as impressive) as 'Would you like extra pressure on your frenulum while I simultaneously stimulate the perineum?' But a little knowledge really does go a long way – especially in the bedroom.

! The average man produces 100 million sperm at a rate of about 1000 a second every day. But don't be too impressed. That's about the same as your average guinea pig!

How the penis works

You'll benefit more from this section if you have a real live specimen in front of you. Yes, I'm serious! Pluck up courage and ask your partner to model for you – it's much easier to identify the parts we'll be talking about by looking at the real thing. Explain to him that you're giving yourself a lesson on how his penis works so you can be better in bed. Assuming it's not your first date, he's unlikely to turn down the invitation. Just remember that the penis you're studying intently is still attached to a body. Your boyfriend will probably feel a little strange and shy to begin with and may be concerned he won't 'measure up'. Allay his fears by talking to him as you're examining and turn it into a lesson for two. Of course he knows which bits feel good when rubbed and which don't, but chances are he doesn't know the proper terms for them either!

Think of his penis in four parts: the *head* or *glans* (the mushroom-shaped top of his penis); the *urethra* (the tiny slit at the top from which he urinates and ejaculates); the *shaft* (the length of his penis); and the *frenulum* (the small piece of skin where the head meets the shaft). Your partner may or may not have a foreskin (loose skin which covers the head of the penis). If he has been circumcised, this skin was probably removed when he was a baby. If he has not, the foreskin naturally pulls back to expose the head during intercourse, giving him the same sensations as a circumcised guy. Approach the foreskin with care: don't yank it back enthusiastically to see what's underneath. Use lubrication and ease it back gently – ask him to show you how he does it.

As a general rule of thumb, the shaft of the penis is the least sensitive part and the head the most. The head is extremely sensitive to stimulation because it contains numerous nerve endings that are close to the surface of the skin. In other words, he'll feel your touch here more than anywhere else. Even more sensitive is the frenulum. It's on the underside of his penis (the side closest to his testicles rather than his stomach). Find where the head meets the shaft and you'll see what looks like a puckering of skin in the middle. That's the frenulum – something you'll become very familiar with if you're interested in giving him pleasure!

'I'll masturbate about four or five times a week on average, every day if I'm horny. No matter how sick or down I am, I still do it a minimum of once or twice a week – I've never been that sick that sex fades totally from my mind. It's no big deal really because it only takes a few minutes. I go into the toilet and imagine some girl I've seen that day and thought was hot. Usually I come when I'm at the bit in the fantasy where she's giving me a head job. Her masturbating herself in front of me is another favourite.'

John, 22, student

Penises vary in size but the average flaccid penis (not erect) is around 9.5 cm long and 3.9 cm in width. When he's aroused, the erectile tissues in his penis fill with blood and it grows and becomes firm. During *orgasm* ('coming'), he'll usually *ejaculate*; that is, propel semen (or sperm) out of his penis through a series of muscular contractions. Contrary to popular belief, orgasm and ejaculation are two separate processes which don't necessarily occur at the same time. Orgasm is the sensation; ejaculation is the discharge of sperm. He can ejaculate without having an orgasm, or have an orgasm without ejaculating. So he can fake it too!

The *scrotum* is the pouch of skin at the bottom of his penis that holds the *testes* or *testicles* (balls). They have two functions: to produce sperm and to produce male hormones like testosterone.

Some men like their scrotum licked, held or gently massaged during sex. His anal region is also extremely sensitive but, again, some men like you to pay attention to it, some don't. The *perineum* is the area between the testes and the anus: it's rich in nerve endings and also responds to being stroked or licked.

Gay and bisexual men masturbate the most – once or twice a day or more.

The *male G-spot,* (see page 106 for more on this), now identified as the *prostate gland*, is found around the urethra at the neck of the bladder. I wouldn't advise cheerfully prodding the prostate gland during this exercise (unless, of course, he's aroused) – he's liable to shoot through the roof rather than find it a turn-on. Explore it during sex by inserting a well-lubricated finger gently into his anus and pressing against the front wall – it feels like a firm mass about the size of a walnut. Massage it firmly or stroke it in a downward direction during oral sex or intercourse, preferably just before he orgasms.

How the vagina works

He's been looking at his penis ever since his eyes were able to focus: your genitals are hidden from view. Just about every woman has given in to curiosity at some stage and looked at their vagina in a hand mirror, but even if you're as familiar with your genitals as he is his, you'll get a lot more out of this exercise if you look at and identify each part. Choose a private place with good lighting where you won't be disturbed. I'd suggest going through this exercise yourself first, before repeating it with your partner. Sure, you'll feel a little uncomfortable with him 'down there', staring at something that's rarely exposed. But if you're seriously interested in good sex, it's a must! Common sense should tell you that if he's never even clapped eyes on your vagina, he's got little chance of discovering exactly how to pleasure you. Genitals are individual and vary greatly from person to person. Your clitoris isn't in exactly the same spot as his last girlfriend's was and fumbling around in the dark isn't the best way for him to find it.

The female sex organs are highly complex but, like his, basically divide into different sections. The external organs – everything you can see outside – are collectively known as the *vulva*. The *mons pubis* is the fleshy mound covered with pubic hair, forming a 'V', that you can see when you stand in front of a mirror. This acts as a 'cushion' during intercourse. Sit or lie with your legs comfortably apart and the first thing you'll see are folds of skin covered with pubic hair. These are called the *labia majora*. Open them and you'll expose the inner 'lips', called the *labia minora*. The size and shape of both lips vary greatly. Usually, the outside lips cover the inside but it's quite normal if your inner lips protrude. The labia minora contain glands which secrete sebum, the fluid that lubricates the vagina. When you become excited, the lips become engorged with blood (just like his penis), increase in thickness and become redder.

'I guess I'm pretty matter-of-fact about it all. I'll get the urge, go into the bedroom and remove my underpants. I sit on the bed with my back against the wall, legs apart and feet pressed together. I've got both the Nancy Friday fantasy books and I've marked all my favourite fantasies, so I flip through, decide which one excites me today, apply some lubricant and off I go. I can be in and out of there in the time it takes to make a cup of coffee!'

Fiona, 22, receptionist

If you're a virgin, you may have a *hymen,* a thin membrane which covers the opening to the vagina. If it's still intact, it usually has holes in it that allow menstrual blood to escape. Don't panic if you haven't had sex but it doesn't appear to be there. Usually it's torn during childhood through activities like horse-riding and gymnastics or from using tampons.

Between the vaginal opening and your anus is a small area of smooth skin called the *perineum*. This area is highly sensitive to sexual stimulation. Like men, some women like a finger inserted into their *anus* on orgasm, though this is individual and depends very much on the woman (and the man who's doing it).

Just above your vaginal opening, you'll see the tiny hole that you urinate from. This is called the *urethra*. The *clitoris*, the most sensitive organ, is found at the top of the vagina (the end closest to your belly button) and looks like a tiny pea covered by a protective hood of skin. The bit of the clitoris that you can see protruding is actually part of a much larger organ that extends inside. In total, the clitoris is about four inches long and when the tip is stimulated (usually with his fingers, tongue or the head of his erect penis), the entire thing engorges and becomes firm and sensitive. The clitoris shares the same components as the penis, they're just hidden from view. Men have what amounts to a clitoris along the upper side of their penis but it's completely covered by skin while the tip of ours protrudes. So while we think of women's genitals as being 'inside' and men's 'outside', the bit on women that is the most sexually sensitive of all is well and truly 'out there'. His penis is used for other things (the transfer of sperm and urine); our clitoris is exposed for no other reason than to give us pleasure. It's the only organ which acts solely to receive and transmit sexual stimulation. So forget penis envy – he's the one who should be jealous!

Find your *G-spot* by inserting your fingers and pressing upward on the front wall of the vagina (the side closest to your front rather than your back). It's a small lump on the front wall that feels spongy (see Chapter 4 for more details).

The *vagina* itself is a muscular tube of about 8 cm that, when adequately stimulated, expands to fit any size penis with ease. When your partner initially penetrates you, the muscles of the vagina contract and grip the penis. As you continue intercourse and become more turned-on, the vagina expands even further – sometimes so much so, you can't feel his penis inside you no matter how large it is. This explains why, for both partners, the initial few thrusts are sometimes the most pleasurable because the vagina feels tighter.

For most women, stimulation of the clitoris is necessary to *orgasm*. Intercourse can indirectly stimulate the clitoris through thrusting but more direct touching with fingers or a tongue is usually more effective. When you do orgasm, your vaginal walls contract strongly and rhythmically, usually about three to five times, causing intense pleasure.

A HANDS-ON GUIDE TO SOLO SEX

The secret to sexual pleasure is at your fingertips. Literally. You've done your homework on the basic biology of how your body works, now we're going to study how your body responds to touch by masturbating. A lot more fun, believe me!

Ⓕ FOR HER

If this is your first attempt at masturbation, it's essential you choose a place and time where you won't be interrupted. Hearing your mother's voice on the answering machine is a tad off-putting when you're hovering on the brink of your first orgasm, so take the phone off the hook for a start. If you share a flat with other people, lock your door. Pull the curtains if you want to and do whatever it takes to make you feel comfortable.

Most women don't remove all their clothes to masturbate but for the first time, do. Look at your genitals in a mirror and reacquaint yourself with your clitoris. Remember it's usually at the top of your vagina and looks like a tiny pea covered by a hood of skin. Stimulating the clitoris is what will give you an orgasm.

Before you start, grab a tube of personal lubricant from the bathroom. You can buy K-Y or something similiar from chemists and supermarkets, and it's better to use that than Vaseline or baby oil which alters the delicate pH balance of the vagina and can trigger things like thrush. You will also need some massaging oil or moisturiser.

Start getting in the mood by massaging the oil into your breasts, arms, all over your body, being consciously alert to what strokes feel good, what don't. It may help if you read an erotic book or watch a video while you're masturbating; alternatively think sexy thoughts – fantasise about past or present lovers, someone you'd like to have sex with or a scenario which excites you.

Lie in a comfortable position on the bed with your legs relaxed and apart. When you feel ready, begin to explore your outer genitals with your fingers – rubbing, stroking, applying pressure, experimenting until you find the techniques which feel the most pleasurable. Now apply some lubricant to the inner lips or lick your fingers and use saliva.

Start concentrating your movements around or directly on the clitoris. This will feel more sensitive than the rest of your vagina so start by gently stroking it while it's still covered by the hood of skin. Keep up a steady rhythm with whatever stroke you've chosen. As you get more excited, the hood will retract. Stroking the clitoris directly may feel even better. Experiment with hard strokes and soft, circular and back and forth strokes to find out what feels best.

After a while, those pleasurable sensations will build and seem to centre around the clitoris. At this point you may want to increase the rhythm or pressure of your strokes or simply continue what you've been doing. You'll know when you orgasm. You'll feel an unmistakeable surge of pleasure – a 'climax' of the feelings you've been enjoying – and your vagina will go into a series of wave-like spasms. You may feel your vaginal muscles contracting. Usually, direct contact with the clitoris is painful immediately after orgasm, so don't be alarmed if it hurts if you continue to stimulate it.

If you're hung up about it

Talk to any good sex therapist about improving your love life and the first thing they'll tell you is this: if you haven't masturbated yourself to orgasm, you haven't even reached first base yet. Sensible advice. But if you come from a strict religious background or had parents who told you touching yourself was dirty and deviant, it's not so easy to shrug off those deep-rooted attitudes, no matter how silly they are. By the time we reach our 20s, most of us have figured that masturbation (a) won't make us blind and (b) doesn't make us perverts. But while most people, particularly women, recognise this *intellectually*, emotionally it's a different story. If you're having problems even reading this chapter, it's probably worth booking in to see a sex therapist to work through your feelings.

Feeling okay but just a little bit squeamish? Try...

Calling it by a different name

Even though we talk about sex as a natural, normal thing to do, it's still not something we do in public. It wouldn't occur to most of us to bonk our partners on the lounge-room floor in the middle of a dinner party with friends, or even nip off into their bedroom for that matter, just because we felt like it. For various reasons – some good, some bad – sex is hidden. And the message that sends to some people is that it's not okay.

Masturbation is even more shrouded in mystery. While we're used to seeing couples thrashing about the bedroom in movies and on TV, masturbation is still reserved for the porn films, reinforcing its 'dirty' image and leaving some people with the impression that it's still not right to touch ourselves 'down there'. Even the name 'masturbation' throws up lots of prohibitions for many women. So, for a start, try calling it something else: pleasing yourself, tension release, your sleeping pill. By normalising it, and using a word or expression your brain doesn't instantly associate with 'bad' thoughts, it will seem less threatening. Sounds simple, but sex therapists swear it's an important step in the right direction.

Taking your time and giving yourself permission to enjoy

When we masturbate, we tend to do it very quickly and get it over with because when we first started, we were worried we'd get caught. Also, a lot of people only masturbate when the sexual tension builds so high, they *have* to get rid of it.

Turn it around from something you only do when you have to and learn to view it as a 'treat'. One way of doing this is to use it as a reward – start masturbating after good things have happened to you. It's fat-free (unlike that bar of chocolate), great for your health (unlike a drink or cigarette) and won't cost you a cent (shopaholics take note). Soon you'll start to associate it with the good things and the whole process will become more positive.

Upping the pleasure principle

Tried masturbating but it didn't do a thing for you? I'll bet you didn't use lubricant. Rub away all you like but if you're dry, it'll feel irritating not pleasurable. Personal lubricants (like K-Y) keep the whole genital area wet and make almost any touch feel sensational. Lubricate your mind as well with sound and pictures. Put a sexy CD on the stereo and hang an erotic print in your bedroom. Alternatively, look at a snapshot of your adored, hunky boyfriend. Make sure your surroundings are as sexy as you want to feel.

Her four most popular techniques

1. Sitting up or lying down with legs apart

This is the most popular and traditional way to masturbate, which is why it's nicknamed the 'masturbation missionary position' by some sexperts.

Position: Lie on the bed with your knees up and legs apart or sit up, cross-legged, with your back against the bedhead or wall. Try pressing the soles of your feet together to increase tension in the groin. You might like to read an erotic book or magazine while masturbating even if you do discard it and let your imagination take over once you're close to climaxing.

Technique: There's no right or wrong way to touch yourself but most of us use our fingers. Some women are so sensitive, they'll stroke themselves through their knickers; some like direct clitoral stimulation, others indirect. All but 1.8 per cent of women (according to the sexperts) use some kind of clitoral stimulation to climax. The middle right-hand finger is often a favourite. Experiment with an up and down movement on the clitoris or do slow circles around the edge if it feels too sensitive. Start by stroking lightly, though you might want to increase the pressure later. Alternatively you can rub side to side or 'flick' the clitoris, strumming it the way you would a guitar.

The rhythm varies – most women prefer it regular, though a few stop and start. Try slow and light or fast and heavy to find the rhythm that you decide is most pleasurable. Most settle on a rhythm that suits and continue right through their orgasm, others bring themselves to the brink and then wait a few moments before recommencing. Some start off slow, then build up to their previous speed, others simply continue what they were doing before they paused. Another popular technique is to simply place one finger on either side of the clitoris and move against them.

Comparatively few women insert things into their vagina, for good reason! The clitoris, which gives us orgasms, is outside the vagina. However it's a good idea to include the odd 'dipping' movement inside, not just because it feels good, but because it helps transfer your natural lubrication from the vagina to the clitoris. The clitoris gets dry very easily, so apply more lubricant as you go along or lick your fingers regularly.

Stimulating the same area constantly can make your clitoris feel numb, so shift your hand slightly now and then to a different area to maintain the feeling and restore sensitivity. If your clitoris starts to feel irritated, stop direct stroking and instead manipulate the little hood of skin that protects the organ. Most women do this naturally anyway since the clitoris is extremely sensitive.

Timing: There's no 'normal' time span to reach orgasm; it depends strongly on your mood, stress level and how turned on you are. Sometimes you'll find yourself climaxing within a few minutes; other times it might take fifteen.

The climax: As you approach orgasm, press the heels of your feet together to increase the tension in the groin. You could also try squeezing your vaginal muscles in and out or deliberately clenching your buttocks to create pressure. Some women find moving sensually or moaning helps push them over the brink; others will sit or lie perfectly still without uttering a sound.

Few of us reach orgasm without fantasy, so let your imagination go wild! Relive a particularly hot session with your boyfriend, what you'd like to do with another person – conjure up a sexual scenario that turns you on. Don't get hung up about your fantasy; it doesn't mean you're odd, gay or secretly want to be raped. Most women fantasise about things they wouldn't dream of doing in real life – that's why we call them fantasies!

2. Rubbing against something

This is the second favourite masturbatory position. Instead of applying direct stimulation to the clitoris with your fingers, you rub against something, using the effect of pressure and friction to climax.

Position: Most women who masturbate this way lie on their stomach with their genitals pressed firmly into the bed with a pillow or cushion between their legs to rub against. Others lie on their backs with a blanket or pillow between their legs and use their hands to hold either side of the pillow to keep the pressure firm. One woman I know thrusts against a rolled up sock, another the arm of her teddy bear. Some women still use their fingers but use a pillow or crunch their legs tightly together to increase the pressure. You can also sit on the floor and thrust against the leg of a chair.

Technique: Remember when you were too young to go 'all the way' but used to hump against your boyfriend's leg and hip for

'I lie down on the bed and keep my legs tight together so my hand is crunched in between my legs. I don't use lubricant – I'm usually pretty wet, especially if I'm horny enough to want to masturbate. I rub directly on the clitoris but very lightly and keep the same rhythm all the way through. I don't put my hands inside myself, but sometimes I'll squeeze my nipples really hard. Occasionally, I'll put a pillow between my legs and grind against that to come. I don't fantasise, but concentrate really hard on getting off, the sensations I'm giving myself. No man has ever been able to masturbate me better than I can do it myself – they're too heavy-handed.'

Anna, 25, bank manager

stimulation? This is the same technique. Generally, you hold the object still and move against it, rather than the other way round, though some women will pull a sheet or blanket through their legs rhythmically. Again, you'll need to experiment and maybe 'arrange' your genitals so the thrusting feels pleasurable. Most women thrust quite hard, keeping up a steady rhythm until they climax. Placing a cupped hand over the entire genital area and moving it while you're pushing against the pillow is also popular.

Timing: Again, there's no 'norm'. Lots of women start with this technique, then move onto direct clitoral stimulation with their hands to finish themselves off.

The climax: Increase the pressure as you approach orgasm by clenching your thigh and bottom muscles. Most women also do 'Kegel' exercises (rhythmically squeezing the same vaginal muscle that you'd use to stop yourself urinating) as they continue thrusting. Again, fantasy plays a large part and because you're thrusting against an object, it's relatively easy to imagine the object is the person you're fantasing about!

3. Using a vibrator and/or a dildo

Roughly 15 per cent of women who masturbate use dildos or insert objects but a huge majority of us have tried, or own, vibrators. Orgasming with a vibrator requires little effort: hold it firmly against the genital area and most of us will climax within minutes! For this reason, many sex therapists recommend you don't use a vibrator to masturbate *every single time*. For a start, it's restrictive since you won't always have it with you. Secondly, it doesn't teach you any of the sexual skills you can use readily with a partner. At least try to masturbate to orgasm by rubbing or using your fingers, even if you use the vibrator most of the time.

! *Women with the highest education are more likely to masturbate. Forty-one per cent of women who completed high school never masturbate, but only 7 per cent of postgraduates don't indulge in solo sex.*

Having said that, vibrators are a terrific, quick and convenient way to orgasm if you're tired or don't have much time. Contrary to what the porn industry believes, most women don't use vibrators inside their vaginas but use them outside to stimulate the clitoris. Even if you've got a penis-shaped vibrator, chances are you use the tip rather than insert it. The most effective vibrators are sold in department stores as body massagers. They work well because they have a flat surface which stimulates the clitoral area effectively – they're also a lot less embarrassing to buy if you're a little shy! (While we're on the subject, don't relegate your vibrator to the back of a cupboard when your boyfriend's around; he'll love using it on you and will also enjoy the vibratory sensation on his genitals.)

Position and technique: If you're using a dildo, you can sit or lie while inserting it or hold it firmly at the base and 'lower' yourself on top – the positions are as varied as they are for intercourse. If you don't have a dildo but would like to insert something, try a not-too-ripe peeled banana; they seem to simulate the hard but soft feeling of a penis and are totally harmless to insert. Since clitoral stimulation is usually necessary to orgasm, you'll also probably need to use your hands to stimulate the clitoral area directly, using any of the techniques listed above.

Positions and techniques with a vibrator are limited only by your imagination. The standard technique is to press it firmly against the closed labia (lips of the vagina) and hold it there, varying the pressure,

'When I was about 13, I put a finger inside me while lying in bed and waited for the fireworks to go off. Not surprisingly, nothing happened. I actually didn't have an orgasm until I was about 22 when I found my flatmate's vibrator. Over the next year or so, I experimented with it: moved it in a circular motion, teased myself, tried different pressure. But the problem with vibrators is that you don't really discover how to give yourself pleasure because the machine does it for you. After I left, I deliberately didn't buy one and taught myself to masturbate with my fingers. It took a while, but now I can orgasm within about five minutes.'

Jennifer, 32, journalist

until you orgasm. Try it standing up, sitting with legs apart, or lying down. Another technique is to stand with your legs apart, hold the vibrator still in front of your genitals and move backward and forward, grinding against it. Moving it in a circular motion is also popular as well as kneeling on the floor and squatting over it.

Timing: If you've only got two minutes to spare, masturbating with a vibrator is the technique for you! Unless they deliberately 'tease' themselves and hold off, most women can orgasm with a vibrator within 60 seconds to three minutes. To make it last longer, try setting it on the lowest vibration speed, applying pressure and moving it in a circular motion, lifting it away if you feel yourself too close to climaxing.

The climax: If you're using a dildo, inserting it right before you're about to orgasm may be the most satisfying. It gives your vaginal muscles something to contract around and makes you feel pleasantly 'filled up'. You might want to thrust deeper or faster when you feel yourself about to orgasm.

4. In the shower

It's soapy, slippery, wet and totally private, which is probably why the shower is the place where many women either masturbate or at least get the urge to!

Position and technique: Unless you have a detachable hand-held shower hose, you probably won't masturbate to climax in the shower, though lots of women will stimulate themselves while soaping their genitals to get in the mood. If you do have a hand-held shower, try sitting in the bath or kneeling (if the bath's full, make sure your genitals are above water level), then turning the shower to maximum pressure and directing the jet so it runs over the clitoral area. You might want to use your hands as well. One word of caution: it's fine to use soap as a lubricant outside the vagina but don't push soapy fingers inside (again, it can lead to an imbalance and cause things like thrush and cystisis). If you're lucky enough to have a spa (or access to one), you'll no doubt have discovered the pleasure of positioning yourself so a strong jet of water stimulates the clitoris.

Number of women under 40 who use a vibrator: 26 per cent (88 per cent buy their own). One of the most popular penis-shaped vibrators sold in Australia: the Fair Lady. The shaft has rotating pearls in it to stimulate her G-spot and it comes with a detachable clitoral stimulator.

Timing and climax: Some women can climax using their hand-held showers but most use it more as preparation, to get themselves in the mood, rather than to actually bring themselves to orgasm. Many switch to one, or several, of the other three techniques to finish the job.

Why not try...

- **Masturbating in semi-public:** want the added spice of danger? Try masturbating in the toilet: at work, on a plane or at a party. Do it while you're driving or under a blanket on a long, boring plane flight. One girl I know can bring herself to orgasm (and continue a conversation) by sitting on the floor with her legs tucked under her, heel pressed firmly against her clitoris.
- **Watching yourself in a mirror:** you'll see how you look when you're turned-on, the sexy expressions you make while you orgasm.
- **Caressing more than just your genitals:** try rubbing or pinching your nipples or stroking your tummy just above your pubic hair as you're about to orgasm.

- **Leaving your underpants on:** instead slip your fingers around the sides – it'll bring back memories of those first forbidden touches!
- **Masturbating while sitting in a chair with your legs over the side:** it's gloriously wanton.
- **Doing it from behind:** lie on your bed on your front and put a pillow under your stomach, masturbating from behind.
- **Standing up or leaning against a wall.**
- **Squatting Indian style!**

TEN GOOD REASONS TO MASTURBATE

1. It feels fantastic.
2. It teaches us about our own body: what turns us on, what doesn't. Masturbation helps you identify what your basic sexual needs are and how best to satisfy them. Pass this onto your partner and you have a solid basis for a sizzling sex life.
3. It releases tension and helps us sleep – a secret sleeping pill without any side-effects!
4. It teaches us to separate love from sex. We're more able to distinguish sex-affairs from love-affairs because we realise having an orgasm doesn't mean we're in love.
5. If you're single, it stops you climbing the walls or sleeping with the first guy or girl you meet.
6. It's totally safe.
7. It's a great beauty treatment. Orgasm improves circulation, combats the effects of stress, makes skin glow!
8. You can concentrate purely on your own pleasure without worrying about someone else.
9. The more you masturbate, the more orgasms you'll be capable of having both with and without your partner. The more you do it, the easier they are to reach!
10. Being able to give yourself an orgasm is true sexual independence.

Ⓜ FOR HIM

The first time

If you're male and old enough to read, you're probably killing yourself laughing at the suggestion that you might need advice in this area. While some women don't start masturbating until their late teens or even late 20s, most men are quite practised at it by age 12 or 13. But even if you've brought yourself to orgasm a thousand times, don't smile smugly and flip the page just yet. The *way* you masturbate could be causing problems in your sex life with your partner.

Because of our illogical but pervasive perceptions about masturbation – that it's 'naughty' and something 'dirty old men do' – your first masturbatory experiences as a boy were probably furtive and riddled with guilt. 'Playing with yourself' was something you got over with as quickly as possible – fabulous when you've only got three minutes before Aunt Gertrude comes knocking, not so fabulous when you're with a partner later on. If it still only takes you a few seconds or minutes to masturbate yourself to orgasm, you're probably intimately familiar with the term 'premature ejaculation' (orgasming too soon, before you or your partner is satisfied). In effect, from a very early age you've 'programmed' your penis to ejaculate quickly by ensuring orgasm follows mere minutes (or seconds) after direct stimulation.

As they get older, most men relax into masturbation. They have more privacy, no longer feel guilty and start experimenting with different techniques and varying sensations. The more you 'hold off' your orgasm when masturbating yourself, the more practised you'll be at delaying it during sex with someone else. If you're still using the same technique you applied when you were 13, it's time to try something new!

Humour me. Pretend this is the first time you've pleasured yourself. Pick a time and a place where you won't be interrupted, don't set any time limits and try one, or all, of the techniques listed below. The aim isn't to see which technique brings you to orgasm the quickest but to experience (and get your penis used to) different sensations. Masturbation isn't and shouldn't be something you do simply to ease tension. It's an experience that should be enjoyed for its own merits.

'It's totally normal to continue masturbating even if you're living with a girl and have a fantastic sex life. Masturbation is one form of sex. It provides different feelings than sex with another person so even if you're getting heaps of it with her, you still crave that different sensation. The only problem usually is opportunity. My (now ex) wife once caught me masturbating in the shower and was horrified. I thought at the time it was because she thought masturbating was dirty but I realise now it was because I wasn't having sex with her. She couldn't understand why I'd prefer to do it myself when she was lying in the next room.'

Gary, 25, lawyer

His three most popular techniques

Contrary to popular perception, most men don't read 'girlie' magazines while masturbating. The men I interviewed weren't too enthusiastic about watching porn videos either ('How often do you get the whole place to yourself to do that?'). Simply fantasising – forming visual images in your head – is the most popular accompaniment to solo sex.

Unlike women, who often have two or three 'favourite' fantasies which guarantee them orgasm, yours vary depending on what's happening in your life, even on that day. You'll build a fantasy around seeing a flash of stocking on a train, replay a recent and particularly hot encounter with your girlfriend, or fantasise about what you'd like to do with the girl you took out for the first time the night before. Some men up the fantasy factor by sitting on their hands before masturbating to make them go numb. The idea is that if you can't feel your own hand, it feels like someone else is touching you.

1. Making a fist

Making a loose fist and running it up and down the penis is the most common way men masturbate, varying the tightness of the grip, speed of the strokes and length of the movement to suit individual preferences. Like women, men discover what feels best through experimentation.

Position: Most of the men I interviewed said about the only prerequisite for where they masturbated was privacy. If your flatmate or girlfriend is away for the weekend, you'll do it while lounging on the couch watching a video. Standing in front of a mirror is also a common turn-on. However the most usual place is lying on the bed, legs slightly apart.

Technique: Most of you reach for some sort of lubricant first, and you aren't too fussy what you use – soap, shampoo, baby oil, handcream, Vaseline, your girlfriend's super-expensive face cream (thanks, guys!) – whatever you can lay your hands on. Personal lubricants like K-Y aren't popular, though once used, men tend to stick with them. While the penis isn't as sensitive to products as the vagina, a personal lubricant works more effectively.

The usual method is to make a loose fist, palm facing the side of the penis, starting at the top and moving down in a pumping motion which runs up and down the length of the penis. Some men go right to the bottom of the shaft, others concentrate more on the head. Most men prefer to increase the tightness of the grip as their hands move over the head, others find their glans too sensitive and do the opposite. Rhythm is most important. No matter what stroke is used, keeping up a steady, constant rhythm is what builds sexual tension.

You might like to stroke, massage or hold your testicles with the other hand or rub the perineum, the area between your testicles and your anus. Some men also like to touch or pinch their nipples.

In the same way that women tend to concentrate on their clitoris, most men eventually focus on the frenulum. The shaft is relatively insensitive and serves more to let your hand move up and down rhythmically. As your hand moves up and over the frenulum, try using a rolling action with your fingers and palm, manipulating the area firmly but not too vigorously. (One man confessed he'd ended up with a friction lesion on his frenulum during a particularly frequent and enthusiastic masturbation period in his life. The pain was secondary only to the embarrassment of being told what had caused it by his family doctor.) You could also try squeezing the base of the shaft to increase sensitivity and maintain the erection.

> 'Sometimes if you haven't had sex for ages and you start going out with someone, you'll stop masturbating in anticipation of the real thing. Masturbation takes the edge off and sometimes you still want it there.'
>
> Andrew, 31, tradesman

As an alternative, use your fingers to gently stroke the penis and testicles until you achieve an erection, then use two or three fingers and your thumb instead of your whole fist to slide up and down. Or try holding a finger still over the frenulum and moving your other fingers and thumb over the front of the penis in a smaller movement.

Timing: Like women, how soon you reach orgasm depends on how horny you are and how vivid the fantasy, but it also depends on factors like whether you feel stressed or tired. Most men reach orgasm fairly quickly – usually within two to five minutes – and deliberately slow it down or stop and start if they want to delay the inevitable. Try reversing your hand movement as you feel orgasm approach. Bend your wrist towards you so your fist is twisted and your palm now faces the opposite side of your penis. This shifts the stimulation to different areas.

The climax: When they feel they're about to come, most men increase their stroke so they're moving up and down the shaft as rapidly as possible. Some grab hold of their testicles as they are ejaculating, claiming it makes the orgasm last longer; others grasp the bottom of the shaft for the same reason. Once the orgasm starts, almost all men either slow down dramatically or stop stimulation completely. This is because the penis, particularly the head, is incredibly sensitive just after ejaculation (something girlfriends often don't understand because lots of women like to be stimulated right through to the last spasm of their orgasm).

What do you do with the little pile of semen you've created? Most men either ejaculate straight into a towel or over their bodies, wiping it off with a tissue afterward.

2. Using a pillow

Rubbing against stockings or something silky is often how young boys first discover they can make themselves orgasm. While 'The

Fist' technique is certainly more popular, particularly if you're *dying* for it, many men said they rubbed against a pillow when they were in a more mellow, sensual mood.

Position: Most men either stand or kneel with a pillow, folded over, in front of them. They then rub the penis in the fold and simulate intercourse. Others stand, place a pillow at groin level and move their penis and testicles over the top in a back and forth motion.

***!** Once every 8 minutes – that's the number of times men, on average, think about sex or have a sexually related thought.*

Just as some women swear they can orgasm simply by squeezing their thighs together, several men I interviewed said they'd been able to mentally will themselves to a climax in certain situations (and they were proud of it too – 'Look Mum, no hands!'). After travelling for a week on the road with his friends (with no opportunity to masturbate), one man said he put a pillow over his lap, squeezed his thighs together, sat on his hand so he could massage his testicles and orgasmed simply by the pressure of his erect penis straining against his (by now rather tight) jeans. Now there's a challenge for the guy who believes he's tried everything!

Technique: You don't need to be a Masters and Johnson pupil to figure this one out. Either pretend to have intercourse with the pillow, rubbing your penis in and out of the fold you've created, or rub your penis back and forth across the top. Use your hands to hold the pillow in place.

Timing: Some men use the pillow technique in much the same way as couples do foreplay, switching to The Fist or more direct stimulation once they approach orgasm. If they don't switch to something else, the thrusting speeds up, just as it does during 'real' intercourse.

The climax: Some men clench their buttocks together as they continue thrusting but most use fantasy to push themselves over the edge. In that instant, the pillow becomes almost lifelike – you'd swear it grows a set of breasts in that crucial moment!

'We used to have a "wank room" in the house that I shared with my friends which had a stack of pornography, which we called "wank books", by the door. When we felt horny we'd grab one from the pile, tell the others "I'm going into the wanking room" and that was that. Most of the time, no-one even looked up from watching TV. We were all very open about it, so much so that when mates came over to our place, they'd do the same thing. In my circle, masturbation is seen as normal as breathing. But I think we're the exceptions rather than the rule.'

Dean, 20, plumber

3. In the shower

Masturbating in the shower is more common with younger men, probably because it's the one place you're guaranteed some sort of privacy as a teen. But even if you live by yourself, all that warm water gushing gently over your genitals, soaped-up, slippery hands washing your penis – the resulting sensations have made many a man forget about those work problems and focus on more pleasurable thoughts.

Position: Most men stand, usually facing away from the door (old habits die hard); others find it more comfortable to sit down. While soap is the classic lubricant, others find it irritating and use hair conditioner instead.

Technique: While with other masturbatory techniques most of you went straight for the goodies, the shower was one place where the rest of the body came into play. Some men started by soaping themselves all over ('like a lover would'), and nearly all soaped and massaged their anus, perineum, scrotum and testicles before even touching their penis. From there, most moved into The Fist technique.

Timing and climax: Possibly because they didn't concentrate exclusively on the penis or head immediately, most men said they took a little longer to reach orgasm this way. Another very obvious benefit? Cleaning up afterwards is a cinch!

HOW MASTURBATING CAN MAKE YOU A BETTER LOVER

If you have trouble reaching orgasm with your partner or if you're a premature ejaculator, masturbation can help. For men, it's invaluable for gaining control over your orgasms. For women, it's about the only way you'll discover what your partner can do to turn you on. Here's how to make it work for you.

F FOR HER

- **Don't use the same method constantly.** Many women can happily give themselves an orgasm but rarely climax with their partners. Assuming your relationship is healthy and you don't have any psychological hang-ups about sex, this usually means you haven't shown him how you masturbate yourself (see 'Why you should do it in front of each other' over) or the method you use to masturbate isn't one that's easily transferred to couple sex. For example, he can't turn himself into a human vibrator and give you the same sensation it does. So if that's the only way you can climax, you've got two choices: use the vibrator when you're with him or learn a more couple-friendly technique. Practise until you can masturbate yourself to orgasm with your fingers and try as many variants as possible. If you can only orgasm one way, you're restricting yourself sexually. The more techniques you experiment and are successful with, the more chance you'll have of recreating them with a partner.
- **Play games with yourself.** Practise control over your orgasms. Set a timer and don't allow yourself to orgasm for five minutes; the next time try and orgasm within one. Read the section in Chapter 4 which talks about the G-spot (page 117) and set some time aside to find it. Practise Kegel exercises (see page 97 for more detail). Pull in your vaginal muscles to the count of three, push out for three. Try masturbating while tensing your muscles; do the same while relaxed.

Ⓜ FOR HIM

- **Do it more often.** If you ejaculate prematurely – you have an orgasm before either you or your partner is ready – masturbate more frequently. The more you masturbate, the less sensitive your penis will be to stimulation. Haven't seen your girlfriend in a week and feeling paranoid that the sex session you've been dreaming about will be all over in three minutes flat? Masturbate at least twice during the day you'll see her, if possible an hour before you have intercourse. This will help delay ejaculation.
- **Time yourself.** Try counting backward as you're masturbating. The aim is to take your mind off what you're doing. Start with a high number, like 500 – the higher the number, the more your brain has to focus on counting. The first time you might only make it to 488. The next, aim to get down to 450, then 400, etc. You can use the same technique during intercourse.

> 'I used to work on a magazine and one of my jobs was to edit an excerpt from an erotic novel. I was stuck reading the book for hours and could feel myself getting all hot and flushed. In the end, I just had to relieve myself so I went to the loo, locked myself in and masturbated for ages. I could hear my workmates chatting a few feet away and that turned me on even more. Since then, I've masturbated in various toilets, once standing up in a dark corner at a party where everyone was out of it but me. The more chance I have of being caught, the better.'
>
> Debbie, 23, writer

WHY YOU SHOULD DO IT IN FRONT OF EACH OTHER

Partners can't read minds. So get rid of that 'If he/she truly loved me, they'd know what turns me on' stuff right now. Body language can speak volumes and talking to each other is essential but, as the saying goes, a picture is worth a thousand words. Watching each other masturbate, you see first-hand what technique you each use – the pressure and speed, how you speed it up or slow it down on approach to orgasm, how you stimulate yourself (or not) while you're actually having an orgasm and what you do with your spare hand. All you need do then is copy each other.

Generally, men are more comfortable masturbating than women are. If your girlfriend's the I'm-game-for-anything type, doing it in front of her may simply be a matter of taking a hold of yourself during foreplay. Chances are, she'll sit back and watch – lots of women are *fascinated*. If she ignores what you're doing, simply say, 'I've had fantasies about masturbating in front of you. This feels great.' If she still doesn't get the hint add, 'This is how I do it when you're not around. Watch.' If you want her to imitate your technique, get her to put her hand over yours so she can feel the pressure and rhythm you're using. Ask her to copy you and give lots of positive feedback – 'Wow! You're better at it than I am.' Uninhibited women can easily apply the same principles.

Your partner's a little shy and so are you? Talk about it first. Say you watched a show/a friend told you/you read about how watching each other masturbate will improve your sex life immeasurably. Ask if your partner agrees and suggest that the next time you make love, you try it. Don't be concerned if it all seems a bit serious and uncomfortable the first time round. Start by showing one technique you use: come on – that's a mere second or two of embarrassment! And get them to do the same. Later, when you both feel more comfortable, you'll be more confident and relaxed about bringing yourself to an actual orgasm. Masturbating in front of your partner or watching them masturbate has always been up there with the most popular male sex fantasies – and the new breed of sexually liberated females are adding it to *their* list.

! Number of women who masturbate: 80 per cent. Number of men: 94 per cent – but they do it twice as often as women. Number of men who continue masturbating after marriage: 72 per cent. Number of married women who do the same: 68 per cent.

Foreplay

Not just the entrée, it can be main course (and dessert) as well!

'Foreplay?' joked a male acquaintance (note, not a *friend*) of mine. 'Isn't that when she says yes?'

Tragically, he's not the only guy to think that way. It takes the average man two to three minutes of direct sexual stimulation with a partner to orgasm. It takes the average woman 20 to 30 – which goes a long way to explain why women are a lot keener on foreplay than men. Unless you're talking fellatio, of course – there's no such thing as a bad head-job. What are the three things men want more of in bed? Oral sex, oral sex, oral sex.

Okay, we've got the message already – only problem is, men don't seem to have got ours. Let me put it very clearly. MOST WOMEN WANT MORE FOREPLAY. Some women would be grateful for any at all. But like everything else attached to sex, there are some outdated attitudes about it that seem to be clinging on for dear life.

Despite the name, foreplay isn't necessarily something you do *before* sex. Stop thinking of it as an 'entrée' that's to be raced through to get to a 'main course' of intercourse and you're halfway to becoming a better lover already. If you're both really aroused, foreplay might be something you do *after* penetration, when you've taken the edge off. Experienced couples do it *during* intercourse – they'll take a break for some oral sex or masturbation to keep the mood hot and heavy for longer. The most inventive lovers of all do nothing *but* foreplay the entire sex session. Not every time, just sometimes. Orgasms through mutual masturbation and oral sex are often more intense for both sexes; for some women it's the *only* way they climax.

'I met a girl at a bar who looked me straight in the eye then said, "I want you inside me," within five minutes of meeting her. This happened at around 9 pm and we didn't sleep together until the early hours of the morning, but I was in a state of high excitement from that moment on. That's what I call good foreplay.'

Simon, 29, sales representative

Foreplay isn't a luxury to indulge in when you've 'got time', especially if you are planning to have intercourse. It's necessary for the woman's vagina to physically prepare for penetration; without it, she'll be left dry but not high. And even men who can get an erection by inserting a coin in a slot machine can't deny that a good, slow, erotic 'tease' dramatically heightens the sensations of intercourse.

Just one tip before you go gleefully poring through the chapter, eager to try out every suggestion: don't try to do everything at once. One of my girlfriends, who'd complained to her lover that she was bored with sex, had ice dripped over her breasts (and up her nose), (prickly) feathers stroked all over her body and a (rather too ripe) banana shoved you-know-where, all while she was blindfolded and tied to the bed, all at once. Full marks for effort but the shuddering climax he'd hoped for didn't happen. She felt shuddery all right – like she'd just been put through the spin cycle of a washing machine.

If there's one rule about foreplay it's this: savour each experience, relax into it and take your time. Anticipation is one of the biggest turn-ons of all. Herein lies the secret of being a truly good lover – and truly hot sex.

> 'My first husband was so predictable with foreplay, I could not only tell you exactly what he'd do, but what order and how long he'd spend on each bit. First he'd kiss me on the mouth, fondling my breasts at the same time. About one minute later, his hand would go straight to my genitals, he'd put a finger inside me and move it in and out a few times, then climb on top. He refused to talk to me about sex and denied there was a problem (he told me I'd been reading "too many books" if I expected more). No wonder I left him.'
>
> Rachel, 32, gym instructor

WHAT EVERYONE WANTS MORE OF – MASSAGES!

In an ideal world, we'd all have two professional massages a week. Unfortunately, few of us have the time (let alone the cash), so that leaves . . . our partners, right? While no-one particularly wants to start every romp around the bedroom with a leisurely massage, once a month is something all of us can aspire to. By all means take turns massaging each other, but not in the same session. There's nothing worse than having to put all those sensual feelings on hold if you have to reciprocate the minute your partner's hands leave your body!

A sensual massage

Schedule it for a Saturday or Sunday afternoon when you have hours to while away. Take the phone off the hook, put something slow and sexy on the stereo and make sure the room is warm. It's more pleasurable for both of you if you're *both* undressed – though he's probably better keeping his underwear on if it's his turn to play masseur (an erect penis tends to get bumped around a bit). If you really want to make his day, leave one thing on (like a pair of sexy knickers or high heels) while you're massaging him. Aim to spend at least an hour sensuously plying him with your hands.

I've written this for a woman to follow, but the same technique will work on her too.

Get him to lie face down and cover all the bits you're not massaging with towels. Start by warming some scented oil or baby oil between your palms. (Don't drop it directly onto his skin – it's cold!) Now gently stroke along his back. Skim your fingertips very lightly over the skin to make it supersensitive (this is the bit where he gets goosebumps) before moving onto firmer strokes. You don't need to be a professional because almost anything feels good, but you could try some or all of the following strokes.

- **Circling:** make firm circular movements with the hands, working outward and away from the backbone (the hand movements mirror each other).
- **Gliding:** put your hands on the lowest part of his buttocks, palms flat and fingers pointing toward his head. Use the weight of your body and push both hands up along the spine.
- **Thumbstrokes:** use your thumbs in a circular motion to ease muscular tension, particularly in tight areas. Similarly, try running your knuckles along either side of his spine for a blissful sensation. Generally, you should always work upward and away from the spine.

Make sure you pay attention to every (non-genital at this point) part of his body during the massage; massage his back and front including his hands, feet, bottom and chest. For the first half hour, make it more relaxing than sexy – for the last, tease him mercilessly! Run your hands between his buttocks and penis, rub his inner thighs and lower stomach, but don't touch his penis, no matter how much it strains toward you. After at least 45 minutes of stroking and kneading, he's ready for the *pièce de résistance:* an erotic genital massage!

***!** Average time two-thirds of couples spend on foreplay: between 6 and 20 minutes. Number of men who agree it's possible to have a satisfying sex life without penile penetration: 43 per cent.*

The knock-their-socks-off erotic version

Genital massage has been around for thousands of years, but has only recently been discovered by western society – and westernised, of course! The true, unadulterated version draws heavily on the Kama Sutra and Tantric sex and is preceded by all sorts of bizarre, complicated rituals. But for our purposes (and because, to be honest, I've never found things like breathing in each other's breath terribly sexy), we'll skip straight to the nitty-gritty. You'll have a bit of a giggle over the names but these explicit techniques are easy to learn and can transform the most mediocre lover into a wow-honey-that-was-*incredible* sort overnight. You may need to have the book beside you the first couple of times to follow the instructions, but when you've mastered it . . . well, your lovers won't forget *you* in a hurry!

Ⓕ FOR HER

Most men assume the 'power position' during sex, so erotic massage will be especially pleasurable for him because it's a totally different sensation. Instead of you lying back and him doing all the work, he gets to relax and experience the sensation of touch while *you* take control.

Most of these techniques work best with him lying on his back on the bed, legs comfortably apart, and you kneeling between them. You'll need lots of oil; a 'water-based' one, sold at most sex shops, is ideal but unscented massage oil or baby oil will do the trick. Ask him to give you feedback all the way through the massage, saying which strokes and pressure he prefers. Watch his face and read his body language for clues. The idea isn't for him to orgasm quickly but to immerse himself in the concept of receiving pleasure. If it seems like he's losing control, stop what you're doing and lay both hands on top of his penis. Hold still, maintaining a firm but not heavy pressure, for about 30 seconds to calm him down. If you want him to orgasm, speed up the strokes.

The roll

Once he's lying on his back, kneel between his legs. Hold his testicles between your fingers and thumb and roll them gently, slowly and lightly using the pads of your fingertips.

After a few minutes, change into a tickling stroke: put your hands underneath his testicles so they're resting gently on your fingertips and, using the pads of your fingers, tickle them. The lighter the pressure, the more exquisite the sensation.

Spiralling the stalk

This is great to use if he's having trouble getting an erection.

Hold the base of the penis with one hand and take a firm hold of it with your other. Start at the bottom and slide to the top using a circular, twisting motion as you wind toward the head. Picture a corkscrew – that's the sort of movement you're imitating.

When you get to the head of the penis, use the palm of your hand to caress the entire surface. Only work upward.

> 'My girlfriend puts a hell of an effort into our sex life. Each time we have sex, she'll introduce something new – whether it's a position, a technique or location. It used to freak me out. I couldn't help obsessing that she'd done all this with someone else (or was having a bit on the side and picking up tricks that way). Then I figured she just had a vivid imagination and was really into sex. She drives me nuts outside the bedroom, but there's no way I'm letting go of her.'
>
> Neil, 19, mechanic

The 12 o'clock stroke

Save this one until he's aroused and has a full erection. It's called '12 o'clock' because you're moving directly upward in a straight line.

Open your hand so your thumb and fingers are separated to make an 'L' shaped space. Slide your hand underneath the testicles until they rest between that space (if you're using your left hand, your fingers would be on the left-hand side of the testicles, thumb on the right). Push up a little so you're lifting them slightly.

With your palm down separate the first two fingers of your other hand to make a 'V' and slide the penis between them, working upward from the testicles to the head and tilting your hand so the flat of your hand brushes up against the shaft of the penis. Only work upward with this stroke. When you reach the head, remove your hand and start from the bottom again. Don't just slide up the middle; try sliding up the sides as well.

Making fire

This is the final technique because he's almost certain to orgasm.

Imagine you have a stick between your hands and are trying to start a fire by rolling it. Hold the palms of your hands straight, facing either side of his penis.

Using a rolling/rubbing motion, start at the bottom of his penis and slide upward, then down again, keeping the motion consistent and rhythmic. His penis will sit naturally between your palms. Start slowly, then build pressure and speed when he approaches orgasm.

Ⓜ FOR HIM

Rather than foreplay, think of her erotic massage as a sensual gift. It may lead to intercourse but she's far more likely to enjoy it if there's no pressure to have sex at the end. As with the male massage, most of these techniques work best if she's lying on her back with her legs apart and you're kneeling between them. Put pillows under her knees and let her legs fall open naturally: it's more comfortable and she'll feel less vulnerable and exposed.

Don't use oil on her vagina; use a thin, liquid lubricant. K-Y is too heavy. Try Astroglide, Glyde, Liquid Silk or Sylk (available at pharmacies and sex shops). Warm the lubricant by rubbing it between your fingers.

Ask her to tell you which strokes feel best, whether she prefers a firm or gentle touch. If you're unsure, err on the too gentle side; she'll probably push against your hand if she wants more pressure. Keep the rhythm regular and don't chop and change techniques too much. Watch her face – if it's relaxed, so is her body.

Remember erotic massage isn't meant to replace foreplay. Use these techniques every single time you make love and sex will, once more, become routine and predictable. Instead, adapt the strokes to suit her individual preferences, combine techniques, invent some of your own – then transport her to orgasmic heaven!

Stroking the thighs

Perform this first to relax and arouse her.

Alternating between using the flat of your palms and your fingertips, lightly brush up the inside of her thigh. Then do the whole length of her body. Start at the ankles, brushing over the genitals and pubic hair, then move up to the breasts, circling around them. Repeat several times.

Focusing on the genitals, stroke the pubic hair and genital area using soft, gentle motions. Use your fingers to gently stroke and 'tap' the outer labia (the outside lips), keeping up a regular, consistent rhythm.

Awakening the clitoris

Lie next to her or kneel between her legs. Using the knuckles of your first two fingers, knead the outer labia lips, moving backward and forward while massaging. Make sure you're kneading, not pinching. Working downward, massage the whole labia with a firm but gentle pressure. Move downward toward the anus, then lift your hand and start at the top again. Alternatively, you can use your thumb and first finger if that feels more comfortable.

The two-finger stroke

Nicknamed 'the bread and butter' stroke, this technique is the easiest and simplest way of giving her pleasure.

Rest your thumb and index finger at the top of the vagina (the end where the clitoris is), on the inside lips. Rotate your fingers around the top of the clitoris, then move your fingers downward. Massage and roll evenly, rubbing up and down on either side of the vagina, settling into an even rhythm.

She's ready for more direct clitoral stimulation when she opens her legs wider, pushes against your hand or raises her pelvis off the bed.

Rock around the clock

It's extremely useful to imagine a clock dial surrounding the vaginal area, the top (near her pubic hair) being the 12 o'clock position and the lowest point (near the vaginal opening) being 6 o'clock. If she tells you what feels good, you can memorise the position (3 o'clock, 9 o'clock) for next time. Plus she can direct you more accurately. This technique was adapted from the Tantric original by the outrageous (but ever inventive) sex guru, Annie Sprinkle.

Using the tip of your finger, move around the clitoris in a circular motion. Using bigger circles continue the circular motion down the entire length of the vagina, alternating with stroking, teasing, caresses with your fingertips.

Now move back to the clitoris and circle directly over it with a fingertip. Some women don't like direct clitoral stimulation, so check with her which area feels best when stimulated, using the 'clock' as a guide.

Try 'pulling' the clitoris between two fingers. It's not actually possible to get a grip on it, but the pulling motion feels fabulous!

Entering the garden

This is a double-action stroke that works on the G-spot and clitoris simultaneously to bring most women to orgasm.

Insert a finger (or two) into her well-lubricated vagina, curving them so you're working on the front wall (imagine you're aiming upward to her stomach). Hold your finger still for a few seconds; she may move against it, but don't apply pressure until she feels comfortable.

The G-spot feels like a small, textured lump. When aroused, it engorges with blood and becomes more sensitive. Once you've found it, move into a 'come here' motion, like you're beckoning someone with your finger. Don't press hard or constantly; a gentle, beckoning, stroking motion is usually far more pleasurable. Try a 'zig-zag' motion so your fingers are passing over the G-spot without concentrating on it too directly.

With your other hand, 'rock around the clock', circling the clitoris with your finger, thumb (or a flat-surfaced vibrator). Also try moving directly backward and forward over it as she's about to orgasm.

ABOVE THE BELT: A GUIDE TO STIMULATING HER (AND HIS) BREASTS

If you're a DD cup, encouraging him to pay attention to your breasts usually isn't a problem (getting him to pay attention to anything else probably is). But for those of us whose grandmothers don't even notice when we go without a bra, our breasts are often bypassed on the way to what men perceive to be the real goodies, the genitals. Yet for most women – and lots of men – the breast area is highly erotic, playing a vital part in sexual excitement.

As with the rest of our bodies, what we like, when and how we want you to touch them is all individual. As a general rule, start off gently and slowly, increasing the pressure in line with your partner's arousal. Watch their body language carefully to see how they respond to different touches – and make sure it's desire that's making the nipples erect, not the cold breeze drifting in through the open window!

Ⓜ FOR HIM

Try sucking, nibbling, licking, stroking or gently squeezing the entire area. The nipples and areola (the pinky brown bit around the nipples) are sensitive but so is the area underneath. Some women feel zilch when you directly touch their nipples, but stroke underneath and, *hey presto*, they'll stiffen immediately. Use your tongue, fingers, whole hand, lips and the head of your erect penis to stimulate the entire area.

! *Men are more likely to reach orgasm during intercourse while feeling your breasts than you are from having them felt.*

Some women like their nipples flicked, pinched hard or bitten. But this very much depends not only on personal taste, her mood and how many glasses of wine she's had, but where she is in her menstrual cycle. Sometimes, even your fingers might feel too rough; other times, what seems like a fierce bite to you might not be hard enough for her. There's no magic way of telling what she fancies on a particular day – just ask her what feels good.

Ⓕ FOR HER

Some men's nipples seem to be directly linked to their penis. Suck, stroke or tweak them and they'll get an instant erection. Other men are lukewarm to the idea – play all you like but he'll still look about as excited as someone sitting in the dentist's waiting room. Again, there's only two ways to find out which category he fits into. Open your mouth and apply it to a nipple to see how he responds or ask him directly.

Use the same techniques he uses on you (or you'd like him to) – nibbling, stroking, sucking the nipples gently to begin with, upping the pressure if he seems to enjoy it.

Try a Tantric technique. Put a glass of water with ice-cubes in it by the bed. Rub an ice-cube on his nipples to make them stand up and get the blood flowing to that area. Now use your fingertips to make a circular motion around the nipple, alternating occasionally with a little pinch. Pull at the nipples to draw them out, watching his face to see which motion arouses him most.

DELICIOUS DETOURS

'Happiness isn't a destination; it's a means of travelling.' This old saying can be applied to foreplay. Rush through the 'travelling' and you might find the destination isn't quite as exciting as you'd expected. Lavish attention on the *whole body* and you can't help but take your time.

Erogenous zones are areas on our bodies that create intense sexual arousal when stimulated. Apart from the obvious bits that we all share (like the penis and the clitoris), each of us has our own secret area that sends frantic YES! YES! messages to all the right places. For some, it's being bitten in the small of their neck. Others go crazy when someone strokes their buttocks. But what works for one lover won't necessarily work on the next, so consider each new lover unexplored territory. There are few places on our bodies that we don't like being touched. Why restrict foreplay to the breasts and genitals when the entire body is itching for attention?

- **Take a body tour.** When you get to a new city, you often take an orientation tour to get your bearings, right? Then what's stopping you doing the same with your new lover's body? You can go all out here and even use a few props. Make him lie down naked on his stomach and close his eyes – make sure the room you're in is private and warm – then trail a scarf slowly and tantalisingly across his naked bottom and back. Then turn him over and stroke a feather around his penis and scrotum. You can then move on to using your hands, hair, breasts and mouth on his nipples and genital area, creating different sensations as you search for his ultimate pleasure zones.
- **Try stroking her face,** the back of her neck, her back. Play with her hair, lift it up from her neck and stroke underneath, slide your palms up and down her arms – and this is just while you're watching TV together. Don't even make it to the bedroom.
- **Massage his feet,** kiss his toes, massage his hands, then take each finger into your mouth and suck it, pretending it's his penis.
- **Don't dive straight for his penis during foreplay.** Use long, sensual strokes up his inner thighs until he's *trembling* with desire.

- **Bottoms up!** Both your bottoms are an arousable area. Try massaging them, stroking, even gentle slapping. Don't neglect the perineum (the bit between your genitals and your anus). Press firmly and massage with two fingers, gently stroking along the entire length; use your tongue to do the same.
- **Use your fingers to rub along the outline of his lips,** then insert a finger into his mouth for him to suck. Do the same with your nipples. He can do the same with his penis.
- **Get into neck nibbling.** Do you know anyone who doesn't enjoy having their neck kissed or gently nibbled? (If you do, they're either incredibly ticklish, or totally uptight.) It's a sadly ignored area that can produce amazing results.
- **Suck her toes,** slide your tongue into her belly button (try diving on her after a shower if you're paranoid about 'fluff') – have fun with foreplay! It really doesn't matter if she laughs instead of sighs – she's still complimented that you find *all* of her sexy, not just 'the good bits'.
- **Kiss all over his body,** not just on his mouth and genitals.
- **Use your whole body to massage his.** Lie on top of him when he's lying on his back or front, gyrate slowly and revel in the simple sensation of skin against skin.

And for my next trick . . .

- **Tie him up.** We've all seen it done in the movies. You don't need to pop down to a sex shop and buy one of those leather numbers to slip on (unless you want to, of course) or crack a whip (ditto) to play the dominatrix. But you *do* need a bedpost (or chair) to tie him to, a couple of long scarves (some old stockings or a few of his ties will do) and a nasty smile on your face. Once he's comfortably trussed (don't cut off the circulation, you need the blood flowing for him to get an erection, let alone keep his heart pumping), you can try out a number of erotic scenarios, like . . .
- **Masturbate for him.** Watching you give yourself pleasure will give him a big kick. The effect will be even more spectacular if you masturbate loudly and theatrically while he's tied up and is utterly helpless. If you want to get him *really* worked up, simply leave him tied up and then . . .

- **Blindfold him.** Even a see-through chiffon scarf can increase the sexual tension tenfold. It also makes you less inhibited about what you do to him because he can't see you. Tie the scarf across his eyes then build the anticipation by withdrawing completely for a few seconds, then caressing him in his favourite places, and a few he's not expecting. This also lets his imagination run wild – you could be a provocative French maid, slave girl . . . you get the picture.
- **Undress each other.** Don't just fling your clothes in a corner and hop into bed naked; let him undress you and vice versa. Stop along the way to lick and caress the body part that's just been exposed.
- **Play the vamp.** Thought the only time you'd use those long, black gloves was on black tie occasions? Put them on now and start masturbating him. Yes, it does come out in the wash.

! *Whipped cream, ice-cream and chocolate spread . . . they're the three foods 30 per cent of women would most like their partners to lick off their body.*

- **Make it good enough to eat.** Whipped cream, bananas and berries aren't just good for fruit salads. Take them out of the kitchen or, better still, stay there and satisfy two appetites at once. Having a feast off each other's bodies is a laugh more than anything else, but even if it simply makes sex more fun, it's worth the experiment. Unless you're talking hot and spicy foods, it's safe to smother or insert most foods in and around the genitals for both of you to devour. While you're at it, grab some ice-cubes from the freezer, put them into your mouth, then suck his penis.
- **Drop it.** Leave the sisterhood stuff outside the bedroom door. If he fantasises about you dressing up as a waitress, serving him exactly what he hungers for, he *is* treating you like a sex object – but isn't that the point?
- **Go for the cliché** – most men love it. Invest in some sexy black underwear. After a night out, take off your clothes to reveal stockings and suspenders. (Even better, flash him a glimpse *while* you're out.)

- **Tease, tickle and titillate.** Brush your lips over his mouth but don't let him kiss back. Put his penis momentarily in your mouth, then withdraw and start kissing his neck. Sit on top of him and let him partially penetrate you, then get up and walk away. The trick is to keep him unbelievably aroused rather than frustrated. At some point, though, you have to put him out of his misery by bringing things (and him) to a fabulous finale!

THE LONG, SLOW STRIP

You probably can't equal (but then again, who knows?) the hot little strip that Kim Basinger did for Mickey Rourke in *9 ½ Weeks*. But you can certainly make up in enthusiasm whatever you lack in professional technique. Here's a wiggle-by-wiggle guide to taking it all off and really turning him on.

- You absolutely must wear stockings and suspenders and sexy underwear. Add a silky, short slip (à la Kim).
- Put on some music. Anything you like to dance to will do (though heavy metal possibly won't create the atmosphere you're aiming for). Try some Barry White or Prince; if you have the original Joe Cocker song 'You can leave your hat on', put it on and hit the replay button!
- Gulp some champagne for dutch courage, sit your partner in the lounge room and tell him if he laughs you'll not only kill him, you'll stop immediately. (He won't even smile!)
- Start by rubbing your hands over your body, letting the slip ride up your thighs and the straps slide down off your shoulders. It's best if you have a slip you can step out of, rather than one you have to pull over your head (and end up getting stuck in).
- Removing your stockings is next. Really work this one, rolling the stockings down seductively, leaving your suspender belt on.
- To begin with, play it coy and keep your eyes modestly lowered, so he gets the impression you're undressing privately and he's not supposed to be looking. As you get to your suspender belt, move into a more dominant role – fling yourself and it around a bit like professional strippers do.

(Practise this in front of a mirror first and keep your distance. Flicking him in the face with the belt will ruin the mood – and he needs two eyes to watch you.)

- Remove your knickers a bit at a time. Play it up a little by almost taking them off, then deciding not to. Put one leg up on the side of a chair as you push them down over your thighs, so he can see your genitals.
- Walk over to him and look him straight in the eye when you undo the final garment (your bra) thrusting your breasts forward. That way you can also finish the show off with an extra most strippers never supply – taking *his* clothes off in the middle of a long, slow, French kiss.

TOUCH UPS

The sexperts call it 'mutual masturbation', a ghastly term which conjures up an image of a group of people, all sitting around in a circle, playing with their own genitals. While mutual masturbation *can* mean masturbating in front of each other, it's usually used to describe you giving him a hand-job and vice versa. In other words, it's 'heavy petting' – what you were (probably quite rightly) accused of doing when you stayed out late with your boyfriend as a teenager.

Like every other sex skill, expertly masturbating or 'touching up' someone else's genitals takes practice. Though it's pleasurable to be touching each other simultaneously, if you're really serious you'll take turns. It's far too easy to lose concentration and focus instead on what he/she is doing to you. This is one area where I'm pleased to be female. The great thing about penises is that they're usually happy no matter what you do to them – the very fact that your hand is 'down there' stroking him, will usually be enough to get his juices flowing – unlike vaginas and clitorises, which are super-sensitive, contrary creatures, highly individual and finicky.

There's another huge difference between the two sex organs. For women, gentle is nearly always best; for men, firm is invariably better. What sends you orbiting into orgasmic heaven can leave him limp; what makes him groan with pleasure can have you yelping in pain. So, if you're a female, you can probably up the pressure a bit. I'm not suggesting you wring his penis with abandon or bend it willy-nilly (it's *attached*, remember, and not made of plasticine), but you can probably go harder than you are. If you're male, tone it down a little. She'll soon let you know if your touch is so soft she's forgotten you're even in the room.

> 'I swear it's true: I've never had a woman try to masturbate me to orgasm. Usually, they'll stroke and play around a bit but they've never taken a firm grip and done it the way I do. It doesn't worry me as long as they're good at oral, but I find it intriguing. Why don't they?'
>
> Shane, 36, small business owner

As with any sexual technique, the best way to get good at mutual masturbation is to ask your partner to show you how *they* do it and imitate. At the very least, guide each other by saying what feels good and what doesn't. Even a 'harder' or 'move up a bit' is better than nothing.

F FOR HER

Just as you hate him diving straight for the clitoris, he hates you pouncing immediately on the penis. Kiss and stroke everywhere, glide up the inside of his thighs, pay attention to his testicles and the area of his tummy his erect penis sits on.

Remember our biology lesson? (If you don't, go back to page 4 and read 'How the penis works' again.) The head of the penis is packed with nerve endings and so is the frenulum (the string of skin underneath the penis where the head meets the shaft). Pumping up and down the shaft alone will do little more than give you a mini-workout.

If he's uncircumcised, don't pull back the foreskin until he's well lubricated (either with pre-ejaculatory fluid – the stuff that comes out when he's excited that looks like sperm – saliva or personal lubricant). Even then proceed with caution. The head of the penis is more sensitive on uncircumcised men; you're better off using the foreskin as a buffer between you and the head, and manipulating that up and down over it.

- Get into a good starting position. Chances are you're lying beside him, but while this is the most usual position it's probably the hardest to work with. If you're serious, get him to stand in front of you or sit astride him. Want to stay lying down? At least prop yourself up on one elbow so you can work properly with one hand; better still shift your weight so you can use both hands and still be balanced. Make sure you're on the right side (that is, if you're right-handed, that's the best hand to use). If it feels awkward your end, it's going to feel less than perfect his.
- Start by stroking his penis until it hardens, then roll it gently between your palms before moving into the basic stroke. Make an open fist with your hand (see page 20 for more detail) and move it up and down the shaft of the penis in a regular rhythm. As you get to the head, try closing your fist and gliding over it, increasing the pressure a little.
- Ask him to put his hand over yours to show you what pace he likes. The three things to keep in mind are: smooth, firm and consistent. Try to make one long, smooth action rather than a number of jerky movements. This shouldn't be too hard because it's a very simple movement – just close your fist as you go over the head, and open it to move down the shaft. Try long strokes taking in the whole length, or short strokes concentrating on the head.
- Start off slow and speed up as he approaches orgasm. The faster and harder you masturbate him, the quicker he'll orgasm. If you want to tease, speed up for a while, then slow down before speeding up again.
- You have two hands. Use the other one to cup the scrotum, play with his nipples, massage the perineum firmly with your fingertips.
- Some women use two hands on his penis – one holding it firmly at the base, the other moving up and down the shaft. Others prefer to make a thumb and first finger ring rather than a loose fist. (While we're on the subject of hands, change them often so they don't become numb.)
- As he's about to climax, he'll tense up and breathe heavily. If you're watching closely, you might notice the head of his

penis becoming dark red and his testes lifting toward his body. Most men prefer you to be working quite fast until they start ejaculating, then to slow it right down or simply stop and hold the penis during ejaculation. Lots of men say they like less pressure on the head the closer they are to coming. It's incredibly sensitive just after ejaculation; resist the urge to do one last stroke for good luck and remove your hands gently. (This is also why he'll wince with pain if you cough while he's still inside you but has already ejaculated. Coughing involuntarily squeezes your vaginal muscles around his – ouch! – oversensitive penis.)

- As an alternative, let him masturbate his penis between your breasts. If they're little, hold them close together with your hands to create a cleavage.

COMMON MISTAKES WOMEN MAKE

- You're either too hard or too soft. Getting the pressure right is simply a matter of asking him which feels best. Men with smaller penises generally like a softer touch (the nerve endings are more concentrated).
- You don't ask what he likes and use the same technique on everyone. (You ask people how they like their coffee don't you?)
- You don't keep up a steady rhythm or do it for long enough. Many guys complain that women are jerky, stop at all the wrong times and don't position themselves properly so their hands go numb way too quickly.
- You don't hit the right spot. The bottom of his penis may feel wonderfully macho and hard to you, but it's stimulating the top that feels best to him.

Ⓜ FOR HIM

Just like 'Monopoly', you can't collect your £200 until you've passed 'Go'. In other words, don't even think about touching her genitals until you've paid your dues on her breasts, neck and tummy, and stroked up her thighs.

- You're probably lying beside her, hopefully with the hand you're most comfortable working with free. If she's not already wet, lubricate the area with saliva or personal lubricant. Her natural lubrication will keep the area moist once she's fully aroused.
- Start by 'warming' and stimulating the whole genital area. Place your whole hand over the closed outer lips and rub in a circular motion. You'll be stimulating the clitoris by moving her lips against it.
- When she starts to become aroused, the outer lips will open naturally themselves. Gently part them a little wider and move your fingertips up and down the inner lips, in a long, slow, soft movement, grazing the clitoris – still covered by a little hood of skin – on your way up and down.
- Wait until she's well lubricated before honing in on the clitoris. Then circle around it with one fingertip several times before sliding back down the inner lips again. Get her to guide you by putting her hand over yours to show you what speed and pressure she likes. Even lubricated, the clitoris is extremely sensitive. If you're too rough, too direct or stimulate for too long, too soon, it gets oversensitive and feels painful. Concentrate exclusively on the clitoris only when she's close to orgasm.

> 'I went out with a bodybuilder whose idea of foreplay was taking his clothes off. I guess I was supposed to get off by looking at all those muscles. It was all over in about three minutes – and he didn't know what afterplay was either.'
>
> Helena, 26, journalist

- An alternative technique is to use vibration. Place your middle three fingers over the top of the vagina (where the clitoris is), press firmly (but not too hard), then vibrate your hand gently but rapidly and consistently or move it in a circular, vibratory motion.
- The three golden rules for men: gentle, slow and regular. Keeping up a steady rhythm for a long period of time, even if your technique isn't perfect, will get you further than switching all over the place with the most adroit strokes.

While she can speed up, slow down or stop completely to tease you, you do the same and she'll end up frustrated rather than turned-on.

- Most women like to be penetrated with a finger (fingernails trimmed, please!). Use one finger to begin with, add another when she's more excited or use your thumb and press deeply. Move it in and out of the vagina, gently to start with. Some women love to be penetrated deep and quite hard but still keep it slow. She'll be wetter inside, so spread the lubrication over the clitoris. Keep stimulating the clitoris while penetrating her by keeping the flat of your hand firmly pressed against it while your fingers dip in and out.
- A lot of the time you'll have one hand working on her clitoris, the other inside her. When you've got one hand free, use it to stroke her nipples. As she's about to climax, she may clench her buttocks, tense up, hold dramatically still and go completely quiet. (Not all women put on a Meg Ryan *When Harry Met Sally* performance.) At this point, it's crucial to keep doing whatever it is you're doing – don't stop or change *anything*. As she's coming, slow down but keep going (gently). She'll push you away when she's had enough.
- Try rubbing her clitoris with the tip of your erect penis as a sexy alternative to using your fingers.

Common mistakes men make

- You're too rough. This is the number one complaint of all women, regardless of age.
- You get offended if we try to guide you and don't read our body language. It doesn't matter how many lovers you've had, each female is different. We're not criticising you when we move your hand, simply teaching you what suits us. Many women say men don't read their body language for signs. If she presses against you, she wants more pressure; if she pulls away, she wants you to be more gentle. ➢

- You don't keep a consistent rhythm. Just as we start climbing the climax ladder, you change techniques and we slide right to the bottom again.
- You push your fingers inside too soon. Stimulate the labia and clitoris a little first.
- You stop at the crucial moment. Our orgasms often last longer than yours do (we *knew* there had to be some payoff for having to suffer through period pain). You might think she can't possibly still be having one, but she may be. If you stop what you're doing while we're still climaxing, the orgasm continues but it's not as intense and we feel horribly robbed.

BLOW THEM AWAY!

If you're not good at giving oral (even worse, can't be bothered learning), give up now on ever graduating from sex school. Nothing will score you more points in the bedroom than delivering mind-blowing fellatio (to him) or cunnilingus (to her).

Oral sex is the one erotic act everyone consistently reports wanting more of. Without it, many women would never orgasm with a partner. Equally adored by both genders, oral sex appears to have universal appeal. If being told 'You're a great lay' is a compliment, you'll be worshipped for performing hellishly good head-jobs.

Why the fascination? The thought of someone's tongue licking your genitals seems naughtier than intercourse; unless you're in the 69 position, it's perfectly acceptable to lie back and receive pleasure without having to reciprocate simultaneously; and tongues are usually wetter, softer and more agile than hands and penises. They're also warm and genitals respond to heat much more than they do cold fingers. Convinced it's a skill worth mastering? You should be. Read on . . .

F FOR HER

Giving him mind-blowing fellatio (the posh term for oral sex) is number one on his sex wish-list, and it's the thing most women feel least confident about. Who better to ask for tips than a sex worker who specialises in it? (If you have something against taking advice from experienced, high-class prostitutes, get over it now. They make a living out of sex and are experts in their field.) I asked Olivia, a skilled fellatrix, to reveal her most intimate secrets for this no-holds-barred guide to giving him pleasure. Prepare to turn from the most nervous novice into an instant expert – and have him begging for more! This is her guide, so I'll let her tell you in her own words . . .

Ten-step guide to the best fellatio he's ever had

1. Learn to love it

'Women who love sex are good at it; it's as simple as that. If you don't like giving him oral, the best techniques in the world won't turn you into a skilled fellatrix. Usually it's the smell, swallowing or gagging that women are scared of and all are easily fixed. Turn a shower into foreplay if he's not scrupulously clean and use the soap as a lubricant to masturbate his penis (if he's uncircumcised pull the foreskin back very gently and wash underneath). Gagging isn't a problem if you use my techniques and you don't have to swallow to be good at oral.

'Fellatio, or 'French' as we call it, is requested and enjoyed by almost all clients, regardless of the prostitute's speciality. Show him that you love doing it – make lots of noise and *'uuumms'*, compliment him on his penis – and he'll be anything *but* putty in your hands! Get to know his penis: examine it, talk about it. Be aware of his body language. Learn how to read his moods and play up to any secret fantasies.'

2. Give him lots of foreplay

'Women aren't the only ones who love foreplay (even if *he* hasn't realised it yet) and your mouth shouldn't be anywhere near his penis till it's rock hard. Pamper him by giving him a massage then a 'body tease'. Oil his body and yours and lie over him, supporting your weight on your hands. Come in close and slide up and down, gyrate your pelvis against his body letting him feel how turned on you are, and push your bottom in the air (especially if there's a mirror behind you). If you've got long hair, use it; lean forward and let it caress his body. Bite his nipples, and tease him by lowering yourself over his penis so your genitals are touching but don't let him penetrate. Give him 'Spanish': put his penis between your breasts and roll and knead them around it using your hands. Stroke, lick and nibble your way down his body while you're telling him exactly what you're about to do to him. Get feedback: ask him what *he'd* like you to do.'

> 'Most girls, they treat your penis like it's a lollypop. Licking alone doesn't do a thing for me and most of the time they'll screw up their faces during oral, like it's some nasty object. You know she's only doing it because she thinks you expect her to. That's why if you meet a girl who gets off on giving you head, you're stoked.'
>
> Danny, 18, gym instructor

3. Vary the scene and stimulate all his senses

'Don't do it in the same position every time. Guys love getting oral just about anywhere but variety's a turn-on. Try him standing up and you kneeling or squatting in front of him; him up against a wall; a '69er'; in the car; in the park while walking home from a restaurant. Different locations add a fresh psychological kick. It doesn't matter what you're wearing but lots of men find it exciting if you're totally naked and he's fully clothed with just his zip undone; alternatively, try you fully dressed and him totally naked. Make sure he can watch. Men are erotic visualists and primarily aroused by what they can see, one reason why they're so into girlie mags. He'll want to see your face, maybe even hold your hair back. Don't close your eyes, keep them open. I hold eye contact with the man while I'm fellating him and make 'horny eyes' – narrow them sexily and make them smoulder. If you're too embarrassed to look at him, look at his penis instead.'

4. Don't just concentrate on his penis

'His anus, perineum, testicles – all are erogenous zones you should pay attention to before and during fellatio. Get him to lie on his back then lick and stroke him on the perineum (the area between his anus and testicles), massaging it with slight pressure. Bend his legs back and lick from the base of his anus through to the scrotum. Cradle his testicles in your hand, lick them, take one or both in your mouth. Massage near the base of his penis, one hand holding it, the other massaging.'

5. Use your hands and start masturbating him

'Always use two hands during oral: one to stimulate him elsewhere (nipples, testicles, anus), the other as a guide. It gives you more control and he can't gag you. I usually keep one hand at the bottom of the shaft of his penis, then it's up to me to control how deeply I take it into my mouth. Lots of men like to put their hands on the back of your head but tell him it's hands-*off* if he won't stop pushing you deeper than you want to go. 'Deep-throating' is a head game more than anything else. If you can do it, great! If you can't or don't want to, rest assured that it doesn't necessarily feel better; it's just what he's seen in a porn film. Most feeling is at the head of his penis not the bottom. If you're really paranoid about gagging, place the penis to one side of your mouth rather than dead centre.'

6. Take control of his penis but handle with care

'Some women are too rough! The best way to find out how he likes being masturbated is to get him to show you how he does it himself then imitate the technique. Don't tug or yank at his foreskin if he's uncircumcised; make sure it slides up and over the penile head. Take a firm grip, then start teasing. Let him see your nice pink tongue and play up the lick movements. Do long, lollypop licks, lick up the side, around the head, cover your teeth with your lips (and keep them that way!) and do 'lip-pinches' (a biting motion without teeth involved) up and down the side of the shaft. Use lots of saliva: the more lubricated he is, the more pleasurable it will feel. Finally, take his penis right into your mouth, swirl your tongue around the head, then withdraw and give a big 'uuummm' of satisfaction!'

! ***Is it fattening? There are around 150 kilojoules in the average ejaculate of sperm, while about 630 kilojoules are burned in an hour of sex.***

7. Technique is all-important

'The basic technique is to slide your hand up and down his penis (closing it when you reach the head, opening it slightly as you slide down the length) as it's moving in and out of your mouth. With your lips covering your teeth, close your mouth around the penis and encircle it so there's a firm but comfortable pressure. You're not actually sucking, more making sure your mouth is a snug fit. Practise on your finger and imagine it's his penis. What sort of sensations seem like they'd feel good? Imagine how his penis feels when it's in your vagina and try to imitate the sensation. When you're confident, move into the 'twist-and-swirl': make a gentle twisting motion with your hand as you're sliding it up and down his penis and swirl your tongue around the rim of the head, paying particular attention to the frenulum (see 'How the penis works, on page 4). Tense your tongue and vibrate it; swirl it around the head and the base – the more tongue movements while it's in your mouth the better! As with women, a steady rhythm is important. Start off agonisingly slow, then increase the pressure and the rhythm as he approaches orgasm.'

8. Tease him mercilessly

'Take him to the brink of orgasm (you'll get better at timing this with practice!) so he experiences that intensely pleasurable pre-orgasm wave several times, then stop fellating him and use your mouth on his testes, the perineum and his anus before returning. Be creative and use different strokes: long slides up and down his penis, taking it deep in your mouth; shorter strokes concentrating on the head and inserting just the tip. Once he's approaching orgasm, however, stick with the same technique and rhythm.'

9. Step up the stimulation just as he's about to orgasm

'The male G-spot is about 3 to 6 cm inside the anus and by inserting a finger, you'll make his orgasm even more intense. If he enjoys anal stimulation, he'll push his bottom toward you or stick it up in the air the minute you start to explore the area. Be gentle and make sure your finger is well-lubricated. If you feel uncomfortable doing this, give him a stronger orgasm by pressing the perineum area firmly with your thumb as he's ejaculating.'

! ***If his sperm tastes bad, it could be something he ate. What he eats and drinks hours before making love strongly affects the way he tastes. For the best flavoured sperm, feed him bland foods like pasta and potatoes; for the worst, serve a curry, washed down with beer and coffee.***

10. Decide beforehand what you'll do when he ejaculates

'It will be obvious when he's about to orgasm: the penis starts to throb, jerk and spasm; some men stop thrusting and stay perfectly still, others thrust harder. Some men are oversensitive when they orgasm so keep your hands away from the head of the penis and masturbate him at the bottom. If you're going to swallow his semen, do it properly. Don't make faces; simply swallow it and say 'yuuumm'. If you don't want to, don't take any sperm in your mouth; spitting it out is rude, unattractive and insulting. Instead, withdraw when he's in the throes of orgasm and continue stimulating him with your hand. A sexy alternative to swallowing is to let him ejaculate elsewhere on your body – over your breasts or your neck. If you rub it into your body afterward, he'll know you enjoyed fellating him as much as he enjoyed receiving it!'

Tricks of the trade

- Drink a hot drink beforehand. The sensation of a hot mouth around his penis is sensational! Smearing honey or cream over it, then licking it off, adds a fun element.
- Play up to the power fantasy. Power – having it or being completely dominated – is a common fantasy for many men. Let him call the shots and kneel before him or *you* take control and let him know you're boss!
- Clean your tongue with a toothbrush every time you clean your teeth. A healthy, pink tongue is a turn-on.
- If he goes limp, slow it down. Ask him why. Either he's stressed or tired and can't concentrate or you're not fellating him correctly. Applying too much pressure – holding him too tightly with your hand or sucking too hard – can make him lose his erection. Also bear in mind that men are individuals with their own preferred turn-ons and techniques. Talk, start again and slow it down.
- To make him come quickly insert a finger into his anus or press the perineum firmly with your thumb. The more extra stimulation you give, the quicker he'll usually orgasm.
- It's what you do before your mouth even touches his penis that counts. The more foreplay and teasing he's had, the more sensitive he'll be. Just about any sensation will feel great!

HIS TOP FIVE ORAL SEX TURN-OFFS

1. **She acts like she doesn't want to be there.** A woman who's performing fellatio only because she has to was listed as the number one passion killer.
2. **She bites.** While some men actually like their penises being 'nipped', most feel faint at the mere thought! Accidentally biting or scraping his penis with your teeth is an absolute no-no. Keep them covered at all times with your lips.
3. **She's too rough.** Yanking back the foreskin on uncircumcised men, holding or sucking too hard, pumping his penis 'like she's trying to draw water from a dried-up well' were all top turn-offs.
4. **She's got no idea what she's doing.** 'Women who do that stupid bobbing-up-and-down head motion might as well not bother,' says Olivia. Not knowing how to pleasure him orally, and not bothering to find out by reading some sex books or asking him what feels good, was a common complaint.
5. **She acts like semen is poison.** You can be a skilled *fellatrix* without swallowing but that doesn't mean you have to race out of the room gagging the minute sperm appears! Accept that sex is messy: if he ejaculates elsewhere on your body is it really such a big deal?

Ⓜ FOR HIM

Cunnilingus is the rather unexotic name for you giving her oral sex, but men who master it rarely lack lovers. Trouble is, it's *dark* down there and you're often forced to rely on touch and feel rather than eyesight. Apart from eating more carrots, there's not too much you can do about the natural lighting around her vagina. But you can persuade her to let you turn the lights on because it's essential you get this technique right. With some women, oral sex is the only way you'll get her to reach orgasm; for the rest, it's often the most intense. Again, I went to an expert to find out how best to perform cunnilingus. David is a male escort and sex worker who only services women. And guess what's the most commonly requested thing on his menu? Here, in his words, are his professional tips. Don't just read this section, *study* it. If you want to make her quiver, this is how!

! Oral sex has officially replaced intercourse as a female's favourite sexual activity – well, it certainly has in one American college. Ninety-six per cent of the 1000 female students surveyed claimed they enjoyed cunnilingus more than penetration.

A ten-step guide to ohmigod-don't-ever-stop oral sex for her

1. Women are slower to become aroused and slower to reach orgasm than men, so time – not rushing her – is the biggest luxury you can give a woman

'If she's stressed, relax her first by massaging or stroking her body until she starts to become aroused. Follow this with lots of kissing on the neck, and stroke and lick her breasts and nipples before moving on to her genitals. Leave her underwear on and stroke her through the fabric until she becomes wet; only then remove it.'

2. Start by running your hands up and down the outside, then the inside of her thighs and at this point, ask her how she likes oral sex: slow, fast, gentle or hard

'While kissing and licking down her body, pull the outer vaginal lips over the inner in a gentle, circular motion to warm the entire area.'

3. Position counts

'If she's shy, it's best if she lies back while you're kneeling at the foot of the bed between her legs. Lots of women love being licked while they're standing and you're kneeling (it appeals to their slave fantasies plus they can control the pressure and rhythm by holding your head) or being licked from behind. Another favourite which gives her ultimate control: lie back on the bed while she kneels above you and lowers her genitals down to your mouth. She may put her hands flat against the wall behind for balance. Some women like to

> 'I stayed with a complete loser of a guy for six months simply because he gave the best oral sex I'd had in my life. I was addicted to it. I couldn't give him up because – and sadly, this is true so far – I knew I'd never find a tongue like that again.'
>
> Mary, 24, secretary

feel completely exposed with their legs wide open, others prefer their legs quite closely wrapped around your head. It all depends on how sensitive her clitoris is.'

4. It's really important to keep her moist, so use lots of saliva to lick the entire area before concentrating on the clitoris

'Don't tense or point your tongue; it's better to use the whole surface of the flat of your tongue rather than just the tip. That's the one thing that most men do wrong. Start with indirect stimulation, gently wiggling your tongue around and over the clitoris: it's toward the top of the vagina and feels like a tiny marble.'

5. Move into longer, wet, gentle strokes with your tongue, keeping up a slow but steady rhythm

'Rhythm is really important; chopping and changing techniques and rhythm all the time doesn't work with women. Read her body language or ask her what stroke feels best, then keep on doing it. If she pulls away, you're being too rough; if she presses her vagina closer or pulls your head closer, step up the pressure slightly.'

6. It's generally best to be too gentle than too rough

'Again ask her what feels best. Try shaking your head from side to side, making circles around the edge of the clitoris as well as up-and-down strokes.'

7. Make sure she knows how much you are enjoying yourself by making noise

'If she thinks you're enjoying it as much as she is, she relaxes and knows she can take her time. Again, you have to be prepared to settle in and keep going until she says to stop. The tongue movements are gentle and if a guy can't keep them up for at least 10 to 15 minutes, his tongue's too tense or he's doing it too fast.'

8. When she's really aroused, insert a finger inside her vagina

'A lot of women like to be inserted with a finger or dildo just before they come but others find it distracting. If she's good at communicating, she'll pull your hand away if she doesn't like it; if she does, she'll usually move her hips against your hand to achieve deeper penetration. Some women like manually stimulating their own clitorises while you're performing oral; others put their fingers down to feel your tongue working on them. If she does either, lick her fingers as well.'

> 'It's weird but I don't really like guys giving me head. I don't know why, I just feel uncomfortable. I'm not prudish about anything else. I've only ever liked it with one guy – and he was so good, he had a reputation for giving great oral sex. Somehow he hit all the right spots. With everyone else though, I can take it or leave it. Leave it really.'
>
> Nikki, 17, student

9. When you're not manually masturbating her as well as licking, use your other hand to knead her breasts and nipples or to stroke the perineum, the area between her anus and vagina

'Some women like a lubricated finger inserted into their anus as they orgasm; try inserting the tip gently and see if she pulls away before going any deeper.'

10. Her body will tense when she's closer to orgasm

'At this point, increase the pressure slightly or move a little faster. The most important thing though, is to maintain the rhythm as best you can even if she starts moving around. As she's actually orgasming, switch back to slow, gentle strokes but make sure you cover the whole clitoral area by using the whole surface of your tongue. Most women's clitorises are unbearably sensitive immediately after an orgasm, so don't be surprised if she puts a hand down to cover it or pushes your head away.'

THE FIVE THINGS MOST MEN DO WRONG

1. **You only do it if we ask and obviously find it off-putting.** A man who turns his nose up and says 'it smells', even when she's fresh out of the shower, is being ridiculous. Assuming she doesn't have any infections, the natural scent of a vagina is musky and sensual. Don't blame her for swapping lovers if you can't be convinced.
2. **You're too rough.** Some women like a very firm tongue but gentle suits most of us. The clitoris is sensitive so while over-enthusiastic licking will have her squirming, it's with pain not pleasure.
3. **You don't do it for long enough.** You might be able to orgasm at the mere sight of her mouth wrapped around your penis, but she takes longer to climax. Tell her she can take as long as she wants because you *love* doing it to her and she's yours for life.
4. **You change techniques too often.** Women need regular, consistent rhythm for an extended period in order to orgasm. While she might be impressed with your extensive repertoire of mouth movements, stick with one or two each session. The clitoris is a funny beast – it can be terribly turned on by one sensation but take ages to get used to another if you chop and change.
5. **You stop at the crucial moment.** You might like stimulation to stop while you're orgasming, but we prefer it to continue, though often softer, right through to the last spasm. If you stop just as we're hovering on the brink, we often don't make it over the fence.

THE UPS AND DOWNS OF A 69ER

A 69er got its name because the numbers are head-to-toe, as you are. It simply means both of you giving each other oral sex simultaneously. The usual position is the female on top of him, her bottom pointed toward his face, genitals lowered so he can lick them. Meanwhile, her mouth is positioned above his penis.

It's the idea of a 69er – giving pleasure to each other at the same time – which is the turn-on for most people. In reality, it's all too easy to get lazy on your end. If your partner is sending you through the roof, you'll forget about them and try to get away with a few lacklustre licks; same goes for them if you're working your magic. On the upside, 69ers are great for variety and work well when you're *so-o-o-o* turned on, just about anything will feel good. If you like the position but have trouble keeping your mind on the job, take turns. He can give her cunnilingus in that position while she uses her hand on him. She can fellate him while he uses his hand to stimulate her.

! ***Number of women who enjoy receiving oral sex: 73 per cent. Number of women who like giving it to him: 24 per cent.***

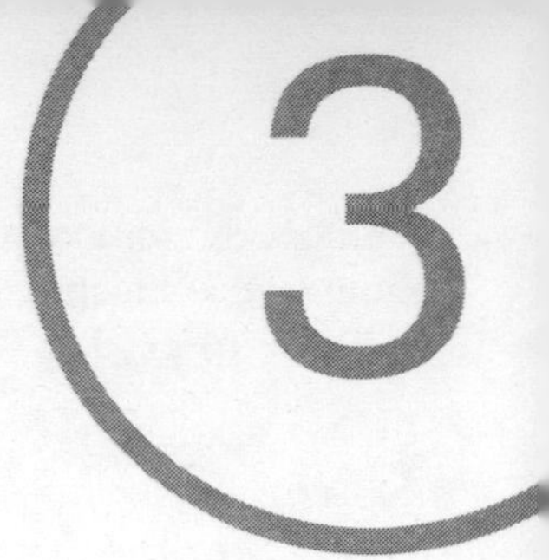

Intercourse

Some new angles on the old in-out, in-out

It's God's fault that couples have so many problems with intercourse. If he really wanted women to enjoy it, he would have put the clitoris *inside* the vagina. I mean, what was he thinking? The only organ in the body designed exclusively for sexual pleasure and it's stuck right up there in penile no-man's land. (Did Adam have an L-shaped one, or has God got a wicked sense of humour?) This simple design fault has caused no end of problems. Because many women need clitoral stimulation along with thrusting, it's the reason why most don't orgasm during intercourse. (If you're male and absorb this point, your Filofax will never be empty again.)

> ! ***The number of synonyms for sexual intercourse in* Roget's Thesaurus: *47***

It's also responsible for the main male beef about bonking. While women mutter about a distinct lack of intercourse orgasms, men are complaining about our lack of enthusiasm. They say females very often consider bonking to be the bit where they get to relax while he does all the work. Like, why should they bother when *they're* not going to hit the jackpot?

Happily, both problems are solved with the one, simple

solution. Remember that dopey saying your grandmother used to sprout? She was right. Busy hands *are* happy hands – and so are the genitals they're busy with.

Clitorises aside, there's a lot more to penetration than you think, and a myriad of ways to vary that one in-out movement. Intercourse is often thought of as the least creative sex act of all. I beg to differ. Hopefully, you will too when you've read through this chapter.

THE FIVE FAVOURITE POSITIONS

There are more than 600 documented positions for intercourse and you'd be asleep within minutes if I tried to list each one of them. Most are variants on the five basic positions anyway, so I'll focus on these and let you use your imagination to discover the other 595!

Despite the endless variety possible, the average couple alternate between two or three positions, most settling on missionary, woman-on-top and rear-entry. There's no such thing as 'the best' position – it all depends on your shapes and height, your individual preferences and mood at the time. Some positions work well if he comes too soon, side-by-side suits lazy, Sunday-morning sex, rear-entry a fast and furious 'quickie'.

For most men, orgasm is guaranteed in just about any (if not all) intercourse positions. For women (sigh!), as I said, it's a different story. Clitoral stimulation is pretty well an essential for most of us to come during intercourse, so I've not only addressed this section to women but included 'Orgasm potential for her' under each position. Having said that, don't be too concerned if your partner's favourite position is different from yours or vice-versa; take it in turns or do both in the same session.

Whatever you do though, do it with passion. Both of you will get a lot more out of all that humping and grinding if you thrust your hips to meet each other's, grab bottoms and pull them close to you, run your hands up and down backs, arms and backs of thighs and lick or bite the closest thing to your mouths. Go for it. Make so much noise, your neighbours consider double-glazing their windows.

> 'I don't come during intercourse but I love it all the same. It makes me feel close to my boyfriend. Our bodies fit together, it's all wet and hard and I feel all filled up. The initial thrust is always the best, especially if we've teased each other to the point where neither of us can wait any longer.'
>
> Naomi, 25, secretary

Missionary

Rumour has it that early missionaries, sent to 'civilise' the colonies, considered this the only respectable way to make love. Hence the name 'missionary' position and its rather staid image.

It was probably the first position in which you had intercourse. I suspect it'll be the last (bodies aren't too agile at 90) and, even if we hate to admit it, it's how most couples have intercourse most of the time. For good reason. The basic position – the woman lying on her back, legs apart with the man between them – requires zero imagination, little effort on her part and is reasonably comfortable for both. It's the position you use when you're both fairly interested in sex but not spinning cartwheels over it. Ironically, it's also the first position to spring to mind when you're so eager for him to be inside you, you don't care how the hell he does it, so long as he does it *now*. Missionary also appeals to the come-on-you've-got-to-admit-I've-put-on-weight girl (that is, 99 per cent of women) because of the flat-tummy thing. We lie on our backs, the flab spreads out and we look extra thin. Bonus!

Why it feels good for her

You're face-to-face and can talk and kiss, so it can be quite romantic. But you also have less control over what's happening and basically can't move very far. Bend your knees for deeper penetration. Stimulate the clitoris more effectively by keeping your legs together (squeezing your thighs) and have his legs open, lying over the *outside* of yours.

Why it feels good for him

He basically runs the show, being in complete control of the depth of penetration, the angle and the pace. For this reason, it's not a bad choice if he's a premature ejaculator because he can stop if he gets too carried away. If the opposite's the problem (he's had one drink too many and having trouble orgasming), reach down and hold back the skin on his penis, grasping at the root of the shaft with your finger and thumb, while he's moving in and out of you. There is one drawback for both of you: neither of you can see any of the real action.

> 'I'd say most guys would nominate missionary or rear-entry as their favourite positions. The first one's easy and no effort; in the second, you're guaranteed to get your rocks off. Doggie was also the position I most enjoyed when I was with a girl I loved. I think I now associate it with her and the good times.'
>
> Steve, 24, gym instructor

Orgasm potential for her

It's not great for manual stimulation of your clitoris but it can make him last longer in intercourse if that's a problem.

How to make it even better

Put one or two hard pillows under your bottom; pull your knees up to your chest or wrap them around his back for deeper penetration; try lifting your legs high and resting one or both feet on his shoulders; lie sideways and move most of your body off the bed, head resting on a cushion on the floor (yes, the blood will rush to your head but that's the idea – some women swear this makes female orgasms scream-material).

One way to make it instantly more exciting for both of you is to put a ban on using the missionary. If you do 'slip up' (and you will – anything 'banned' becomes immediately desirable), it'll seem naughty, forbidden and anything but boring.

How to vary it

Get him to stimulate your G-spot. Rather than thrusting in and out, you half sit up, lift your bottom, then slowly lean backward, repeat until one (or both) of you climax; let him lift your legs up and hold them; roll over completely and end up with – you on top!

Comfort rating for him
His arms can get tired supporting his own weight.

Comfort rating for her
Unless he rests his weight on his elbows or hands and knees, even breathing can be difficult. If he's the size of a Sumo wrestler and you're a waif, forget it.

Woman-on-top

Any woman worth her stuff, in or out of bed, has to revel in this one, even if it's just for the connotations of the name. You on top, you in control – it's deliciously *liberated*, not to mention a hell of a turn-on for both of you. For best control and balance, most women sit on top of their partner, who's lying on his back, then lower themselves onto his penis, legs bent at the knees and folded backward. You can also try squatting. In the basic position, you're usually facing him. Don't try woman-on-top unless he's very hard – it's incredibly easy to bend a semi-erect penis and cause injury.

***!* Number of positions in which most couples have intercourse: 2 to 5. The favourites: missionary and woman-on-top. Number of lovers who use more than 20 positions regularly: 5 per cent.**

Why it feels good for her
It's the opposite to the missionary: instead of him calling the shots, you have complete control over the depth of penetration, angle and speed. You're in the power position and can show off all you like. Exhibitionists don't do it any other way but even if you're not, it's still fantastic. (If you don't feel confident about showing off your body, simply lean forward.) If deep penetration sometimes hurts – your cervix is sensitive for instance – this is one position you can relax in, without fear of pain. He can only go as deep as you let him.

Why it feels good for him
He gets off on watching your body and what's happening – this position lays it all right in front of him. He can see your body clearly and watch the expressions on your face as you approach

orgasm. *You* might think breasts look ridiculous wobbling up and down, *he* thinks they look sexy. Not only that, he gets the double bonus of watching his penis disappear into your vagina while *you* do all the work. The pressure's off. You're looking after your own pleasure (at least in terms of penetration), and he doesn't have to worry about timing or depth.

> **'I *hate* getting on top. My legs seize up, I feel stupid and it hurts my back. I also hate doggie. It makes me feel cheap and undignified.'**
>
> Louise, 32, real estate saleswoman

Orgasm potential for her

Both his hands are free to caress your breasts and stimulate the clitoris (lean forward and lift up a little for easier access). If you're a fan of the G-spot, this position is likely to hit it (lean backward). It's also pretty easy for you to touch your own clitoris and bring yourself to orgasm while he's inside you.

How to make it even better

Try moving in small circles as you're lifting yourself up and down; tease him a little (or a lot) by rubbing his erect penis over your vaginal lips, letting him enter just a fraction then denying him full penetration by lifting tantalisingly higher; turn him on by playing with your own breasts or your clitoris.

How to vary it

Face his toes instead of his head (resist the urge to do a 180-degree turn while impaled unless you warn him first); get him to hold your waist to help you move up and down; lean forward or backward to experience the sensation of stimulation on different parts of your vaginal walls; lie (instead of sitting or crouching) on top of him with your legs outside or inside his; try him sitting in a chair with you on his lap; try him sitting up with legs straight out in front of him, you lower yourself onto his penis and sit with your knees bent and feet flat on the floor.

Comfort rating for him

Ten out of 10 – what's *not* to like? Women are usually lighter than men, so he's unlikely to complain about you being too heavy.

Comfort rating for her
It can be tiring if you're using your legs to move up and down but think of it this way: you can skip the squat machine at the gym the next day.

Rear-entry (or 'doggie-style')

This position allows *deep* penetration and ignites the animal instinct in anyone with a libido because it's so primitive. It's a firm favourite with any couple who really get into sex, and is avoided by couples who think walking hand-in-hand along a beach is racy. A warning for women with men who come too soon: don't even let him think about this one unless you're both happy with a quickie. With the combination of deep penetration, the unleashing of the 'beast' in him because he's 'taking you', fantasies soaring right off the pleasure scale because he can't see your face and could be having sex with anyone . . . He'll last, *ooohh*, two seconds if you're lucky.

! *Men used to initiate sex 75 per cent of the time, now women are the first to suggest it 40 per cent of the time.*

Why it feels good for her
Uninhibited women love rear-entry – anyone with a slave fantasy can let their imagination run riot (rear-entry is him at his most dominant and you at your most submissive and vulnerable). Because you can't see him, he could be anyone (the guy on your favourite soap, the wonderfully *built* workman you saw on the street, your boyfriend's best friend). Your breasts are often hanging down so the blood flows to the nipples and makes them extra-sensitive.

Why it feels good for him
It allows him to penetrate as deeply as he possibly can and he's visually stimulated (turned on by what he can see more than what he can feel). The sight of his penis pumping in and out of your vagina is, well . . . his idea of heaven really. Your bottom presses against his testicles for extra stimulation and speaking of bottoms, most men *love* being able to see yours. (No, he's not looking at how 'fat' it is.)

Orgasm potential for her

Orgasms often feel more intense because he's hitting the sensitive bits (the front wall of your vagina). His hands are totally free to stimulate your breasts from behind or your clitoris. This is by far the best position to stimulate the G-spot since the penis hits the front vaginal wall directly.

How to make it even better

Give in totally and let him penetrate you from behind while you're on all fours.

How to vary it

Rather than kneel: you lie face-down, flat on the bed, legs spread, he lies on top of you and penetrates from behind (great for indirectly stimulating the clitoris). Try him standing behind you, you stand then lean forward until your hands touch the floor. Attempt 'the wheelbarrow': he stands behind you, then lifts and holds your straight legs like a wheelbarrow while you've got your weight supported on your elbows on the bed.

Comfort rating for him

He's a prime target for carpet burn on the knees if you're doing it on the lounge-room floor but does he care? Nah!

Comfort rating for her

Rear-entry positions allow deep penetration – too deep sometimes, especially if he gets completely carried away and starts thrusting like he's trying to find oil. If it feels too deep, lift your bottom. Better still, simply ask him to hold back and go shallower.

Face-to-face positions while sitting or kneeling

Close and intimate, many people find these positions a relaxing variation on the norm. Positions where you're sitting on the end of the bed, he's kneeling in front of you on the floor; you sitting in his lap while he also sits up – these are all examples of what the sexperts call 'face-to-face'. They're good for adding variety and are relatively easy to move into from missionary or woman-on-top since most are derivatives of these anyway.

Why it feels good for her

They're versatile, there's good eye contact and he's in the ideal position to hold his penis and use it to manually masturbate your clitoris and vaginal lips.

The shower, the kitchen table, the lounge room floor and behind a locked bathroom door at crowded parties – these are the places 500 women said they'd prefer to make love in. Anywhere but the bedroom.

Why it feels good for him

You can put your hands behind him and pull him to you by grabbing his buttocks. He'll like the visual stimulation of watching your genitals do their stuff.

Orgasm potential for her

In most positions, he can see and touch the clitoris easily, making it easy for him to masturbate you to orgasm.

How to make it even better

Try rocking as you're thrusting, using your legs as leverage to maintain a steady rhythm.

How to vary it

Use it to spice-up your 'favourites'. Change into a face-to-face sitting position from woman-on-top or missionary, even if it's just for a few moments.

Comfort rating for him

Your heights and sizes can make some positions difficult, even impossible. Don't choose a position that he feels 'twisted' in if he's got back problems or if you're a bigger person than he is.

Comfort rating for her

Some women complain of leg cramps but if you share the work – sometimes he thrusts, sometimes you do – it shouldn't be a problem.

Side-by-side

It's comfortable, cuddly and sensual – perfect for those languid days when you're nicely turned on but not frothing at the mouth to get it. The favourite is the Spoon (nicknamed because the shape the two of you make is rather like a pair of spoons nestled together). You lie on your side, he enters you from behind, arms wrapped around you. Draw your knees up to allow him to penetrate, then keep your bottom stuck out toward him and the top knee forward.

Why it feels good for her

There's lots of body contact, and both his hands are free to play with your breasts, neck, clitoris. It's very cuddly and effortless if you're tired or not very well.

Why it feels good for him

It's great for premature ejaculators because it's less 'full-on' but also comfortable enough for him to settle in and take his time orgasming. There's maximum body contact and it's easy for her to reach behind and caress your buttocks, testicles or perineum.

Orgasm potential for her

Hit the G-spot by getting him to lean back and away from you diagonally. It's easy for him to reach around and use his fingers to stimulate your clitoris.

How to make it even better

Turn it into an 'X': your heads are at opposite ends of the bed and you're making an X with your legs, he's inside you, each of you has one leg underneath each other's, one above. Clasp hands for control; this is great for slowing him down if he ejaculates too quickly.

How to vary it

Grind your bottom against his penis; bending from the waist and moving your upper torso downward. Reach around to fondle his penis while it's moving in and out of you.

Comfort rating for him
For relaxed, unhurried lovemaking it's a winner all round.

Comfort rating for her
Ditto. It's also more comfortable than him-on-top positions if your partner is heavy. A bonus for both of you – you can fall asleep in exactly the same position you made love in.

LOSING IT: A GUIDE FOR THE FIRST TIME YOU HAVE SEX

There's a school of thought that says how and who you lose your virginity to will not only affect your sex life forever but your future relationships with the opposite sex. Heavy stuff, but quite logical when you think about it and certainly well worth bearing in mind if you are contemplating taking the plunge.

If losing your virginity is a positive experience, you're more likely to view sex as something that's healthy and enjoyable and lovers as nice people who can be trusted. The reverse happens if it's a nightmare. That clumsy, five-minute fumble can have extraordinary repercussions so *no-one* should take losing their virginity lightly.

Even if it's no longer something we save for our wedding night, it's still a huge changing point in our lives. It's the initiation ceremony which we think will transform us from gangly schoolgirl to alluring woman, from spotty youth to macho man. Because of the double standard – women who lose it early are sluts, men who lose it early are studs – most women pick their first partners carefully (if not sensibly). Most guys can't *wait* to 'pop their cherry' and do so with the first girl who'll say yes. Regardless, there are things both sexes can do to make the first experience more enjoyable and much less traumatic.

Ⓜ Ⓕ FOR BOTH OF YOU

Accept that practice makes perfect and your first time probably won't be all that wonderful. Most people are eager to experience what, on TV and the big screen at least, looks like damn good fun, but are horribly disappointed the first time round. It helps if you're sexually educated – have read a few good sex books, experimented with foreplay and have a vague idea of what's going to happen – but even then you should prepare yourself for surprises. When I first had sex, I knew all about clitorises and orgasms, but boy did I get a shock when the guy actually started *moving*. Somehow, I'd imagined that once in, you both just . . . I don't know, *lay there*, clamped together!

> 'I always thought it wouldn't worry me if he was a virgin but a guy asked me out recently who I was quite keen on. He was 24 and we got on really well but when he told me he was a virgin, I just couldn't look at him the same way. I kept wondering what was wrong with him. Was he gay? He said he'd been too busy to worry about women – but seriously, for the last eight years? Come on! In the end, I just couldn't be bothered.'
>
> Deborah, 22, receptionist

Ⓕ FOR HER

- **Don't do it until you're absolutely 100 per cent convinced you want to.** The guy who says 'Unless you have sex with me, I'm not going out with you anymore' should be ditched immediately. The boyfriend who's eager but lets *you* decide when is a sensible choice.
- **Tell him you're a virgin.** It doesn't matter how old you are, it's always best to confess. The first time round, you need lots of time to get aroused and you need him to enter you gently. A good lover will do this automatically the first time you make love, but lots of guys don't fit into this category.
- **Be prepared.** If you're both around 15 or 16, you're extremely fertile. Don't kid yourself: you can get pregnant doing it 'just once' if you don't use contraception. If both of you are virgins, you don't need to use a condom for sexually transmitted infection (STI) prevention but they're often the easiest, and most accessible, method of contraception if you're not on the contraceptive Pill. If you want to go on the Pill, see a doctor or go to a Family Planning clinic and ask for a prescription. Remember with most Pills you have to wait for a while before they start to work. (See Chapter 6 to help you decide which

contraception is best for both of you.)

- **Choose the time and place as carefully as your partner.** Some women do lose their virginity while carried away in the heat of the moment, but most plan the event. If it's at all possible, do plan it. The first time is real butterflies-in-the-tummy material. You'll not only be experiencing new physical sensations, you'll be struggling with a few psychological issues as well. Will he still like me afterward? What do I do if my parents find out? Think through all these questions beforehand and if you still want to go through with it, try to find a time and place where you can both take your time without getting interrupted. In a perfect world, you should snuggle up into each other's arms afterward and spend the night together, but this isn't always possible.

> **'I planned my first time down to the last detail. I was going out with the cutest guy in school and we had lots of foreplay. Sure, it wasn't as great as I thought it would be, but we did it again the next night and I started to see what all the fuss was about.'**
>
> Amelia, 30, teacher

- **Don't be surprised if you're not as 'turned on' as you have been in the past.** Chances are the two of you have 'heavy petted' before (he's had his fingers inside you, fondled your breasts, maybe even performed oral sex). But while previously you were nearly sliding off the couch with excitement, now nothing much is happening at all. Relax – it's normal. You're just a little tense and apprehensive. Take your time and let him know he may need to spend longer on foreplay than usual. If you find you're still not lubricating (or 'getting wet'), apply some personal lubricant (you can buy things like K-Y from the chemist or supermarket). Don't even attempt intercourse unless you are wet – it will hurt.
- **Gently does it.** It's easiest to stick to the missionary position the first time round. That simply means he'll lie on top of you. It's a good idea if you use your hand to guide his penis into your vagina. This gives you control over when he penetrates, so it's less of a shock. You may have a hymen – a

protective membrane over the opening to your vagina – but you probably won't. Things like using tampons, gym and riding horses usually break the hymen way before you're even *thinking* about intercourse. If it hasn't broken, him pressing his penis gently against it will break it and allow you to have sex. When he first penetrates you, try 'bearing down' slightly with your vaginal muscles (push them 'out', using your tummy muscles). He should thrust very slowly and gently at first and stay shallow. He can move deeper as you both relax but it's best if he doesn't really 'go for it' the first time.

- **Don't expect to have an orgasm.** He probably will, usually very quickly; you probably won't. This doesn't mean you're not capable of one, just that women usually have to 'learn' how to orgasm; with men it's much more automatic. You might like to read Chapter 1 on masturbation, before or after you've had intercourse, and teach yourself to orgasm that way.
- **If he's a virgin and you're not, be a little tactful.** He'll already be feeling nervous and worried that you'll think he's hopeless (even if he is, tell him he was great). Expect him to orgasm in about one second flat and you won't be disappointed. Guide and help him along but not in an 'I know what to do, you don't' way. If he wants to take control, let him. Most of all, keep in mind that even if he's an abysmal lover at first, as long as he's willing to learn, time (and you) can turn that around pretty quickly.

Ⓜ FOR HIM

- **Admit that you're a virgin even if you're embarrassed.** Be realistic: it's unlikely you're going to be the best lover she's ever had if you've never even had intercourse before.
- **Use a condom.** If you don't know her well, they're protection against sexually transmitted infections (STIs). If she's a long-time girlfriend, you're both virgins and she's on the Pill, fine, don't use one. Just make sure she hasn't

! *A man's pulse doubles its usual rate just before orgasm.*

got some starry-eyed idea that it would be romantic if she got pregnant. If you have any doubts at all that she's not taking the Pill even though she says she is, wear a condom.

> 'I lost my virginity to a girl I loved deeply. But after we'd done it, I wanted to get out there and do it with other girls, try out what I'd learnt. I was a complete bastard and did just that. I still feel ashamed about it now and that was 10 years ago.'
>
> Trevor, 24, shop assistant

- **Decide how 'special' you want it to be.** If you really don't care who it's with, you just want to do it, then there's no problem – just make sure you've always got condoms and will be able to cope emotionally if it's a horrible experience. Doing it with a girlfriend you love (and who loves you) is obviously less frightening and a lot more fulfilling, but not always possible. Don't be pushed by your friends into having sex before you're ready. For starters, you don't *know* they've already done it (often the biggest boasters haven't) and there's no magic age that you must do it by.
- **Don't freak out if it's all over quickly.** You'll feel more comfortable and confident about intercourse if you've had some experience with foreplay *before* you go barging in there, so to speak. But while it's important for female virgins to have lots of foreplay on D-Day, for you it's probably a case of the less you have, the better. Don't panic if you ejaculate before your penis even enters her, or if you thrust only once or twice then orgasm. You're as turned on as hell at the mere *thought* of finally being able to do it and this is completely normal. If she's willing, wait for a little while then try it again – you'll last longer the second time round, even longer the third, etc.
- **If she's a virgin and you're not, recognise that it's an emotional experience for her.** While you can't wait to 'get rid of' yours, she's probably thought carefully before 'giving' you hers. It really is a gift she's bestowing on you and you should be incredibly complimented. Return that respect by taking it slow and easy and don't do it unless

you're prepared to stick around for at least a little while afterward. If you only want sex, not a relationship, have it with someone who isn't a virgin.

> 'When we're doing it missionary style, I get him to move really slow and close my legs around his penis. I squeeze my vaginal muscles tight then get him to use one hand to rub my clitoris. If he's penetrating me hard and stimulating my clitoris at the same time, I climax really deeply and it seems to go on for ages.'
>
> Mandy, 18, fashion student

PUSHING ALL THE RIGHT BUTTONS

Women can only orgasm from clitoral stimulation. Casually slip *that* statement into any conversation about sex and you're virtually guaranteed a brawl. If you think there's controversy over the G-spot, the debate over whether women can have vaginal as well as clitoral orgasms burns twice as fiercely. It didn't even occur to our parents that intercourse might not be the be-all-and-end-all when it comes to coming. But when Masters and Johnson, the highly influential sex researchers, told us *categorically* that the origin of *all* female orgasms was in the clitoris, it divided men and women – and women and women.

For a start, most men are loathe to give up on the myth of the almighty penis as the ultimate satisfier. A survey by sex researcher Shere Hite showed that the overwhelming majority of men would like their partners to reach orgasm from their penises alone, without additional clitoral stimulation. Then there's a group of people that won't, and feel they can't, admit that clitoral stimulation is the only way they climax. These are the women who've 'faked it' during intercourse for sometimes years. It's a little hard to turn around to a long-term partner and say, 'Yes darling, it's true. And I've lied to you approximately 500 times over the last five years.' The rest of us divide again, this time into women who've *only* had orgasms via the clitoris and will happily admit it, and those who swear on their mother's life that they've also had them vaginally.

While the hard facts of sexual research lean toward the 'clitoris-only' side, there are so many personal accounts from women who say they have vaginal orgasms that sexperts are now pretty convinced that there's a kind of orgasm that originates in the vagina. Most probably, it's linked with the G-spot or the A-spot (see Chapter 4). Women who have vaginal orgasms say they're not as intense as the clitoral kind but feel 'deeper', more prolonged and appear to be accompanied by contractions of the uterus and the vagina, as clitoral orgasms are.

> 'I can't relate to those guys who get all uptight if a girl wants you to masturbate her during intercourse. My first serious girlfriend said to me, "You're not going to like this but it's the truth: most women fake orgasm during intercourse and the only way I'll come is if you play with my clitoris at the same time." I assumed all women were like her and have always done it since. A lot of women have said to me, "You know, you're the first guy that's ever done that without me having to ask." '
>
> Peter, 36, small business owner

Regardless of what theory you believe, there's little doubt that even if you *can* have vaginal orgasms, stimulation of the clitoris during intercourse makes them even more intense. Who knows? Try the following tips and maybe you'll join the select (and small) group of lucky women who claim there's such a thing as an out-of-this-world, OHMIGOD orgasm where both vaginal and clitoral orgasms happen simultaneously!

- **Talk about it first.** Be honest with your lover. If you can only come during intercourse if he's stroking your clitoris as well, tell him. Explain that it's not his fault but that lots of women are built that way and it's a matter of biology, nothing to do with his sexual technique.
- **Make sure he knows where your clitoris is.** Show him and let him take a good look in daylight. Then while you're having intercourse, guide him with your hand to where it is. Different positions can make him lose his bearings.
- **Choose a position that allows easy access.** If you skim through the intercourse positions, you'll find which are best for clitoral access under the 'Orgasm potential for her'

section. It takes more than a few seconds of stroking, so make sure his hand's not twisted and cramped. He should be comfortable while he's doing it so it doesn't detract from *his* enjoyment. Occasionally, climax before or after intercourse instead through oral sex or masturbation.

- **Share the workload.** In other words, stimulate your clitoris yourself sometimes so he doesn't have to. Or put your hand over his while he's stroking it. You can guide his strokes better and it seems more of a together, two-way thing.
- **Tell him to be more gentle than usual.** Often the act of thrusting makes it hard for him to keep his hand movements soft.

! ***Number of women who've faked an orgasm: 56 per cent. Number of women who enjoy intercourse: 94.7 per cent. Number of women who claim to orgasm every time they have intercourse, without additional clitoral stimulation: 29 per cent.***

ROCK'N'ROLL YOUR WAY TO ORGASM: A RADICAL NEW WAY TO HAVE INTERCOURSE

The coital-alignment technique (CAT) is the brainchild of American psychotherapist Edward Eichel and it's an entirely new approach to intercourse. Even the most jaded sex therapist sat up and took notice when Eichel published his findings back in the early 1990s because they were so astounding. Not only did CAT increase the chance of intercourse orgasms for women, he wrote, it upped the odds of experiencing *simultaneous* orgasms. (Despite common perception, the chances of both of you screaming 'Yes! Yes!' at exactly the same time during intercourse are rare – that is unless one of you is faking.)

Eichel tested his theory on 43 men and women. Before using his technique, 23 per cent of the females said they orgasmed during intercourse; this jumped to 77 per cent after using CAT. Not one woman had had a simultaneous orgasm with her partner; more than one-third did after using the technique.

The theory behind it is quite simple. Eichel is of the school that believes clitoral stimulation is necessary for women to orgasm. He decided the in-out motion of thrusting was pathetically hopeless at achieving this and invented an alternative 'rocking and rolling' motion. CAT puts rhythmic pressure on the clitoris and keeps it there. Trouble is, it's not an easy technique for couples to master. You have to think very much 'outside the square' to stop doing something that's become second nature after years, so while some devotees now don't have intercourse any other way, most go back to the old in-out-in-out simply because it's easier. Want to give it a try? Here's how to do it . . .

The position

He gets on top of you, lining up his pelvis over yours. His penis is inside you but he's riding 'high' so the shaft of it is outside the vagina and pressing against your mons pubis (the fleshy mound covered with pubic hair). He rests his full weight on you and doesn't prop himself up on his elbows. His weight makes him slide forward, toward your shoulders and head. Make sure he doesn't slide back; his pelvis shouldn't slip below yours. Wrap your legs around his thighs and rest your ankles on his calves.

The movement

You're using your pelvis, not your legs and arms, to move. This is the moment you regret not enrolling in those Arthur Murray dance classes because coordination is everything. The aim is to establish an identical rhythm – both of you moving in exactly the same way at exactly the same speed.

The woman leads in the *upward* stroke: push up and forward to force his pelvis backward. He allows his pelvis to move back but continues to press against yours. The penis disappears into the vagina during the upward stroke. For the *downward* stroke, reverse the process. He forces your pelvis backward and downward. You press against him as he's doing it, pressing your clitoris against the base of his penis. During the downward stroke, his penis rocks forward and presses against the mons pubis, sliding into a shallower position inside the vagina. You're using pressure and counterpressure, not thrusting in and out.

To orgasm

Instead of speeding up, as most couples do during thrusting, the idea here is to maintain a steady, even pace. Don't speed up, don't slow down. If you've got it right, orgasm will happen naturally – for both of you.

CAN I STOP NOW? A WORD ON THRUSTING

Position isn't everything, and if you haven't gathered *that* by now, you haven't been paying attention. But quite apart from things like clitoral stimulation, you can ruin the best-laid plans for the world's greatest bonk simply by thrusting wrongly.

Thrusting – the act of his penis penetrating the vagina and moving backward and forward – seems simple enough. Just a case of put it in there, (almost) take it out again and repeat until white stuff comes out, right? Not quite. There are some misconceptions (aren't there always with sex?) that both of you should be aware of. Since he's often the one in control of thrusting, I've directed most of my comments to the male. But that doesn't let *you* off the hook. If there's one thing you can do to make thrusting more pleasurable for him, it's to thrust back, pushing your pelvis up to meet his. Don't just lie there, do something! If you're on top, some of the comments below apply to you too, so read on . . .

- **We don't need a marathon session every single time.** Some men pride themselves on being able to have intercourse for hours on end. If by this you mean prolonging intercourse by switching positions, stopping for oral sex and mutual masturbation (maybe even a bowl of Cornflakes to keep the energy level up), congratulations. But if you're boasting about thrusting, in the same position, for hours on end, well . . . it gets a bit monotonous really. Most women I know find 'will-he-ever-finish' men boring. Besides, being pumped for too long can hurt. We stop enjoying it, lubrication slows down and our vagina gets dry. Despite this, most men I know worry themselves sick that they don't go on for long enough. Granted, it is nice if the act takes more than three minutes, but don't get *too* hung up on the time thing. Ask your partner how long she'd like you to last – you might be surprised.

- **Keep your thrusting consistent and rhythmic.** There's nothing worse than that constant stop-start technique some men use. Often it's because you're worried about coming too soon, but sometimes you think it's a turn-on for us. By all means tease – it can be exciting if you deny us the long, hard thrust we're dying for – but don't do it too often or too regularly. Then it's just frustrating. Most of the time, aim for continual, regular thrusting and don't go too fast; men who thrust as fast as a jackhammer never make it onto the good-lover list.

> 'A girl that says, "Harder, harder," gets me every time. There's nothing better than letting go at the end and just going for it.'
>
> Doug, 19, labourer

- **Ask her how deep she wants you.** Sometimes women want their partners to thrust *very* hard and *very* deep. Other times shallow, gentle thrusts feel better. It depends not only on the position, but our mood and for some women, what stage they're at in their menstrual cycle. Here's a no-fail, magical way to find out what she's in the mood for today: ask her. You may find your girlfriend never wants deep penetration because it hurts. If even the mildest thrust sends her shooting through the roof, she needs to see her gynaecologist. Otherwise, it's probably because her cervix is in a position where it's getting bumped. Try aiming to the side instead of dead centre.

BOTTOMS UP! A GUIDE TO ANAL STIMULATION

Our bottoms are 'forbidden' zones, so the naughty element (if-I-can't-do-it-I-must) makes anal stimulation automatically exciting for many people. Quite apart from the psychological kick, the anus and rectum in both sexes are packed with nerve endings. For some, it's their most highly charged erogenous zone.

But for every couple who adore adding anal stimulation to their lovemaking, particularly during intercourse, there's another that turns pale at the mere idea of someone touching them in their most 'private' spot. For that reason, I wouldn't advise anyone to pounce on their partner, airily promising the best sensation they've

> 'The first time a lover put his finger up my bottom, I was absolutely horrified. He gave no pre-warning, just shoved it up there with no lubrication. I hated it but it's a different story with the guy I'm seeing now. He knows when and how to do it properly and now I can't orgasm unless he penetrates me anally.'
>
> Sue, 26, mother

ever had, without telling them exactly where they plan to stick their finger first. If your partner blanches at the prospect, that's their choice, and it's not up to you to change their mind. However you *can* gently point out that if they're worried about it being messy, they needn't be. The lower rectum is normally empty and as long as fingers are clean and well-lubricated with nails trimmed, they're not going to cause any damage. (Inserting *objects* into the rectum is another story. We don't want you the laughing stock of the hospital emergency room, do we?) Washing your hands thoroughly afterward, *before* touching her vagina or his penis, protects against any transference of bacteria.

The feelings produced by anal stimulation are quite different to what you're used to and it's great for heightening sensations you're already experiencing. Combine it with intercourse and your orgasms will feel exquisitely erotic; you can also use it during oral sex or while mutually masturbating each other. Simultaneous clitoral and anal stimulation makes both feel even better; insert a finger during intercourse to give him an exceptional climax.

If this is your first time, I'd try the following exercise during oral sex or mutual masturbation first, then introduce it during intercourse. It's a bit hard to keep thrusting away *and* ask questions and gently explore the area at the same time. Get to know each other's 'yes' and 'no-thanks-very-much' spots first, then try it just as your partner approaches orgasm.

 FOR HIM

Move from stroking and caressing her genitals, and start stimulating the perineum (the smooth area between her anus and vagina). Stroke first, then use three fingers and massage firmly.

Let your fingers brush across her anus and see how she reacts. If she pulls away, or clenches her bottom together, she's either not interested or nervous. If you haven't discussed what you want to do before now, you're playing with fire if you proceed any further!

If she lifts her bottom or presses against your hand, that's a pretty good indication that she'd like you to continue. Before you do, you *must* apply some lubricant to your finger and her anus. Continue stroking the opening until she's relaxed, then insert the tip of a finger into her rectum. Hold still for a moment or two, then try circling or moving your finger gently in and out. Keep the heel of your hand pressed on the perineum.

Ask her if she's enjoying it before pushing your finger further inside. If you stimulate her clitoris at the same time, she'll get double the pleasure.

Ⓕ FOR HER

If his erection's a little half-hearted, this can firm him up in no time. Apply the same techniques listed above on him then . . .

Finger massage his entire rectum, moving in slow circles. Then insert one or two *well-lubricated* fingers about 5 cm into his rectum. Hold them still until he relaxes, then feel the front wall of the rectum until you find a firm, walnut-sized mass. That's his prostate gland and G-spot (see 'How to find his G-spot' on page 106 for more detail). Stroke or press it with a downward movement, using the heel of your hand to press behind the scrotum for extra *uuummmm*.

Ⓜ Ⓕ FOR BOTH OF YOU

If you can't have sex (don't have a condom on you, don't want to have intercourse during your period) or simply want to try something new, give gluteal sex a go. This simply means him using the valley created by her buttock cheeks as an alternative 'vagina'. It's different, quite exciting and dead easy. She clenches her buttocks together and rotates her pelvis; he thrusts between them.

A QUICK FIX

If you don't have time for a prolonged sex session or don't particularly want one, give in to the oh-so-sweet pleasures of a 'quickie'. A 'quickie' is fast, hasty sex of any form. Done at the right time with the right partner, it can be equally, if not more, satisfying than those long, drawn-out sex sessions. The trick is both of you being in the same gloriously turned-on mood simultaneously. This is one instance where you can forget everything I've told you about spending time on foreplay. The whole appeal of a quickie is that it happens spontaneously and the only foreplay you need is 'Let's do it'. Just remember one thing: a quickie quickly turns from erotically exotic to furiously frustrating if it's the way you have sex *every* time.

'My boyfriend and I were out to dinner with some friends. I went to the toilet, he followed me and we both thought "quickie" at the same time. We opened a side door and found an area where the rubbish bins were kept. We had the best sex but it was over in minutes and I figured no-one could possibly suspect what we were up to. When I came back to the table, all my friends were killing themselves laughing. They pointed out the window – which had a wonderful view of the rubbish bins below.'

Tracey, 29, public relations

A quickie works best:

- When you're both semi-clothed. If you're prepared to take your clothes off, you're not impatient enough to enjoy one. *Ripping* them off is a different story.
- When they're spontaneous. Both of you have a sudden urge at the same time.
- When you're both working hard, are too tired for extended sex sessions but want to keep the fires hot.
- When the female initiates it. Men often feel like fast sex, so he'll be *excrutiatingly* turned on if you're the one to suggest it.
- If your sex life is dull and needs an instant lift.
- If one or both of you are a little anxious that you're not performing up to par. It takes the pressure off and lets animal instinct take over.
- When you're *dying* to have sex but you're in public or can't justify disappearing for ages. You're in a park where families are playing ball not so far away? If you've got a short skirt on, pull your panties to one side, sit on his lap (he can unzip under the cover of your skirt) and give him a loving kiss. The people at the next picnic table will think you're wonderfully romantic!

Some more 'quick advice':

- Try doing it in a chair – even better, his or your office chair when no-one else is around (don't even think about it if there's a chance of anyone interrupting – it's not worth losing a job or reputation over). You lie back in the chair, he kneels in front of you. Wrap your legs around his bottom.

! *Find sex a bit of a giggle? It's perfectly normal. The sudden release of emotion and tension during or after orgasm can make us laugh. It's all part of the sexual response.*

- Don't restrict 'quickies' to intercourse. Give her oral sex as she's about to walk out the door to meet a girlfriend (leave her clothes on, just pull her knickers to one side); give him the best fellatio he's had in the same situation.
- Start wearing stockings and suspenders rather than pantihose. They look sexier and allow faster, easier access for quickies.
- Rear-entry positions require minimal undressing. You standing up, facing him, against a wall is another alternative (if your heights match up okay). Stand on one leg and hook the other around him for balance and deeper penetration.
- Give into that *melting* desire, even if you are both dressed to go out and your friends are waiting patiently at a bar. Quickies are quick: you could have *done* it in the two minutes you spent hesitating, one hand on the door knob.
- Try elevators, the beach, parks, planes, trains or automobiles. The venue possibilities are endless!

SIZE *DOES* MATTER

Our genitals are as individual as every other part of our body. Take a look at how many different nose shapes and sizes there are and you'll get a good idea of the numerous variations in vaginas and penises. As usual, what one sex wants the other doesn't. Men stress out that their penis is too small (I've yet to meet a man who worries about the opposite), women worry their vaginal canal is too big. There are ways to get around too big or small in both, but let's look at the emotional side first.

Being different from the norm in anything is difficult, but it's how you respond to the situation that counts. You can make a big deal out of it and become paranoid, or accept what nature has given you, work with it and get on with having a good sex life. You *can* get penises enlarged and vaginas tightened through plastic surgery but it's a pretty drastic (not to mention expensive) solution. Experiment a little first with the following suggestions and you may discover the size of your genitals isn't really that important. People don't fall in love – or lust – with body bits; it's the person they're attached to.

Ⓕ FOR HER

If sex is extremely painful or penetration impossible, you could be suffering from *vaginismus*, a condition where psychological factors cause a muscle spasm in the vagina, closing it tightly. If this is you, go straight to Chapter 7 for help.

If your vagina is too small

Women who don't have major problems but whose vaginal canals are small sometimes feel 'stretched' or uncomfortable during intercourse. Fortunately (or unfortunately, since it can often go too much the other way), giving birth through natural labour usually cures this well and truly. Don't panic! Having a baby isn't the only option. There are other ways you can help make things more enjoyable.

- **Always use a lubricant.** I'm a strong advocate of personal lubricants so you're probably sick of hearing me mention them, but adding extra lubrication is the single, most effective thing you can do to make sex more comfortable. If you're too embarrassed to have the tube by the bed, go to the toilet before you have sex and insert some deep into your vagina. Warmth and your natural lubrication will spread it to all the right places.
- **Don't attempt intercourse until you're really turned on.** Explain to your partner that you need lots of foreplay for your vagina to lubricate and expand. If he still doesn't spend time stroking, arousing and exciting you before penetration, switch partners.

- **Choose positions that allow you to spread your legs wide.** Make it easier for him to penetrate by spreading your thighs open and bending your knees. As he penetrates, bear down slightly (like you're trying to push something out of your vagina). You'll feel more in control and it loosens the vaginal muscles. Instead of penetrating in one, quick movement, ask him to slow it down and insert his penis in stages, a little at a time. You tell him when you're ready to accept deeper penetration. A sensitive lover will let you call the shots. If you trust him to wait until you're ready, you'll relax, and so will your vaginal muscles.

If your vagina is too big

Some women are just built this way, others find their vaginal muscles become slack after having babies. Either way, if you're not 'gripping' his penis, the sensation is less pleasurable for both of you. Luckily, this problem's relatively easy to fix if you're prepared to do some homework.

- Do your Kegels daily. Dr Arnold Kegel developed the following vaginal 'workout' way back in the 1950s. It's a series of exercises designed to strengthen the muscles surrounding the pelvic platform, which contract during orgasm. First, you need to isolate the pubococcygeus (PC) muscle. Do this by inserting a finger into your vagina and tightening your muscles around it. It's the same muscle you use to stop peeing when there's no loo in sight. Got it? If you can feel your muscles squeezing your finger, you're in good shape. If you can't, you will be!
- Contract and relax the muscle, 25 times, twice a day to begin with. Start off doing it slowly and work up to the number of repetitions. When you get to the point where you can do 25 *fast*, you're ready to move on – to 50, twice a day! Mastered that? Okay, now try holding each contraction to the count of three, before releasing. Do 25 repetitions, twice a day and again, work up to 50. Once you're at this point, which should only take a few weeks, you'll notice a huge difference during intercourse. Not only will your vagina feel tighter, you can 'massage' his penis by doing Kegels while he's inside of you.

- Put one or two firm pillows underneath you while he's on top. It alters the angle of the vagina, making it seem tighter. Don't open your legs wide in any intercourse position; the closer your thighs, the tighter your vaginal canal. Choose positions which 'slant' your vagina – rear-entry and any position where he's entering from an angle.

Ⓜ FOR HIM

If your penis is too big

You probably feel ten-foot-tall when you're changing in the male locker room, but not so good when new partners look frantically at the door every time you unzip your trousers. The good news is the vaginal canal is elastic enough to deliver a baby, so it's well and truly capable of accommodating even the largest penis (90 to 95 per cent measure 13 to 18 cm when erect). The trick is to:

- **Make sure she's fully aroused and her vagina is physically ready for you.** You need to spend more time on foreplay than the average guy, and use extra lubrication. Even if she's a little bit wet, it'll still hurt. Squeeze that tube of K-Y and don't be stingy.
- **Choose a position that doesn't allow deep penetration.** Try side-by-side or one where she's in control, like woman-on-top. When you first penetrate, start by inserting a third of your penis, and get her to 'bear down' (push her vaginal muscles 'out') at the same time. Hold still until her vagina gets used to you, then you can go a little further. Once you're fully penetrated (if you're extremely big, she might never want the full length), you can very gently start moving in and out. Deep, hard or fast thrusting is out unless she's used to you and can cope.

If your penis is too small

You cringe every time someone makes a joke related to penis size and *hate* changing in the locker room. The first time you're with a new partner, you're terrified she'll say something like 'Is that it?' when you undress or 'Is it in yet?' during intercourse. But if she's got good PC muscles (encourage her to do the Kegel exercises described earlier), you can both still be a good, snug fit. Here's how to make the size of your penis irrelevant.

- **Do not make intercourse the main event.** If you've made her come three times already through oral sex, genital masturbation or indulged her with a sensual massage, intercourse becomes part of love-making rather than the whole show. This takes the pressure off both of you. Most women find it difficult reaching orgasm through intercourse alone so she'll welcome the shift in emphasis.
- **Choose deep-penetration positions or positions where her vagina is 'closed'.** Rear-entry, her-on-top but leaning backward, anything which alters the slant of the vagina and 'closes' it up a little will make you feel larger to her and increase friction. During missionary, put one or two firm pillows underneath her bottom. Rather than opening her legs wide, get her to keep her thighs pressed close together with your legs *outside* hers.
- **Thrust hard and deeply.** If your penis is smaller than average, you can usually thrust harder and deeper than usual (though still check with her to find what feels best).
- **Masturbate frequently to avoid premature ejaculating.** It's highly unfair but unfortunately true that men with small penises very often have problems coming too soon. This is because all penises have roughly the same number of nerve endings in the head. If your penis is small, they're concentrated over a smaller area which makes you more sensitive. The more you masturbate, the less sensitive you'll become, especially if you practise controlling your orgasms while you're doing it.

SEX DURING PREGNANCY

'Oh, it's so *romantic*,' people say, patting your tummy and watching you and your partner exchange soppy, loving looks.

Having a baby together is romantic – and that's partly the reason why sex gets put on the backburner. Your partner loves you to death right now but he may see you differently: you're no longer his gorgeous, sexy girlfriend but a mother-to-be. You're also struggling to reconcile your 'new' (more responsible) self with the 'old' you (who loved hot, furious sex in the very room the cot's now in).

As one of my pregnant friends told me, 'My hormones have sent my libido through the roof but everytime I feel horny, I feel guilty. It's like, I'm meant to be a future mother and all I want to do is screw all the time. The two don't go together.'

But they can. After the first few sickly months, a lot of women find their energy soars and that the hormones sparked by pregnancy give their libido a huge kick. If your partner is supportive, reassuring you that you don't look fat just pregnant, this can be one of the most sexual times in your relationship. Most pregnant women cram their bookshelves with texts on kids and conception so I won't go into specifics about health or harm to the baby here. But you might like to keep the following in mind.

- **How sexy you feel depends very much on your partner's reaction.** If he embraces the whole pregnancy thing and is as excited about the first kick as you are, chances are your sex life won't suffer too much. This is the time when you'll feel most vulnerable about your body. If you usually run around in sprayed-on jeans and tight sweaters, you'll start to hate anyone who still can. The perfect partner will convince you that your 'new' look is just as erotic and you'll both revel in those nice, full breasts and that wonderfully big belly.
- **Mothers have sex too.** Let's be honest here: motherhood doesn't have the sexiest image and he's been as brainwashed by society as you have. If you think he's starting to treat you too much like a Madonna figure (the religious one not the singer), have a chat. Tell him as much as you love the thought of the baby growing inside you, you're the same person you were before you got pregnant. Mothers have sex. So do mothers-to-be.
- **No, the baby's not listening.** 'You have this weird feeling that the baby is listening and hearing everything,' said one expectant mum. It isn't. Can you remember *your* mother screaming, 'Oh Harold, that's *fantastic*'?
- **Don't be surprised if your sexual tastes change.** Before falling pregnant, you loved oral and were so-so about intercourse. Now you hate oral and love bonking or vice versa. Sometimes, you won't want sex at all. Your body feels heavy and awkward, your doctor's always poking and

prodding, complete strangers keep putting their hands on your stomach. Sex can feel like just another intrusion at times like this.

- **What if I feel more turned on than ever?** It happens – a lot. Surging hormones can cause as many erotic episodes as teary ones. While your friends are obsessing what colour to paint the baby's bedroom, *you're* obsessed with what you're going to do in your own when Daddy-to-be comes home. Don't waste a second feeling guilty. Enjoy! Lots of women find they orgasm more quickly and more intensely than before. Delight, don't despair, when your body does all sorts of weird things – like spurt milk out of your nipples in the middle of a climax!

'When my first wife got pregnant I hated it. She was even more uptight than she was before. She made me watch the birth and I couldn't relate to her sexually after that. Every time I thought of her vagina, I thought of the baby and all that blood coming out. With my girlfriend, it's different. We had a baby girl last year and she made me feel part of the whole thing. We had some sort of sex right up until the very end and she was happy for me to stay up the right end for the birth.'

Martin, 30, plumber

- **Will I hurt the baby?** This is his top concern. All that bashing around with a penis, he figures, has to push the baby all over the place. A bit of wishful thinking on his part – it's not *that* big! Your gynaecologist or any good pregnancy manual will tell you which positions are safe and when it is safe to have sex when you're pregnant. Get professional advice when you first find out you're pregnant to allay all your fears.

4

Orgasm

The 30 (if you're lucky) seconds we go to *so-o-o-o* much effort for

A group of scientists once electronically wired up a mouse so every time it pressed a lever, it triggered off an orgasm. The mouse died within 24 hours – from orgasm overdose. While the researchers were tucked up in their beds, he was pressing that lever, over and over and over again until his little body could take no more. That's what I call dying with a smile on your face.

The first person to dream up a *human* instant orgasm trigger will shoot up and off the Rich List within weeks. And no prizes for guessing which sex will be first in line to buy it. For him, orgasms seem to require the same amount of effort it takes to switch on the telly. *With* a remote control. For women, just learning how to have one often involves a long, laborious mission of self-discovery. And even when we do master it, the little buggers sometimes still refuse to materialise on command when we're with a partner.

Perhaps it's because, unlike men – who ejaculate life-giving semen when they orgasm – there's no obvious biological reason for women to have one. Some researchers believe they do have a role in procreation because orgasms encourage us to have sex more often (upping the chance of our eggs being fertilised). Other studies show the contractions during orgasm make the cervix 'dip' into the seminal fluid, giving the sperm a 'leg-up' on the way to meet the egg. Whatever, for women, climaxing sure as hell isn't as easy as painting by numbers. Which is why it's not realistic or sensible to expect you'll both be able to tick the 'Yep, I had one' box *every single time* you make love.

Sometimes he'll have one and you won't, other times you'll strike it lucky and he won't score, and on some occasions neither of you will climax. Orgasm shouldn't be the ultimate aim. Having said that, it's always rather nice if you *do* have one which is why this chapter is entirely devoted to making both your orgasms more likely, frequent and intense. Who knows? If you study hard enough, you might even beat the tally of one multi-orgasmic woman who astonished sex researchers by having 50 orgasms in a row, stopping only when they ran out of male volunteers. (Shame the mouse wasn't around!)

! *Orgasms promote cardiovascular conditioning, make the skin glow, improve overall body tone and can cure menstrual cramps. The emotional release makes us feel less irritable and more relaxed.*

WHAT DO ORGASMS FEEL LIKE?

The first time I had an orgasm I thought I'd wet myself. I was staying with my sister and discovered a personal massager, shoved in the back of a cupboard, while they were out. I looked at it for a while, turned it on and watched it vibrate, then thought, 'Hmmm, I wonder what would happen if I just held it pressed against here for a second. Oh! That feels quite nice, I'll just do it for a little bit longer and . . . OH MY GOD! What the hell was *that!*' I looked down at the floor in astonishment, convinced I'd had some totally bizarre bladder attack. I had no idea I'd just orgasmed but I knew *something* had happened.

Which is why when women ask me, 'How do I know if I've had one?' my answer is always this: if you have to ask, you haven't had a *clitoral* orgasm, though you may have climaxed vaginally. Vaginal orgasms feel wonderful but they're sometimes vague and undramatic. Clitoral orgasms are peel-me-off-the-ceiling stuff. The feeling is so powerful and unmistakeable, you've got as much chance of 'missing' it as you have of not noticing a bright green alien sitting in your living room.

But even if they know they orgasm (and do so frequently), most women and men are curious about them. Do they *feel* the same for everyone? Are theirs different from other people's? Biologically, everyone moves through the same stages. We become *aroused*, then move to a *plateau* phase (highly aroused), onto *orgasm*, then *resolution* (when the body returns to normal). Psychologically, it's unlikely everyone experiences the same sensations since orgasms appear to be as individual as the people who have them. Nevertheless, in an attempt to answer the questions, here's what one representative of each sex said when asked to describe what *their* orgasms felt like – from the very first, tentative flutter right through to the passionate finale.

Number of women who think it's important their partner has an orgasm during sex: 34 per cent. Number who think it's important they have one: 50 per cent.

What she feels

'Sex with someone new, that I've fancied like mad for ages but haven't slept with yet, is different to sex with a long-term boyfriend. I'm usually wet the whole time I'm around a new guy – sometimes even thinking about him makes me lubricate. I'm more turned on but, ironically, I'm often *too* turned on to orgasm clitorally because when we finally get down to it, all I really want is penetration. I have a dull, aching feeling in my lower belly and a need to be "filled up".

'No matter where he touches, it all seems directly linked to my vagina, making it throb until I can't wait for him to be inside. Inevitably, the initial thrust is the best because it satisfies that need immediately.

'If he's big and thrusts long and hard, the aching feeling builds and then peaks, spreading into mild, pleasurable waves which I feel deep inside. My vagina seems to spasm, but less fiercely than with a clitoral orgasm. Vaginal orgasms affect a larger area – like waves of pleasure are crashing all over my body. Clitoral orgasms all radiate from the clitoris. They're more a euphoric explosion, an eruption.

'I can masturbate to a clitoral orgasm within a few minutes but I need to know and relax with a partner before he can give me one. That's because I have to concentrate, block him out of the picture and focus entirely on the sensation. In other words, I have to think about me, not him. Oral sex orgasms are the best – really intense, strong and powerful. When he starts, I feel incredibly sensitive and everything feels great. That sensation then becomes sharper and isolates around the clitoris. It's weird but sometimes it feels as though the rest of my body disappears and all that's left is that tiny little area. If someone chopped my arm off at that point, I wouldn't know; all I'm aware of is what's happening to that centimetre or less of flesh.

'At that point, I deliberately tense up the muscles in my legs and bottom. I start to feel really hot, almost like I'm burning up, then, as I climax, my vagina starts jerking and pulsating and there's a few seconds of exquisite sensation. Even if I don't make any noise, I can't help breathing heavily and faster. Sometimes, I'll have three or four intense spasms, then nothing. Other times, especially if he continues licking softly, they're followed by smaller waves, spaced less closely. Sometimes I'll ejaculate fluid – or at least it feels like I do but I've masturbated and checked the sheets and there's nothing there. After orgasm, I push him away immediately – I'm way too sensitive to be touched. The orgasm itself lasts about 10 seconds but it feels much longer. I'm completely exhausted afterward and don't want him anywhere near me. I feel a bit faint, so lie back for a minute or two. I guess that's why French women nickname orgasm *le petit mort*, the little death.

! ***Men aren't the only ones who have 'wet dreams'. Between 10 to 20 per cent of women have woken in the throes of orgasm.***

'I don't think most women have orgasms. Lots of women think they have them because sensations build then ebb away but that's not an orgasm, that's just desire. In some ways, I'd like to be a male because it seems so easy for them. Men try to put off their orgasms for as long as possible but women are always trying to induce theirs. I don't know any woman who, when she feels an orgasm coming, tries to stop it. Why would she? Women have to be in a certain head space to come; they're not that easy to achieve. I guess the equaliser is men's orgasms seem quicker than ours and they can't have them as often.'

What he feels

'Penises have a mind of their own. If I'm seeing a girl that night and know I'll be having sex, I'll look down during the day and find I've got an erection even though I'm not aware of it. Obviously my subconscious is having a heyday.

'Despite what women think, the more teasing and foreplay the better. The feeling of your penis filling up with blood and becoming erect is fantastic. It happens really quickly – one minute it's flaccid, the next ready for action. I'm not conscious of my nipples becoming erect or anything but I feel quite tingly everywhere. I'll put off the moment of penetration for as long as possible – the anticipation is almost as good as the real thing.

'Girls, if you're with a guy who's trying to rush things at this point, you can bet he's trying to hurry everything up in case you change your mind! Spontaneous, fast sex is great but usually, the more touching and caressing she does the better.

'Just before I climax, I can feel the sperm travelling up the shaft in a rush of fluid. Once you feel that happening, ejaculation is inevitable. If I try and stop it because I want it to last longer, the sperm still comes out but it feels all rushed and I don't feel fulfilled. It's a bit like being fed chocolate cake intravenously: the end result is the same but there's no pleasure in it. My brain has to be conscious of me having an orgasm before it registers the nice part; your body and mind have to be in tune.

'Orgasm is a release. It feels like you've been holding onto something forever and are then allowed to let go. The sperm pumps out in jerky spasms and you feel this body-shattering intense pleasure. My orgasm seems to last about six seconds though my friends have told me theirs last only two to three. I'm either lucky or my sense of timing is shot!

'If I haven't had sex with a girl for a while, it's best if I masturbate a few times first, otherwise I come too quickly and it doesn't feel as good. I think most men are always trying to think of ways to make their orgasms last longer because they're usually so short. They feel different when she fellates me, more acute and protracted. I'd never knock it back, but there's something about being inside her that I prefer.

'Sperm is such an integral part of coming yet most women say they can't feel it shooting into them. That's kind of disappointing for men.

'I lose my erection within seconds when my penis is removed from the vagina and hits cold air; once I've come, it's like *all* over, that's it. Then I need quiet time to chill out, even though I do feel close to my partner if I love her. Unlike women, our orgasms don't seem to vary as dramatically in a physical sense, but some do feel different to others. What makes them stand out isn't what's happening to your body but your head and your heart. If you're with someone you want to cuddle afterward, that's what makes them special.'

FAKING IT

If the Oscar judges were serious about finding award-winning acting performances, they'd look to the bedroom rather than the big screen – there's some pretty convincing acting going on out there! Pretty well all of us have faked an orgasm at some point and if *you* never, ever have, you're in the minority (or telling fibs again).

Why aren't we more honest? Sometimes, it's just *easier* to go with the flow. Did cavewomen enjoy being hit on the head and pulled around by their hair? Hardly. They simply figured it was easier to placate their partner than be eaten by another, more dangerous, wild beast. In the super-stressed, super-fast-paced 90s, both women *and* men resort to play-acting. We're not only too tired to have orgasms, who's got the energy to go through the hassle of explaining why we didn't?

Why women fake

Because we don't want to hurt him and it's easy to get away with

Men rarely notice when we fake it. Whether this is because we are really good actors or because the female orgasm is so easily hidden, we could sneak one in on the bus and no-one would look up from their newspaper, is open to conjecture. The truth is more likely this: women fake so often that most men have no idea what the real thing is anymore.

Usually, we'll time it just as he's about to climax and, as one sex therapist put it, 'Who can be bothered looking for giveaway signs when you're in the throes of experiencing your own pleasure?' Besides, outwardly visible signs of female orgasm aren't that obvious. Sure, our breathing gets heavier and quicker, and sometimes our whole body jerks with each spasm, but not always. Some men say they can feel our vaginas 'quivering' with their tongue if we orgasm during oral sex, but that doesn't help much during intercourse.

Probably the most telltale sign is how sensitive our genitals are afterward. If you can touch her clitoris quite firmly immediately after she's gasped out the last 'Oh yes', chances are she's telling porkies. A few experts claim a dark red flush appears across the chest and shoulders for a split second, just after either sex orgasms, but again, who's together enough to notice?

We'd rather act than tell the truth because we don't want to dent that fragile male ego

Being the caring, nurturing souls that we are, women are loath to admit he's anything but perfect in bed. If he's trying his hardest to last and you're nowhere near coming, you'll fake it to put him out of his misery. Ditto when he's been down there licking for an hour but you just know there's no way you're going over the edge.

To get sex over with

If you're tired and longing for sleep, faking an orgasm gives him the signal it's okay to let go. The tragic part is a lot of women don't mind if they don't have one every time. Just because we don't climax doesn't mean we haven't enjoyed it. Sadly, men often react to being told this with disbelief. Because they orgasm most of the time, they think we're saying it 'just to be nice'.

To save face

Some women feel like a failure if they don't orgasm at the touch of a breast (like our celluloid counterparts). That's the reason fibbing about orgasms isn't confined to the bedroom. If all our friends are owning up to multiple orgasms, why should we admit to none at all?

'I can't decide if men are really stupid or really egotistical. Honestly, they think you've had an orgasm even if you haven't faked one – the slightest sign of excitement and they think they've hit the jackpot. He looks at you all self-satisfied and smug and you're thinking, "What a loser."'

Anna-Marie, 36, bank manager

Why men fake

To explain a limp penis

His reasons aren't that different than ours. If he's tired, had a few too many, worried about work or just not interested in sex right now, he'll pretend he's had an orgasm to explain why he's lost his erection.

'If you feel it going down, you quickly let out a few grunts and moans, pump a bit harder, then pull out,' said one guy.

How does he explain the lack of 'evidence'? 'If you've been giving her heaps of oral and she's already wet, she doesn't notice there isn't any sperm,' he claims.

I'm a tad sceptical because semen has a pretty distinctive smell, but, according to the experts, ejaculate isn't a true indication that he's orgasmed anyway. Masters and Johnson and Miriam Stoppard both maintain orgasm and ejaculation are two separate processes and one can occur without the other. In other words, he can ejaculate without having an orgasm or orgasm without ejaculating.

He's worried he'll hurt you

Men say women take it very personally when a man doesn't come, much more than he does if you don't. Because we think men's orgasms are automatic and inevitable, he's supposed to have one every single time or something's really wrong. We're not attractive enough, didn't turn him on enough, he's in love with the girl in his office . . .

'Yes, I've faked one . . . well, more than one actually. Women get so paranoid if you don't come every single time, it's like we're expected to be these sex robots.'

Jake, 21, bodyguard

What if I suspect my partner's just faked it?

If you suspect she's faked it and accuse her outright, she'll deny it and clam up. Instead say something like, 'Darling, I love making love to you and want to give you as much pleasure as possible. What are the things I do that turn you on the most?' She'll be more comfortable focusing on what you do right rather than what you do wrong to begin with. When she's opened up, ask her to guide your hand (or tongue) in future to show you the techniques which work for her. Say you read somewhere that lots of women like their clitorises stimulated during intercourse. The idea turns you on and you'd love to try it – what does she think?

If you suspect he's faked it, make light of it. If you think he did it because he was stressed or tired, when you come back from the bathroom say, 'That's weird, there didn't seem to be much sperm this time. Maybe men are a bit like women and sex isn't so great when you're really tired.' He probably won't confess, but it gives him the green light to say no to sex in the future.

If he never seems to have a genuine orgasm, he might be what's called a *retarded ejaculator*, an unfortunate term which simply means he can stay rock hard all night but can't ejaculate or orgasm. The cause is usually psychological – maybe he got a girlfriend pregnant in the past and is terrified it'll happen again. Alternatively, he may suffer from *retrograde ejaculation*. He feels an orgasm in his brain but the semen goes back down the urethra. Whichever, if he's *never* orgasmed with you, you've both probably acknowledged the problem by now. Suggest he books himself in for a medical check with a GP to see if there are any physical causes. They'll refer him onto a therapist if psychological factors are at play.

Is it ever okay to pretend?

Some sex therapists (interestingly, all female) say if you have real orgasms with your partner 90 per cent of the time, it's *not recommended* but acceptable if you fake 10 per cent. It's a bit like telling your girlfriend she looks great in that new dress, when it really does nothing for her. If he's doing everything right but you can't orgasm for your own reasons, sometimes it seems kinder to pretend.

There's another theory which actually encourages you to fake it. Called 'fake it till you make it', it's based on the assumption that if you act out the thing you want to happen, sometimes it will. Psychologists use the same technique on depressed patients: the act of smiling triggers hormones which make us feel happier so a forced smile eventually turns into a real one. If you want to orgasm, quicken your breathing, make noise, move your hips – do whatever you do when you really do have one. By re-enacting the lead up to orgasm, you may be able to push yourself over the threshold to the point where orgasm becomes involuntary.

However the overwhelming majority of sex therapists give faking the thumbs down – for a very good reason. If you *never* have an orgasm with your partner, it's pretty pointless pretending to. How are they ever going to learn to give you one if they think they're doing it already? The worst time to fake an orgasm is in the beginning of a relationship, which is, of course, when most women (and some men) do it. Keep *on* doing it and you've set up a pattern of behaviour that's based on deception and dissatisfaction. He'll keep on using the same ineffectual techniques because he thinks he's turning you on; you'll remain frustrated and irritable every time you make love. Having the courage to open up and say 'Actually, that does nothing for me' is difficult, but you really must.

! *Approximately 40 per cent of men admit women have faked orgasm with them; 40 per cent aren't sure; 20 per cent swear it's never happened. Ninety-two per cent of women admit to faking orgasm at least once in their life.*

Communication is the key to good sex – and that's a fact. In a recent survey on people's sex lives, every single couple who rated their sex life as 'very happy', also ticked the 'yes' box to a question which asked if they talked to their partner about their sexual needs. Faking orgasm isn't necessary if admitting to not having one isn't a problem.

THE LONG AND SHORT OF IT

Some orgasms are so intense, your legs aren't the only thing that turns to jelly. 'Marry me,' you beg the guy who bores you silly outside the bedroom. The very next night, with exactly the same

'Orgasms through oral sex feel more intense. If she's using her tongue and is a good fellatrix, she can do more than she can with her vagina. But the very best thing about them is you're completely in her control. In intercourse, you can vary the thrust speed and depth to control your own orgasm; with oral, she gives you one when she feels like it.'

Ian, 33, small business owner

person, you come and it feels more like a sneeze.

Orgasms, like most things in life, vary depending on your mood, your partner, how turned on you are, how tired you are and, of course, on how you're having them. You might experience three massive contractions when he gives you oral sex, a dozen little ones when you masturbate. His orgasm intensity fluctuates too. One night, he'll ejaculate enough semen to artificially inseminate a small town, writhing about for what seems like hours; the next, there's a small sigh and not enough sperm to even warrant washing the sheets. Here's a brief guide to all the different orgasms both of you can experience.

The male orgasm

As he orgasms, engorged reproductive glands empty their contents into his urethra, expanding it to produce an erotically intense sensation. He ejaculates through a series of four or five contractions, usually one every 0.8 seconds. The male orgasm is straightforward biologically and it certainly sounds like there's not much room for variation. But there is. If he hasn't had sex for a while, he'll produce more semen than normal, making his orgasm more prolonged. He'll 'feel' the orgasm in his brain more intensely if his mind's not on other things, and if a lover brings him almost to the peak, over and over, before letting him ejaculate, all his senses will be heightened and the orgasm may feel fiercer. Alternatively, if he's having a quickie, it's a shorter but sharper feeling.

***!** Twenty-five to 33 per cent of women climax without additional clitoral stimulation. Experts believe these women may have a larger clitoris than usual so it's more easily 'rubbed' by a thrusting penis.*

Vaginal orgasms

Because the inner walls of the vagina have nerve endings (not to mention highly sensitive points like the G- and A-spots), one third of women say they can climax this way. In contrast to clitoral orgasms, vaginal orgasms produce a more widespread, 'warm wave' sensation. He can give you one through manual masturbation, fingers deep inside you, or through intercourse.

> 'I only ever orgasm with a partner through oral sex and only if he's really good at it. Lots of my girlfriends claim they come during intercourse but to be honest, I don't believe them. I'm sexually educated and have a high, healthy libido and if I don't have vaginal orgasms, I can't see why they would.'
>
> Gabrielle, 25, journalist

Clitoral orgasms

There's an assumption that vaginal orgasms are 'inferior' to clitoral ones. They're not, just different. But the attitude stems from the fact that clitoral stimulation tends to produce more intense climaxes. Most women build to a high peak of pleasure that triggers a series of intense spasms and vaginal contractions. Unlike men, the degree, number and time between the spasms varies dramatically from woman to woman.

Oral sex orgasms

Both sexes say orgasms achieved through oral sex feel different. Mouths and tongues are soft, gentle and handily agile at stimulating a small area (like your clitoris or his frenulum). As a result, oral sex orgasms can feel stronger and more focused.

Masturbation orgasms

Some people maintain no-one can give you a better orgasm than you can give yourself; others say masturbatory orgasms are short and perfunctory. Usually we climax more quickly, probably because our attention is focused on our own needs. Regardless, most people stop at one and few try to achieve . . .

Multiple orgasms

This is a term everyone uses differently. For some people, multiple orgasms simply means having more than one in a single sex session. Other people (more accurately) mean riding the wave of an initial orgasm until they've had two or three immediately in succession. Like simultaneous orgasms, a lot of couples are in desperate pursuit of multiples, thinking they've 'failed' as lovers if they don't happen. Sensible couples break open the champagne if they do result, but don't worry too much if they don't.

Researchers predict that about one-third of women are multi-orgasmic. Women are slower to climb to an orgasm peak, so remain at the highly aroused 'plateau' phase for longer than men do. If he continues gentle stimulation throughout our initial orgasm, it stops us moving to the 'resolution' phase (when our body goes back to normal) and we're able to climb back up and have further orgasms. While our sleep hormones are released about half an hour after our first orgasm, men's kick into the bloodstream almost immediately after ejaculation.He peaks quickly and usually needs rest to build up semen (and energy) for further orgasms. Though new research suggests he can have multiple orgasms, it's unlikely he'll ejaculate each time. Sexpert Miriam Stoppard cites an American study which documented multi-orgasmic men who had between two and nine orgasms per session. The trick seems to be to separate the process of ejaculation and orgasm. His body might not be able to physically ejaculate several times in succession but his brain seems capable of registering the feeling of orgasm over and over. One technique to try: he (or you) press hard on his perineum (the area between his testes and anus) just before orgasm. This can sometimes stop ejaculation while he orgasms 'mentally' and keeps him hard so he can go on to have another.

Simultaneous orgasm

This simply means both of you have an orgasm at exactly the same time. People on soap operas have simultaneous orgasms more often than they eat breakfast but it's a little different in the real world. The chance of both of you reaching a peak at exactly the same *second* is low but it is not unachievable. In other words, it's romantic to aim for simultaneous orgasms but unrealistic to expect them frequently. Because women take longer than men to build to the pre-orgasmic phase, you can up the chances of coming together by stimulating her until she's almost there before even starting whatever's necessary to make him come.

THE G-SPOT: MYTH OR MARVEL?

Simultaneous orgasm is a must for 25 per cent of men and 14 per cent of women.

The G-spot (Grafenberg spot) was a bit like God. We wanted to believe in it even though we weren't really sure if it existed, and were scared to say 'What a load of hogwash' in case we were the only person at the dinner party who wasn't having G-spot orgasms every five minutes. Men, particularly, seemed reluctant to admit they'd never found it on a woman.

'Have you ever found the G-spot?' I asked one man during an interview.

'Oh yes,' he said confidently.

'Where is it?' I asked him.

'Oh, it varies,' he said. 'On some women it's just underneath the clitoris, on others it's underneath their breasts.'

Somehow, I don't think this is quite what Grafenberg had in mind.

Ernst Grafenberg started all the fuss in Germany in 1944. He published a paper claiming there was an area in the upper wall of the vagina so erotically charged a woman was guaranteed to orgasm if it was stimulated. Fellow researchers pooh-poohed the idea so Grafenberg closed his mouth and kept it shut. About four decades later, a team of American psychologists also argued that women could have multiple orgasms, without clitoral stimulation, if the same area was stimulated. Again, the idea met with little support.

Since then, modern science has proved that our vaginal walls are pleasurably sensitive and there seems little doubt that there is definitely a 'hidden area' which produces intense excitement when aroused in *some* women. But not all females appear to have one. The male G-spot (he had to get in on the act, didn't he!) is less controversial: it was identified almost immediately as the prostate gland. As for women, post mortems on females have failed to find a G-spot, leading some experts to believe in the only-the-lucky-scored theory or that it is only visible when stimulated. Some still claim the G-spot is simply the whole of the front vaginal wall.

So, the debate still rages. Most sex therapists are convinced it does exist, a few fix you with a 'not that old myth' withering stare if you even mention it. If you've found it, or what seems like it, you're the one jumping up and down whenever the conversation moves toward sex, waving the G-spot flag like crazy. If you've tried and failed, you're the one saying wearily, 'Nice for some.' To be honest, I didn't think I was a proud owner until quite recently. I don't know whether my lover found my G-spot, but he certainly hit on something in the general vicinity which made me want to shout '*Eureka!*'

How to find hers

The G-spot is a small cluster of nerve endings and glands near the woman's urethra or urinary tract. Because it only swells and stands out from the vaginal wall when aroused, the G-spot usually can't be felt unless it's stimulated.

The easiest way to find it yourself is to squat – maybe even sit on the toilet. Now, insert a finger into your well-lubricated vagina, curving it so you're hitting the front wall (imagine you're aiming toward your belly). Feel around a little, hopefully causing the G-spot to swell so you can pinpoint it, until you find a raised area that feels textured. Most experts say it's around the size of a large pea.

Some women find their first stimulation of the G-spot distinctly uncomfortable. It can produce similar feelings to wanting to pee. Empty your bladder first or sit on the toilet when you first try. If you relax into the sensation, the feeling will pass.

Hold your finger still to begin with, then experiment. Don't press hard and constantly – a gentle, stroking motion is better. Try stroking left to right and back again or in circles; in other words, so your fingers are *passing over* the G-spot without concentrating on it directly. G-spot orgasms feel different from clitoral orgasms. If you have one, you may find you ejaculate a small amount of clear fluid (which isn't urine, by the way).

It's best if you lie on a bed, with pillows underneath your bottom, for your partner to find it. It makes the area more easily accessible for him to follow the instructions above. Once found, he can combine G-spot stimulation with oral sex or while he's masturbating you. The best intercourse positions to hit the spot are woman-on-top or him behind (doggie style).

How to find his

Just because you haven't found yours, doesn't mean you shouldn't try to find his (it might even give you some clues).

Like the female G-spot, the male's is situated near the urethra. Unlike ours, his has a medical name – the prostate gland – and it has an organic function. There's another point of difference: while we can find our own, it's rather difficult for him to stimulate his because it's up his rectum. He can try (by lying on his back, knees bent and feet flat on the floor or knees drawn up to his chest, inserting his thumb and pressing against the front wall), but it's simpler if you find it for him.

> 'I was with an extremely liberated young lady once who inserted a vibrator into my anus. I felt intimidated at first, but when I let go, it was like wow! It was definitely the most fierce, overwhelming, total body experience I've had. I remember feeling an unusual "full" feeling and thinking, "This is what it must be like for women."'
>
> Anton, 25, broker

Apply some personal lubricant to your finger (nails trimmed and clean) and get him to lie on his back. Gently insert the finger into his anus, then feel up the front rectal wall until you find something that feels like a walnut. Hold your finger still until he's relaxed, then start massaging firmly in a downward direction. He can draw his knees up to his chest once you've found it.

It can take a little while for him to orgasm (so make sure you're both comfortable) but it's worth the effort. If it works, you'll be in the unique position of having given him an orgasm without even touching his penis! Male fans claim not only are G-spot orgasms more intense, they ejaculate in a continuous stream rather than in spurts.

Once you're an expert, try massaging his G-spot while you're giving him oral or stimulate it during him-on-top intercourse positions.

One note about hygiene: always wash your hands after inserting fingers into rectums. If you touch your own genitals you can inadvertently transfer bacteria into your vagina.

THE *A(HHHH)*-SPOT

Just when the search party finally returned from the G-spot expedition, scientists came up with another supposed instant orgasm button. This one's called the A-Spot. A hot spot accidentally discovered in early 1996, it's officially called the 'anterior fornex erogenous' and is located on the front wall of the vagina, a third of the way down from the cervix.

> 'When I first went out with Scott, he was always fiddling around inside me and I thought, "What's he doing?" The third time we made love, I found out: he was looking for my G-spot. And he found it. I can't orgasm from that alone but if he has one hand stimulating that and the other on my clitoris, I'm putty.'
>
> Marie, 20, secretary

Stumbled upon during an experiment to find a cure for vaginal dryness, scientists were amazed to find an astonishing 95 per cent of women became massively turned-on when they stimulated this particular area. Many had their first orgasm or found it led to more frequent and intense climaxes. I'm obviously one of the five per cent. Despite faithfully following the instructions, nothing much happened to me at all. But that's not to say *you're* not going to think it's the best invention since tampons.

According to the research team, stimulating the A-spot not only made women wet within 10 minutes, it led to multiple orgasms. Because their vaginas were more lubricated, the women said they felt more excited, both mentally and physically. Usually, our lubrication slows down or stops after one orgasm. Theirs continued – so they did too.

To find your A-Spot, wet two fingers and slide them inside your vagina, stimulating it until you (hopefully) hit a small mass of spongy material a third of the way up the front wall (curve your fingers and aim toward your stomach). This is the G-spot.

Continue upward to find your cervix. It feels like the very round end of a nose. Move back until you're about halfway between your G-spot and your cervix. That's the A-spot. It's a smooth area that's extremely sensitive to touch. Now slide a finger up and down over the A-spot or try moving in a clockwise then anticlockwise direction.

If you want to strike it lucky during intercourse, opt for positions where the penis hits the front wall of the vagina: him behind (doggie style) or you sitting on the edge of the bed and him kneeling before you.

DEEPER, LONGER, BETTER, MORE . . .

Up the number and intensity of your orgasms by trying any (and all) of the following.

- **Don't race to get to the finish line.** The longer you've spent on foreplay, the more enhanced it will be for both of you.
- **Slow his down, speed yours up.** You envy the fact that he can orgasm with one hand behind his back (literally); he's jealous of your ability to hover in the oh-Jesus-John-I'm-just-about-there stage for ages. Anything which delays his orgasm will increase his enjoyment; anything which makes her more easily orgasmic will increase her pleasure potential.

> ***!** Partner sex often follows a 3-2-1 pattern: three minutes of foreplay, two minutes of intercourse and one orgasm – his.*

- **Teach him control.** As you're stimulating him, get him to tell you how he's feeling by rating it on a scale of 1 to 10 (10 being the can't-go-back-now point). Drive him to distraction by revving him up to a seven or eight, then slowing it down again, several times over, before letting him go all the way.
- **Alternate oral sex with intercourse.** If he's too close to coming, change activities. Get him to give you oral sex until he feels more in control.
- **Touch his penis frequently.** The more often your hand, tongue or vagina touch it, the less sensitive he'll be and the longer he'll last.
- **Don't be a clockwatcher.** Stop wondering whether his tongue's gone numb, wipe the 'If I don't come soon, he's going to miss the football' thoughts. The best lover in the world is the man who says, 'Take your time honey – I love doing it to you as much as you like receiving it' (and means it). You can't fight biology; both of you should accept that it's more complicated for you to have an orgasm than him.

- **Give her a head start.** Give her an orgasm through oral sex or masturbation *before* intercourse. Give him one orally, so his second intercourse orgasm lasts longer.
- **Don't try too hard and don't freak if you don't have one.** Remember when you were a kid and tried to touch a rainbow? Orgasms can be just as elusive. Reach just a little higher, you think, and you'll have one but the next minute it's slipped through your (or his) fingers. Lots of women move steadily toward the point of having an orgasm then, out of nowhere, something intrudes. *I forgot Jane's birthday last week*, your brain inappropriately throws up, or you hear your flatmate's key in the door or remember you have to confront your boss in the morning. Your orgasm potential's disappeared, not forever, but certainly for that session. The same thing can happen if he changes technique or rhythm at the wrong time; everything that has built up fades away. Trying harder will only make things worse. Instead, accept that you will have one next time you make love (making sure it's sooner rather than later) and you will. Stress out about it, start tormenting yourself with thoughts like 'That's it. This is going to happen every time and I'll never have one' and you'll set up more psychological roadblocks than the average detour.
- **Masturbate with him rather than alone.** If you don't have an orgasm during intercourse, give yourself one afterward. He can watch or place his hand over yours.
- **Don't treat her clitoris like it's a lift button.** Some men think the more they press it, the quicker you'll zoom to the top. Most women climax if you work around the base of the clitoris rather than touch it directly.
- **Prime yourself for sex by turning yourself on beforehand.** When he's talking to friends, think about what that tongue will do to you later, how much better his fingers would feel inside you rather than wrapped around a beer glass.
- **Stop worrying about what you look like.** If your partner isn't someone you can let go with, without fear of criticism, they're not the right choice. In, or out of, the bedroom.
- **Show each other how to do it.** Not like an army commander where you're shouting 'Left' and 'Right' but 'Hmmm, that

feels fantastic when you do it really slow,' or 'God, that's great. Do it harder.'

- **Masturbate more.** Researchers claim it increases your sexual appetite because the more sex we have, the more our bodies expect.
- **Make noise.** It sounds and feels sexy.
- **Get wet.** It doesn't mean you're not turned on if you're not lubricating like crazy; you might just be at a different stage of the menstrual cycle, stressed or tired. Accept that sometimes you'll need to add artificial lubricant like K-Y.
- **Both do Kegel exercises.** Women do them to tighten their vagina and give them more control over orgasm; men can use the same genital workout to orgasm more frequently. (See page 86 for details – the same technique works for both.) The experts maintain male masters of Kegels can become 'multi-orgasmic'. He can try contracting his PC muscle hard, for five seconds, as he's hovering on the brink of orgasm. Reputedly, this delays ejaculation but he'll 'feel' an orgasm in his brain. Potentially, he could climax several times before having an ejaculatory orgasm.
- **Give him a squeeze.** Squeezing the base of the penis firmly for a few seconds can delay ejaculation.
- **Fantasise guilt-free.** Many women and men use fantasy to launch themselves into orgasmic orbit; some can't achieve one without it. Quit the guilt trip. Your partner can't read minds, remember?

HOW TO MAKE YOUR ORGASM LAST 1790 TIMES LONGER

Imagine an orgasm that lasts a full 30 *minutes* instead of seconds, with bonus, occasional deep contractions occurring up to 24 hours afterward. This is the extraordinary promise of two American sexologists who've pioneered and perfected the Extended Sexual Orgasms (ESO) technique. Psychiatrist Alan Brauer and psychotherapist Donna Brauer claim if you faithfully follow the four steps of their sexuality program, *every* woman is potentially capable of experiencing a continuous orgasm of ever-increasing arousal lasting 30 minutes to an hour or more.

Of course, there is a catch. The 'training' that ESO requires will make your gym regime pale by comparison *plus* your partner has to be motivated, sexually educated and capable of following explicit, often complicated instructions. On top of that, not all of us *want* to experience an impromptu orgasm while admiring the roses with our 87-year-old neighbour, 24 hours after doing it, but . . . for those who want to give it a whirl, here's how to.

The ESO technique

You 'prepare' for a female ESO orgasm by working through stages 1 to 3 on your own and involving your partner in stage 4. It's not something you can pick up and try tonight; allow at least one month. (I've only detailed the female orgasm here. If he also likes the idea, ask your bookshop if they stock the ESO book or flick through a Tantric sex guide which has similiar techniques.)

1. Change your attitude about sex

According to the Brauers, everyone resists pleasure. Some of us are plagued by a deep-rooted fear of sex (the legacy of over-strict parents or a religious upbringing perhaps), others have more superficial sex worries (like suddenly wondering if we've fed the cat or if our thighs look fat). Either way, intrusive thoughts during the act need to be challenged with 'cognitive restructuring'. Every time you think a negative thought, suggest the Brauers, replace it with 'I'm calm' or 'Relax. I'm having a good time.'

2. Develop your PC muscle

See the Kegel exercise guide on page 86 to find out how to exercise your vaginal muscles. The Brauers also suggest you do 'slow clenches' (squeeze and clench to the count of three before releasing), 'flutters' (squeeze and clench as quickly as possible) and 'push-outs' (bearing down as if trying to go to the toilet using your stomach, anal and PC muscles). Do this for two weeks before starting stage three.

3. Masturbate regularly

Concentrate on what strokes suit you, the speed, pressure and rhythm. When you're convinced your attitude toward sex is positive, your PC muscle is toned and you know your body's responses intimately through masturbation, progress to stage four.

4. Train your partner

This is the fourth and final stage of the program, and the most complicated. It is divided into three steps:

Step one. You lie down, he sits or kneels cross-legged beside or in between your legs. He applies a personal water-based lubricant (like K-Y) to the whole of your vaginal and perineum area (the section between your vagina and anus).
He 'teases' you by lightly brushing and stroking all the genital area *except* the clitoris and inside the vagina.
Stimulation moves to the clitoris. He strokes, slow and steady, circling the clitoris with his finger once per second, while you tell him what feels good, what doesn't.

Step two. He continues clitoral stimulation while you use your PC training to 'flutter', 'slow clench' and 'push-out' as he's arousing you. Concentrate on your breathing. Don't hold your breath and aim to breathe at least six times a minute, breathing deeply from your stomach rather than shallow breathing from your chest.

If you're doing everything right, an orgasm isn't too far away. As you feel the onset of a climax, he should watch for regular two-second contractions in your genital area which means you're about to orgasm. Once the contractions start, he switches from stimulating your clitoris to the inner vaginal walls. Using his fingers, he can either push them in and out or sweep them in circles and in and out of the entrance. If he can locate your G-spot, stroking with his fore or middle finger is another option. Again, it's imperative he maintains a regular, slow rhythm.

Step three. After your orgasm subsides *but before the contractions stop entirely*, he'll feel the vagina start to draw back or 'pull away'. This is the 'coming down' period, usually the point where most couples stop. But in ESO, your first orgasm is only the beginning and the aim is to continue the contractions. He lightens his strokes inside until you give a signal you're ready for more before again upping the frequency and pressure. At the first sign of a pause in the vaginal contractions, he moves quickly back to the clitoris and continues stroking as before. This should trigger further contractions, at which point he moves back to stimulating the inner walls of the vagina.

Your partner continues switching back and forth from vaginal to clitoral stimulation until your contractions occur every 1 to 5 seconds. He then continues for about 15 minutes until the 'coming down' periods (where the vagina 'pulls away') occur less and less frequently and the contractions start to become continuous. When the vagina pushes out in a continual wave-like motion, you're in the final phase.

Now he needs to get into a position where he can use both hands (and keep his balance) to stimulate the clitoris and the vagina *simultaneously*. The result, claim the Brauers: wave after wave of orgasms, the like of which you've never felt before!

IF YOU'VE NEVER HAD AN ORGASM

Personally, I've never met (or even heard a whiff of a rumour about) a man who's *never* had an orgasm. But I can list at least six women off the top of my head who did (or, miserably, still do) fit the bill. For that reason, this section is devoted to females. While an extremely small percentage of men do suffer from ***anorgasmia***, the inability to have an orgasm, the causes are usually physical (see 'Faking it' page 96) or deeply psychological (and therefore best dealt with by a professional therapist).

> **'I've never ever heard of a guy who's never come. If a guy told me that, I'd be like "What?" and pack him off to the nearest doctor. I don't think I'd believe him; it sounds too weird.'**
>
> Peter, 42, vet

A tiny percentage of women do 'miss' orgasms. Their vaginal muscles contract but they don't register any sensation in their brain. It's rare, and the cause is usually psychological and best solved by a professional therapist. For most anorgasmic women, however, it's more likely caused by a lethal combination of a strict (particularly religious) upbringing and a lack of understanding about their own bodies. For that reason, it's a good idea to read about masturbation in Chapter 1 first. This will give you a basic idea of your sexual response system and guide you, step-by-step, through masturbation, the surest route to orgasm. Armed with the facts, you can then work through the following action plan – and be well on your way to working out what all the fuss is about!

1. Change your attitude by educating yourself

In one survey of 400,000 women, 50 per cent said they found it hard to reach orgasm with their partner.

The most common obstacle to having an orgasm is your attitude to sex. If you've been brought up to believe it's 'bad' or 'dirty' or even 'unladylike', you probably feel uncomfortable touching your genitals, or letting your partner touch them. The 'good girls don't' inhibition factor is covered in the masturbation chapter (see page 10). If this doesn't help, book a few sessions with a female sex therapist (call the British Psychological Society for referrals – see the Yellow Pages). The therapist will help you work through your feelings.

2. Accept that you have to 'learn' how to orgasm

Female orgasms aren't automatic. In other words, you're not going to accidentally have one while doing the ironing. It's also extremely unlikely that you'll have your first orgasm with a partner. Practically *all* women have their first *on their own*. So if you're waiting for some magical lover to transport you to heaven, stock up the cupboards – you're in for an awfully long wait. Instead, invest in a few good sex books. This book will give you lots of practical information but you might also want to scour the shelves for books that focus specifically on the emotional barriers to orgasm. Keep reading and researching until you feel good about sex, confident that you understand how your body works and know the basic techniques most women use to orgasm.

3. Accept responsibility for your own pleasure

Do you think it's his responsibility to 'give' you an orgasm? No-one can 'give' you an orgasm; you have to 'take' one yourself, by guiding and telling him how to do it. It's not like a five-course meal where he slaves in the kitchen and you get to do nothing but lie about until you're ready to savour the results. Orgasms happen when both of you know what you want and how to get it.

4. Teach yourself how to masturbate

Chapter 1 describes how to masturbate for the first time and outlines other techniques to try. You'll learn more about your body and its response system if you use your fingers but using a vibrator is also a good idea. Any good department store sells personal massagers, ostensibly designed to massage shoulders but more often bought to massage clitorises. The saleswoman won't know what you're buying it for, so just let her babble on in the background while you check to make sure it's got some sort of flat, small, round attachment. You're not putting it inside but holding it against the *mons* (the fleshy bit covered by pubic hair).

Once you've bought it, refer to Chapter 1 for instructions on how to masturbate using a vibrator. If you don't orgasm with this technique, see a gynaecologist to check for any physical problems (physical impairments to orgasm are rare and treatable so practically all women are capable of them). Otherwise, let rip and have as many orgasms as you can handle before collapsing in a happy heap.

Experts estimate that between 10 and 15 per cent of women never reach orgasm during sex or masturbation. The same number can only climax through masturbation.

Sorry, but the vibrator is now banished to the back of the cupboard until you can teach yourself to climax using your hands. Unless you want to always use a vibrator with your partner, you need to know how to do it manually. Again, turn to Chapter 1 for details on techniques.

5. Teach him how to do it

Once you've masturbated yourself to orgasm, it's time to tell *him* how to do it. Chapter 2, on foreplay, is peppered with suggestions about how to talk to him about sex, as are all the chapters in the book.

6. Change your mindset about your body

Many women don't orgasm because they think their partners can't possibly find them attractive. Let's get one thing straight right now: an overwhelming majority of men are turned on by a naked woman's body, no matter what shape it's in. However, if *you* aren't happy with yours, do something about it. Join a gym, get a make-over, eat healthily, then splash out on some new clothes. But accept what nature has handed out: ignore the faults, play up the good bits and learn to love every centimetre.

7. Stop trying so hard

A watched pot never boils. Your mind should be focused on how pleasurable the sensations are, not on 'Please God, let me have one'. The more you worry about it, the more your body will tense and make orgasm impossible. Try a bit of reverse psychology. When you masturbate or make love, tell yourself you're *not allowed* to have an orgasm, that this session is strictly for 'research' purposes. You'll relax more and may well end up scoring a goal.

! ***In the quest for orgasm, 75 per cent of women rate foreplay as more important than intercourse. More than half the male readers of*** **Penthouse** ***say they don't get as much foreplay as they'd like to make their orgasms more intense.***

8. Make time to pleasure yourself

My friend Sarah was trying to teach herself to orgasm through masturbation but to no avail. When I asked her when she masturbated, she answered, 'When Ben [her 2-year-old] is finally asleep, the washing's on but not ready to hang out yet and the baby's been fed.' Sarah's body didn't need an orgasm, it needed sleep!

For her birthday, a few of us (including her husband) all clubbed in and sent her away for the weekend, solo, to a luxury resort. Tucked in her hand luggage was a smuggled-in vibrator. A blissful 48 hours of peace and she'd not only had one orgasm, she clocked up a dozen.

9. Rethink your relationship

'You're fat', 'No wonder you can't have an orgasm, you're no good at anything', 'You're not a real woman', 'You're frigid' – if your partner says or insinuates negative things about you, your body or your inability to climax, getting rid of *him* is the simple solution to your problem.

IF YOU USED TO REGULARLY ORGASM BUT DON'T NOW

- **Have you built a mountain out of a molehill?** Most men, at some stage in their life, hit an occasion when they can't get an erection. Those that shrug and think, *So what? I was tired,* usually have no problems next time round. Those who think the end of the world has arrived find it's the beginning of a period of impotence. Women are the same. If you don't orgasm when you expect to, consciously dismiss it as a one-off. Thinking you won't have an orgasm is a self-fulfilling prophecy.
- **Are you happy with your partner?** Is it all men or just this man? If you've recently found out he was unfaithful, your body is protesting as much as your heart is. If you generally aren't sure of him or don't trust him, you won't relax enough to climax. Mr Nice Guy can also be an orgasm dampener. Are you frightened he'll think you're a 'slut' if you let go of your inhibitions?
- **Are you particularly stressed or tired right now?** Your body can't orgasm because it's too busy struggling with other issues – like keeping your heart pumping or your brain from exploding. Skip the orgasm mission; take a holiday instead.

5

Sexual Etiquette

Searching for Mr or Ms Compatible without making a complete fool of yourself

The old sexual etiquette book's a mess – things crossed out and things added in all over the place – and quite frankly, I think it's the job of whoever invented the Pill to do the rewrite. Pre-Pill everyone knew exactly what was expected of them: no sex before marriage (and not too much after it either). Then along came that tiny, innocent looking tablet and quicker than you could say 'flower power', those nice, orderly sexual mores were scattered to the wind.

No longer watching for a bun in the oven, women got out of the kitchen and raised temperatures elsewhere. Everyone flopped around on lumpy beanbags, and gazed through dope-dulled eyes at globs of wax floating about in lava lamps, trying to remember who they *hadn't* slept with so they could experience the free love phenomenon yet again. The advent of AIDS sent most scurrying back to the relative safety of monogamous relationships, but the damage was done. The rules of old no longer existed and no-one's had the foggiest as to what's 'normal' or 'expected' since.

Not that it's stopped us bonking away. Only 5 per cent of western brides today walk down the aisle as virgins. The rest of us are sexual veterans by age 21. In fact, we're encouraged to experiment with several or lots of different partners to avoid a *new* no-no – settling down before we're 'ready'. If you do defy your friends and get hitched, husbands and wives are urged to go out separately and see friends solo. 'Space' is the new buzzword. So we go out alone, end up with someone else, get caught, then divorced and it's back to square one, the singles bar – bruised, battered but determined not to miss out on what everyone else seems to be having.

It's astonishing any of us bother dating at all given the minefield of potential disasters that go along with it. Because there really is *no one right answer* to today's between-the-sheets dilemmas, most of us seem to invent our own rules as we go along. But there *are* some broad guidelines emerging. Here, some hopefully helpful solutions to a selection of the most common questions asked by men and women in, or contemplating, a new relationship.

The most treasured memento of past relationships apart from photographs for men: her underwear. For women: his T-shirt.

DATING DILEMMAS

How do I tell if she's interested but just playing hard to get?

Even if she is test-running the 'treat-'em-mean-keep-'em-keen' theory, she's probably giving out *some* signals. Does she look you straight in the eye when she talks to you? Does she always seem to be near you even though she pretends she'd rather not be? Do you catch her looking at you when she doesn't think you're looking at her? If you're not even close enough to put any of these theories to the test, there's nothing for it but to pick up the phone and ask her out. If she's busy the night you suggest, she'll suggest another if she wants to see you. She didn't? She's not playing hard to get, she is hard to get (that is, give up now).

Is it okay if I call to ask him out? Don't men always like to be the one who conquers?

Some of the most confident women I know still won't pick up the phone to ask a man out on a date, which isn't very fair when true equality between the sexes means sharing the male pressures as well as pleasures. The first move – which means facing a possible slap-in-the-face rejection – is still usually left up to him (even though most men I know said they'd be thrilled if a woman rang to ask them out). So, strike one for sisterhood and pick up that phone if you fancy someone. If he instantly thinks you must be (a) desperate to bonk him, (b) hard up, or (c) one of those 'ball-breaking career women', it's better to find out he's a jerk *before* you waste time waxing your bikini line.

Who pays on the first date?

Whoever asked who out. If that's him, he'll usually expect to cough up the cash, but that doesn't mean you shouldn't offer. Forget the notion that letting him pay for your meal means you owe him something (sex, for instance). If during the date you start to think he *is* assuming that, feign sickness and leave. Otherwise, graciously accept his offer to pay even if you're twitching because you earn *twice* as much as he does. He's not being a chauvinist or playing power games, just doing what he thinks he should. Split the bills from then on or take in turns paying. Most couples split expenses proportionate to their respective salaries. The poorer partner can even the score by doing things that require less cash (cooking dinner at home, supplying the wine, etc.).

What if I really don't like her after the first date. Do I have to take her phone number?

No, though lots of guys do because it's far easier to say 'I'll call you' then disappear into the night. (Look up 'bastard' in the dictionary and you'll find their picture.) If you haven't enjoyed yourself, take a deep breath and say something like, 'Thanks. It's always nice meeting new people. Perhaps we'll run into each other again.' She won't wait by the phone, and you won't feel guilty for making false promises.

What if he said he'd call then doesn't?

Give him a little time to gather courage (he'll often take longer to call if he's really keen) but as a general rule, the old theory that if he hasn't called within three days he isn't going to, is pretty accurate. If you went out on Saturday and he hasn't called by Wednesday, he's not calling. Either accept it or ring him. If you slept together and he doesn't call the next day, it's also unlikely he's going to. He hasn't had an accident, his mother's not dying in hospital and there's nothing wrong with your phone.

I'm too scared to make the first move in case I'm accused of date rape. How do I get her to?

Be honest. Say, 'This whole date rape issue has really upset me. I'd hate to think a girl thought I was putting the hard word on her when she didn't want me to. So, I'll leave it up to you to call the shots.' Any girl who doesn't think you're a sweetheart after a speech like that isn't worth dating. She probably won't unzip your jeans within the next 60 seconds, but she may give you an unmistakeably passionate kiss that hints she wants more. If you think she does, ask, 'Can I take things further?'

! ***Number of men who think it's a sexual come-on when a woman asks them back for coffee: 68 per cent. Number of men who interpret a hello kiss planted full on the lips the same way: 50 per cent.***

How do I initiate sex with a new guy without coming on like I'm desperate?

Most men will love it if you *do* seem desperate for sex. But I identify with your dilemma. The old 'I'll just slip into something more comfortable' routine goes down a treat in a James Bond film, but the only time I've ever said it in real life, I meant it – and came out in trackpants and slippers.

If you're stuck at the quick peck on the cheek stage, he's either gay, wants the two of you just to be friends or he doesn't think he has the green light to progress any further. Are you sure you're sending the right signals? Women who are ready for sex go further than holding eye contact – they move closer, touch the guy a lot, linger over that goodnight kiss.

One way of getting the message across loud and clear but in a subtle way is to ask him over to dinner (complete with candles, romantic music and sexy outfit). Give him a cuddle in the kitchen then a sexy snog; afterward, sit next to him on the couch and put your legs on his lap. Later, initiate some passionate kissing – most men won't need more than that to take things from there.

If he still sits there with his hands shoved between his knees, behave like the liberated woman you are: tell him outright you want to make love to him. If he reacts as if your invitation is promiscuous or 'unladylike', he'd be a bore in bed anyhow.

When is it okay to sleep with him so he won't think I'm easy?

Plenty of people regret sleeping with someone too soon, not too many people regret waiting it out. There's no magic formula but there is a sexual double-standard. Some guys will think you're 'easy' if you sleep with them after dating every weekend for six weeks, others won't judge you if you sleep with them the first night. The 'norm', if indeed there is one, is probably after at least three or four dates. (But what constitutes a date? Is a Friday through to Sunday stint one or three?)

When you sleep with each other depends very much on what you want from the relationship, how well you're getting on, your sexual pattern, morals, upbringing – a whole host of issues. Don't make the decision if you've been drinking heavily and don't do it until both of you feel comfortable with each other.

Whose responsibility is it to provide the condom? Will he think I'm a slut if I do?

Both of you should always carry condoms. It's a shared responsibility. If you're single, it doesn't mean you sleep around; it means you're sensible and (like a good Girl Guide) prepared for anything. If you're married with six kids, on the Pill and produce the condom, it's a little fishy but even then (especially then), prudent. If he does give you a withering 'What sort of girl are you?' look when you grab one, put it back in your handbag, put your clothes *on* and exit right.

I start out with every intention of using a condom but it all flies out the window if I've had a few drinks and get carried away. When is the right time to bring the subject up and the condoms out?

We've all woken up the morning after and felt sick from more than just the hangover. 'Did I or didn't I?', your groggy brain tries to deduce, then you find it, there in your bag, still in the wrapper.

Many people righteously carry enough condoms to solve the world's population problem; not so many actually use them. Unfortunately, a condom won't protect you against HIV (the virus that can lead to full-blown AIDS) unless it's actually on his penis. You'll be more inclined to practise what you preach if they're within reach, so keep some near the bed as well as in your handbag.

When's the best time to talk about safe sex? Somewhere between the first drink and taking your clothes off. Make it a personal rule to discuss – and produce – condoms while you're still fully clothed. You'll be far less likely to get so turned on, you conveniently forget.

Don't say, 'You might have AIDS, I think we should use a condom,' but 'God, I'm so turned on. I think we'd better get a condom out now because once we start, there's no way we'll want to stop.' In other words, don't *suggest* using a condom, take it for granted that you will be. If he tries to talk you out of it or refuses to wear one, give sex – and him – a big swerve.

! An unfaithful boyfriend can do more than break your heart – he could give you cancer. If he's playing around and not using condoms, he ups your chance of contracting a strain of HPV (human papilloma virus), which is strongly linked to cervical cancer.

When is it acceptable not to wear condoms?

Many couples decide to get tested for AIDS when they've been going out a while, don't want to have sex with anyone else but their partner, and don't want to continue using condoms. Before being tested, make sure you haven't had unprotected sex (sex without a condom) for at least three months; the result will be inconclusive otherwise. Keep using condoms until the test results come back. If you both test negative and are committed to being monogamous, you've reduced your risks substantially.

Note I said *reduced* your risks. Unfortunately, there's no way of telling whether your partner will be faithful or if he or she will use condoms if they do have sex with someone else. (Make sure you organise alternative contraception if you don't want to get pregnant.)

I want to ask my new lover how many lovers they've had so I can determine how risky they are as a sexual partner. How do I approach it?

Are you serious? It's not worth wasting your breath. For a start, how do you know he or she is telling the truth? How do they know all their previous partners were telling the truth? Even if they have only slept with their childhood sweetheart, it doesn't mean they're not carrying the HIV virus. You can become infected from just one encounter of unprotected sex and the risk doesn't necessarily increase with the number of partners you've had. The guy who's slept with 1000 women but used a condom every single time is safer than the man who's had unprotected sex six times. Skip the pointless chit-chat; put on a condom instead.

! ***Average number of sexual partners most men (30 or under) admit to: 8. Sexperts' estimate of how many they've probably had: 18. The number most women confess to: 4. What's more likely: 10.***

I have genital herpes. How do I tell my new man?

Start by reading the ''Fessing up: How to tell a lover you've got an STI' section in Chapter 6. It's not that difficult. Honest.

TEN WAYS TO GUARANTEE A SECOND DATE

1. Forgive each other for being clumsy. So he knocked wine all over your new suit or your potato shot straight off the plate and flew across the restaurant. So what? You're looking for a partner not auditioning for a Swiss finishing school.
2. Fill the silences. You're both fiddling with serviettes and frantically searching for something, *anything,* to say. Those silences can be unnerving but (I hate to say it) women are usually better at filling them up. Put him out of his misery by making small talk; the more relaxed you are, the more comfortable he'll be. Now's not the time to launch into a history of your gynaecological problems or how that bitch in the office is making your life miserable. Also steer clear of a long list of criticisms of your last boyfriend. Other than that, you don't really have to censor your conversation too much. There's not much point in pretending to be someone you're not – they're going to find 'the real you' at some point!
3. Have a sense of humour. If he stumbles over his words, she trips up, make a joke of it. Laugh your way through those difficult, awkward situations. If she's talking to you with a piece of spinach lodged charmingly between her front teeth, tell her. And don't be scared to say, 'God, don't you wish we could fast forward to our second date? I'm a bit nervous.'
4. Tell them they look nice: 'What a great jacket,' or 'Wow, you look fantastic.' You've both spent *hours* examining your reflection; make each other feel it was worth it.
5. Be honest. Say, 'I was really pleased you called,' or 'I'm so glad you accepted my invitation.' There's nothing wrong with admitting you like someone.
6. Help choose the venue so you can share the blame if it's awful. The service is laughable, the food inedible – does it really matter? Tell a funny story about the time *you* chose a restaurant that everyone hated. It's not the ➢

customer's fault if the venue doesn't live up to expectations.

7. Don't judge them too much on what they say. You're both nervous and likely to say something silly, or maybe give impressions that aren't accurate. Don't criticise or pull each other up first time round. Ease up a little.
8. Enjoy yourself. If you're starving, order an entrée, main course and dessert, even if your partner orders a salad. If you hate red wine, say so. Be yourself. It's a date not a job interview.
9. Ask them out at the end of the night if you've enjoyed yourself. There's a weird date protocol out there that decrees you're meant to say, 'I'll call you' instead of 'Can I see you tomorrow?' even if you're both desperate to. If you really got on well, there's nothing to stop either of you making arrangements there and then. Besides, it saves that post-first-date, pre-second-date panic which everyone struggles with if they've had a fantastic time. She thinks, 'He's far too attractive/intelligent/cool to want to see me again.' He thinks, 'She's figured out I'm not rich or sophisticated – especially since I dribbled spaghetti down my chin/left a meagre tip/spilt the wine.' Deal with it by making the date on the spot.
10. Don't finish the evening with sex. Sometimes it seems to be and is the natural thing to do. If this applies to you, you'll know it. Most of the time, though, it's a mistake. If you're madly attracted to each other and getting on well, what's the rush?

CASUAL SEX

We don't always have sex with people we love. Sometimes we'll quite happily do it with someone we don't even want to spend a whole day with. Why? Because we can lust after someone without necessarily wanting to get involved. While one- (or two- or three-) night stands aren't terribly satisfying long-term, sometimes, for a number of reasons, sex without romantic involvement is all you want. If you're in that head space right now, these are a few of the etiquette trouble-spots you may have to negotiate.

If I'm only interested in having sex, should I say something *before* sleeping with them?

Yes. It's wholly unfair, disrespectful and unforgiveable to whisper sweet nothings which really are nothings. As you're having dinner or drinks say, 'Look, I thought you should know I've just come out of a long-term relationship/ I'm really busy at work right now and I'm not interested in a serious relationship. I think you're gorgeous and I'd love to have fun with you but if you're looking for more, I'm the wrong person.' If you end up in bed together after that, fine. You both knew the score.

> ***It might feel good to snuggle up to a warm body at night, but research proves we sleep better when we sleep alone.***

Whose place should we go back to?

If you're a guy, it probably doesn't matter. If you're a girl, it matters a whole lot. Don't even think about letting some guy you've just met at a bar or a nightclub take you home to his place, even if you *do* fully intend to have sex. He might seem harmless but you can't judge by appearances or by chatting to them for a few hours if someone's violent or psychologically unstable. (If you're tempted, just remember that serial killer Ted Bundy was described by all who knew him socially as 'a nice guy'.) If you take him back to your place, make sure your flatmate is home and alerted. Also remember he now knows where you live. If you check into a hotel or do go back to his place, call a friend first and leave the address and phone number. Ask them to call you in half an hour to check all is okay.

What if I don't want them to stay the night? How do I leave without offending them? Somehow, I always end up cooking breakfast for people just to be polite.

Regardless of whether you're talking about a one-night stand or the future father or mother of your babies, it's rude to jump up and into your clothes before the sheets have even settled. If you're at their place, a good way to work up to leaving is to suggest a nightcap (a drink or a cup of coffee). Then, get up and get dressed while they're making it and move into the lounge room. Even if you drink it in bed, it's still a pretty easy way to break the mood. When you've finished, just yawn and casually say, 'I should be going.' If they ask you to stay, say 'I'd love to but I have a huge day tomorrow and really need some sleep.' If you *do* want to see them again, you can follow it through with, 'But on Friday night, I'd love to stay over.' If someone's settling in to *your* bed, try the nightcap trick again (dressed, in the lounge room). They really have no choice but to put their clothes on and join you. If they still don't get the hint say, 'My flatmate and I have an arrangement that no-one sleeps over,' or 'I'm really sorry. I can never sleep with some-one in my bed and I have to be up really early. Can I call you a cab?'

What if I'd like to see him/her again for sex but don't really want a relationship?

If you were honest *before* you got into bed, all you need to do is call. If you weren't, you'll need to say something like, 'That was fantastic and I'd love to do it again but I think I should tell you I'm not interested in anything serious. Are you happy just with a casual relationship?'

My best male friend and I are both single and have high libidos yet neither of us wants to sleep around. I think the ideal solution is to sleep with each other as friends until one or both of us gets involved. What do you think?

It can be the very best or the worst idea you've ever come up with. I know one couple who carried it off successfully but I suspect they were the exception to the rule. They were both able to separate sex from love and neither had ulterior motives. I know of another couple who now don't speak because of it. It's incredibly difficult to sleep with someone regularly and not become emotionally attached. After all, you already like the person as a friend, so if you also have great sex it suddenly seems *logical* to become a couple. Sometimes people do. Other times, one wants to, the other doesn't and 'my friend Mary' becomes 'that heartless bitch'. Is it worth risking the friendship?

If I always use condoms, do my partners need to know if I have more than one lover?

Yes, it's called being honest. But once you've made it clear that the relationship is not monogamous, there's no need to dwell on it. They don't need to know when you've slept with someone else or who the person was. So long as they're aware it's not an exclusive relationship, it's really none of their business.

It's over but I'd like to be friends. Does that ever work?

Yes. Many ex-lovers are now very special friends, but there are a few factors common to all these friendships. It usually doesn't work if one of you is still in love with the other, if the trust between you was broken (by an affair, for instance) or if the break-up was particularly nasty. It works best if the split was mutual, you live close or share lots of mutual friends (so it's easy to see each other), you've got common interests and *no longer want to be a couple*. That's the magic ingredient: if one of you is secretly hoping the friendship will lead to you getting back together, it can only end in more tears.

I'm pregnant but have only been going out with my boyfriend for a few months. While the relationship is nice, it's not serious and I fully intend to have an abortion. Do I have to tell him?

I would. Not only is it the decent thing to do, he has a right to know for fertility reasons. If he has trouble fathering a child later on, it may help to know he was fertile at some point. Besides, a pregnancy – even an unwanted one – involves two people. Both of you had sex, both knew the risks. He doesn't have the right to tell you what to do about the pregnancy but he does have the right to know he's fathered a child. You're concerned he'll force you into keeping the baby? Play your cards close to your chest. Tell him you're pregnant and thinking about having an abortion, calmly explaining the reasons why you don't want to keep the baby. If he starts threatening you, tell him you'll think about what he's had to say, then leave. Make your appointment with a termination clinic as soon as possible and don't tell him where or when. Legally, he can't stop you but it could be messy if he turns up.

Why do I only find 'bad boys' sexually attractive? I've been out with nice ones but they leave me cold.

Women who like bad boys fall into two categories. There are girls who wouldn't dream of settling down with one but thoroughly enjoy the odd sex fling. Then there are women who only go out with bad boys and spend most of the time miserable because they desperately want them to love them. Several 'popular' psychological theories attempt to explain both cases.

If you fall into the first category, I bet you describe your family and childhood as 'eccentric'. Think about it. What do bad guys give you that good guys don't? Excitement. Drama. (They can only cause you heartache if you let them.) Now think back to your childhood. Would you describe it as quiet, peaceful, serene? *Are you kidding*? I can hear you say. You're attracted to the drama of bad-boy relationships because you're recreating what is familiar. If home was frenetic – your parents had strong personalities and argued constantly, one (or both) had an affair, or you had a brother or sister whose antics turned the house into something resembling the set of a soapie – then you were brought up to believe that constant tension is normal. It's not and if you're only treating bad boys as a fun toy, you've already figured that out.

If you're in the second category, the tension at home was probably more sinister than exciting. Maybe your parents fought viciously, ignored you, or perhaps there was violence or even abuse. Our parents' relationship is often what we base our relationships on: subconsiously, we try to recreate them. If you have a history of always hooking up to guys who are bad for you, book in to see a good therapist, even if you don't identify with *any* of the theories listed here.

SEX FOR SEX'S SAKE: THE RULES

If you've just come out of a long-term relationship (and can't bear to dive into another), haven't got time for a love affair because your career is all-consuming, or have simply met someone who makes you boil down under but leaves you cold above, a lust affair could be *just* what the sex therapist ordered.

Men have been having sex affairs since God said, 'Let there be light' (even if their partners didn't realise). Now, lots of confident girls with raging libidos and a guilt-free attitude to satisfying them are also able to separate sex from love. They're not searching for Mr Right or even a commitment for a date on Saturday night: all they want is good sex and a good time.

Women who stay single are more likely to be among the most intelligent and highly educated of their sex, and to have reached top levels of achievement. Never-married men tend to be the exact opposite.

If that's you, go for it! But be careful, not just with your sexual health and personal safety but with your emotional health as well. Just because there's no commitment to be monogamous doesn't mean either of you have the right to treat each other badly. If you're going to indulge, here are the rules:

- **Refuse to feel guilty.** If you suffer even the faintest twinge of guilt, sex-only affairs aren't for you. If you find you're waking up feeling depressed or bad about yourself, don't do it again. People in casual relationships are exploiting each other – which is fine as long as that's what they both want. Just remember there's a huge difference between having sex and making love. He's not going to send flowers, she's not going to call to say goodnight. So there's no reason to pretend you 'don't usually do this sort of thing', even if you don't. If he thinks you're a bit easy, who cares?
- **Use condoms every single time.** If I have to explain why, you're not a candidate.
- **Use back-up contraception.** Again, for obvious reasons.
- **Do it for the right reasons.** Casual sex may make you feel sexy, attractive and desirable but it won't make you feel special or loved. If you're having sex just to get the hug at the end, stop kidding yourself. Lust affairs are conducted for sheer pleasure. Don't sleep with someone simply to reaffirm your attractiveness.

- **Let go of any inhibitions.** A lot of women find they're much less inhibited with a guy they don't care about. After all, does it matter if he thinks you're fat or kinky? If you've always wanted to have someone tie you up and lick cream off your body, this is your man.
- **Don't broadcast your affairs.** Some women will brand you just as readily as some men will. It's your business, not theirs.
- **Stay in control by being honest with each other.** Establish upfront that you want uncomplicated sex and not a relationship. If you feel yourself falling for them, let them know. They might feel the same. If they don't, stop seeing them and find someone else. Great sex isn't worth a broken heart.
- **Be nice to each other.** He's got a body that makes you wet just looking at it? Tell him. She's so erotic, you're convinced she'll be in your fantasies forever? Ditto. Compliments don't equal commitment.
- **Pick your partners carefully.** If you feel like sex and don't meet someone who measures up, go home and masturbate instead. Choose partners whom you like and who make you feel good about yourself. Other people's husbands, wives, girlfriends and boyfriends are off limits; and don't sleep with friends of friends unless you can cope with the rumour mill.
- **If you're female, don't put yourself in risky situations.** Be super-safety conscious and trust your gut reactions. If you feel it's wrong and the guy's a bit dodgy, don't do it. It's safer to take him back to your place (with a flatmate home and in the next room) than it is to go back to his. If you've seen him a few times and trust him enough to go to his place, leave his address and phone number with someone *you* trust.

THE 'I AM WHO I GO OUT WITH' TRAP

Because women are naturally caring and nurturing, there's a tendency for some to get 'lost' in relationships. Instead of going out, they *merge* with their boyfriends, losing their individuality in the process. This is not healthy.

It's easy to tell if you fit into the 'women who love too much' category. Did you become a sports nut even though you *hate* football, just because your last boyfriend was one? Did you ditch the suits for floaty numbers and grow your hair when you went out with the herbal type? Are you prepared to do just about anything to make him happy, even if it means forcing down steak and three veg when you'd really rather have pasta and a salad? Given time, you'll spend so much of your life pleasing your boyfriends, you'll completely forget what pleases *you*. You become what you think they want you to be – and that's dangerous.

The fact is, if you lie down like a doormat, people will walk over you. *You* think you're being supportive and easygoing, he thinks you're a push-over and treats you like one. Your self-esteem plummets when he loses respect and you find yourself putting up with inexcusable behaviour just because you're now too frightened and vulnerable to be alone. Don't let yourself get to this point. The more you retain your individuality – your friends, your career, a life *apart* from him – the more successful and satisfying your relationship will be. Men respect confident women. Confident women attract confident men, men who'll treat you as an equal. He can't treat you like dirt if you don't let him.

SECOND-TIME ROUND

Relationship break-ups *hurt*. It doesn't matter who dumped who, whether you're heart-broken or relieved that it's over, the end of any serious relationship means a dream is shattered. You loved each other once, you probably thought it would last forever, now it's over. The most confident person is plagued by insecurities for at least a little while afterward – and if you aren't, you should be.

There's a certain amount of 'cleaning up' that's necessary after a serious split. You may need to sift through any accusations thrown at you – some trivial (Is my nose really too big?), some serious (Do I have a problem with commitment? Am I a good mother/father?). You also need to reestablish yourself as 'one' rather than part of a couple. This takes time. Rush through the recovery process, kid yourself you're over it and ready to start a new relationship too soon, and you'll carry the baggage from the old one all your life.

The first few months will be painful, maybe it'll take years for the sharp pain to recede to a dull ache, but eventually you *will* wake up one morning and forget to be miserable. It's usually around this time that the blinkers fall off and the world suddenly seems full of gorgeous, yummy (*Gosh! Check that out!*) people. Your libido kicks back in with a vengeance and hovers dangerously high. You start masturbating like crazy and even the fat little man in the newsagent or the woman pushing the stroller in the supermarket seems possible dating material. Congratulations! Months ago, you never would have thought it possible but you're not only ready to date again, you're ready for sex, maybe even another relationship! Here's a few of the common dilemmas second-time-rounders have to deal with.

! Number of men who've cried themselves to sleep over relationship problems: 55 per cent. Women who've done the same: 65 per cent. Number of men who think sex is the best way to make up after an argument: 35 per cent. Women who agree: 23 per cent.

I split from my husband six months ago. My girlfriends have dragged me out to singles places a few times but everything's changed. I don't know the 'rules' anymore, sex seems different – and I feel lost.

I remember walking past a particularly dreadful singles bar one night, arm-in-arm with my husband, thinking, 'Thank Christ I don't have to do *that* again.' A few years later, we split and (*groan!*) there I was, back on the dating scene. The first few times I went out, I felt truly tragic. I'd forgotten how to do all that silly get-to-know-you talk and everyone seemed younger, prettier and more together than I was. It felt different because I was different. Pre-marriage, I was the quintessential nightclub queen: capable of chatting up men, sinking a G and T, smoking a cigarette and keeping an eye on my friend's handbag, all while I was on the dance floor. Post break-up, I felt about as groovy as the shiny disco balls that had magically disappeared from the ceiling of every nightclub.

Things appear to change fast in dating land but, believe me, it's mostly surface stuff. Your girlfriends could write you a long list of the 'new rules for the 90s' but if you looked closely you'd see they'd just be rewritten versions of the rules you already know. The only thing that has changed is the danger factor. If last time round you feared getting herpes, this time you're dealing with AIDS. The only real new rule is this: you *must* use condoms.

You feel misplaced not because 'the scene' has changed, but because you have. It's like tackling that previously mastered tricky soufflé again when you haven't made it for years. You're apprehensive because you're out of practice. Being single is great fun when you're feeling fabulous, not so great when you're vulnerable, and everyone is after a break-up. The prospect of finding a partner amongst all those strangers seems about as likely as finding a match to half the dinner service you're now left with. Do yourself a favour and avoid the pick-up places for a while. Avoid them permanently if you like. Stick to parties and dinner parties with friends or nights out at restaurants until you feel a little more in control.

How soon is too soon to take a new lover?

It's probably not a good idea to bring the girl you picked up at a nightclub to a friend's dinner party the week after you split from your wife, but it's really up to *you* to decide when you're ready. Just be aware of your real motivations. Lots of people who quickly jump feet first into a new relationship are really just wanting a warm body in their now cold bed, trying to ease the pain or loneliness. If that helps you get through and your new partner is aware of it, fine, but you still have to confront the issues and this is probably best done alone.

When you date again depends on how long you were in your previous relationship, how serious it was and the nature of the break-up. It takes some people years to get over those awful feelings of hurt, vulnerability, pain or anger. Others find they did their grieving while still in the relationship – it ended emotionally years before they physically moved out – and are ready to date within weeks.

If the split was sudden, bitter and painful, you'll probably want to shut the door and hide away for a while. If you've got kids, you'll need to devote time to helping them get over the split. In other words, there's no acceptable time frame that applies to everyone.

Also recognise that there's a difference between taking a lover and getting involved again. Every person you go out with doesn't have to be a prospective long-term replacement. If you meet someone who's fun, who you can rediscover sex with but not much else, great! Don't feel guilty, just enjoy.

Another word of advice: you've probably been leaning heavily on your friends and family during the split-up, letting them know how you feel at every waking moment. If you're ready to have sex again, you're ready to wean yourself and stand on your own two feet. By all means, have a laugh with a mate or a girlfriend over what you've been up to but don't feel obliged to confide all the intimate details. You don't need their permission. You're an adult.

I can't imagine stripping naked in front of a total stranger. I'd be far too embarrassed. My body was great last time I was dating, but now I'm older and I've had a child.

I don't think too many people *would* feel comfortable stripping naked in front of a total stranger! But the man you *want* to take your gear off for won't be. Forget any preconceived notions you have about having to climb into bed on date three. Have sex when you feel ready – when you know, trust and feel comfortable enough to sleep with him without being judged. Unless you're planning on dating a 16-year-old supermodel, your new lover's body isn't going to be perfect either. While you're frantically sucking in your stomach or worrying about how big your bum is, he's nervous the light's hitting that not-so-well-concealed bald spot and that the arms you're grabbing onto aren't as muscular as your ex's were.

Accepting that our bodies age is just another ikky fact of life. Eat healthily, exercise often, dress to conceal your faults and make the most of what you've got, then relax about the rest. Besides, would you swap that gorgeous child of yours for your previously flat tummy? Not in a million years!

My old partner knew my body inside out. I don't know if I can be bothered teaching someone all over again.

Oh, I agree. How boring (yawn)! What an absolute pain in the proverbial to have some gorgeous new lover rediscover all your known sensitive spots (and some you never knew you had). How tedious to have to guide his or her deliciously sexy tongue to all the right bits. How positively awful to have to spend all day in bed, fuelled by champagne and oysters, taking them on a guided tour of your body. I'm with you – it must be dreadful to have to say 'Oh yes, that's it, right there' . . . get my point?

I was ho-hum about sex with my husband, now I can't get enough of it with my new lover. The ironic thing is, technically, my husband was probably better in bed. I feel guilty, like maybe if I'd tried harder with him, we wouldn't have split.

I bet you *did* try hard with your husband, at least at some point. But there's something decidedly unsexy about being married. We 'live in sin' as 'lovers', but once that band of gold's slipped on our fingers, we become 'husband and wife' – respectable people granted official permission by society to have sex. No wonder lots of people don't want to! Spending all Sunday in bed making love somehow seems frivolous when you're married (and really should be up working on that renovation). Add to that problems in the relationship, which you obviously had or you wouldn't have split, and you can start to see why sex maybe wasn't that wonderful.

You can't have great sex with a long-term partner unless your relationship's also great. You broke up for a reason. Whatever that reason was, it had to affect your sex life somehow. Sex with your new lover is wonderful because he's not your husband and you're not struggling with relationship problems. Plus he's new (and anything new always seems more exciting) and, I bet, more passionate. Lust and enthusiasm can beat the hell out of technical skills (though it's always nice to get all three). Stop feeling guilty. Even if you did make some mistakes, it's over. Let go of the past and let yourself enjoy what sounds like an enviable sex life with your new man.

I've just started dating again and a guy 12 years younger than me has asked me out. I like him but fear he sees me as a desperate, older woman.

I'll let you in on a secret: the single, older woman – yesterday's 'old maid' – magically transformed herself into the new sex goddess while you were playing couples. There are lots of young men out there who've discovered that dating an attractive, well-preserved older woman can be a lot more fun than seeing someone who still works a shift at McDonalds. The guy who asked you out sees you as confident, experienced and worldly. He's hoping like hell you'll sleep with him because he's heard (quite rightly) that older women take control in bed, are more sexually adventurous, less inhibited and more likely to let him lie back and enjoy for a change. Go out with him. Turn all his fantasies into reality. Enjoy him as an ego-boosting, marvellous affair. He probably won't be sitting next to you in a rocking chair when you're 60 but he could be Mr Right For Now.

What do I tell my kids when I meet someone? When should they meet him? Can he *ever* stay over?

It all depends on how old your children are, when you split, how well they're coping with it, their personalities, their relationship with the estranged spouse, the person you're dating and how serious your relationship is. Phew! For some time after the break-up, your children will probably be more clingy than usual. They'll be feeling as insecure as you are and worried you'll 'abandon' them as well. They've only seen you act romantically with Daddy and seeing you hold hands or kiss someone else will be upsetting initially – especially if they're secretly hoping for a reunion (and they nearly always are).

Personally, I wouldn't tell them about, or introduce them to, people who you know aren't going to be long-term material. What's the point? Tell them you're going out to have fun with some friends and let them play havoc with the babysitter. Once you decide you've met someone special, introduce your new partner the same way you would any friend. Get him to pick you up from home initially, then maybe invite him around for dinner with other friends. Don't be overtly affectionate if they seem upset, give them time to get used to the person as a friend rather than a father substitute.

Accept reality. You can control kids only to a point. Tell them it's naughty to wander into your room late at night and they'll still wrap that little hand around the doorknob and do it ('Are you hurt Mummy? Why are you groaning?'). Snogging in the kitchen where they can see you or letting your lover sleep over when they're still at the stage of crying themselves to sleep over the loss of a parent isn't on. Take it slow. You know your children; you'll know when they're ready to accept that you have a lover. Don't force him down their throat and insist they like him but don't let them dictate your life either. Your kids are important but your happiness is equally so.

What if my children disapprove of who I'm going out with?

They probably don't dislike the person you've chosen, just resent sharing you and, of course, would prefer you to be back with their *real* mum or dad. They're hurting and highly vulnerable after the split. One person has left them so they want all your attention and if you're giving it to someone else, they feel threatened all over again. Reassure them until you're blue in the face, load them up with so much affection they *can't* feel left out. Make them feel involved when your new lover is around and insist he or she treats them with respect and kindness (even if they are being difficult little buggers). Explain that this person won't replace Mummy or Daddy but that you enjoy their company. It's especially easy for teenage kids to sit in moral judgement of what you're doing – remember how superior *you* used to feel at 15? Let them know you love them desperately but this person also makes you happy.

! Women spend their 20s wanting a caring, sharing man in bed – just when men are only interested in bonking, say psychologists. The opposite happens in our 30s. Women become more sexually adventurous and insatiable, men turn sensitive. A good argument to match older women with younger men.

What if his or her kids don't like me?

You can't make children like you. They'll be especially hostile if you try too hard or (God forbid) try to become a replacement for the parent who's left. Be nice, be kind, spoil them a little. Talk to them even if they ignore you, refuse to get angry if they treat you badly. Ask your partner if there's anything you do that upsets them, and for hints on how to win them over. She or he should also be making an effort to ease the situation on your behalf. If, in time, they're still hostile, there's nothing much you can do but live with it or move on.

Do I have to tell every new lover I've got kids? I find it turns guys off.

Not if it's just for sex, but otherwise why not? Are you going to lock them in the attic whenever he's around? Remove all evidence (just try, bet you can't do it) every time he visits? It's unrealistic and illogical. If your new lover's going to turn white and start shaking because you tell him straight off you've got a child, he's going to run *screaming* into the sunset when you do tell him later, feeling (understandably) duped. And it'll hurt you a lot more then. You come as part of a package – you and your kids. If he can't accept that, it's *his* problem. What are you going to do? Give them away to charity?

> ! *If couples held a weekly meeting to sort out their problems calmly and rationally, the divorce rate would go down by 80 to 90 per cent, say psychologists. Instead, most of us resort to nasty bickering – and one cruel insult erases 20 acts of kindness.*

How do I tell if I've fallen for my new lover out of fear of being alone? I don't feel I can trust my feelings. What's this I've heard about 'transition lovers'?

If you feel you can't trust your feelings, you can't. You're at the stage where you're ready to go out with someone but probably not at the point where you want to (or should) commit. You won't know if your feelings are real until you feel confident again, happy with your own company and capable of making it alone; in other words, when you're at the point where, while you might *want* a relationship, you don't *need* one. Handle the situation in the meantime by letting your new partner know you're still working through things and while you think they're fantastic, you're a little unsure of your feelings. Don't let anyone pressure you into committing before you're ready.

'Transition lovers' is a term some psychologists use to describe the first relationship after a big split. Often, we hook up with people before we're really ready and while we might *think* we're madly in love with them, subconsciously we're using them to get over insecurities and to fill the well of loneliness left by our last relationship. It's not until we feel more ourselves that we realise we don't love them after all. This doesn't mean *all* relationships that happen straight after the split will end; some people do find a new partner quickly and stay with them, happily, forever.

My new girlfriend has the ex-husband from hell. I'm sick of hearing about him and he's now causing problems with us.

Your girlfriend's marriage is finished. *Kaput*. There's obviously no chance of friendship so her ex should be out of her life completely if they're divorced and don't have kids. If they do, it's not an amicable split, so she should see him only when he picks the kids up or drops them off. Better still, she should arrange for him to pick them up from a sympathetic friend's place. In other words, if he's still causing her trouble a year or years down the track, she's letting him – probably because she feels guilty. If he's bitter, chances are she's the one who left. She figures if he treats her badly, it's her punishment for walking out. Tell her you're sick of talking about him and she needs to let go, to get him out of her life and get on with hers. If she can't, pack her off to a good counsellor for some therapy or tell her you're not interested in continuing the relationship until she's sorted out the problem.

FIRST-TIME SEX AFTER A LONG-TERM LOVER

You've been out to every restaurant in town, they've been to your place, you've been to theirs and now it's crunch time. Which is why you're in the bathroom, ostensibly cleaning your teeth (for the last 20 minutes) while your about-to-be-lover waits in the bedroom, wondering if you have any gums left. *Don't be ridiculous*, you lecture yourself in the mirror, *you've had sex hundreds, probably thousands of times before*. *Yeah*, says another little voice, *but with the same person for the last 10 years.*

First-time sex with a new lover, after years with an old one, *is* heart-thumping stuff. Part of you can't wait to give it a whirl (no prizes for guessing *which* part) but the thinking bits would stay happily celibate for another 100 years to avoid any embarrassment. But come out of that bathroom you must (the window's usually far too little to escape from). Just keep the following points in mind.

- **Don't panic if you feel as nervous as a virgin.** In a sense, it is like losing your virginity all over again. Don't fall into the same trap you did back then and expect that it's going to be wonderful. You've fantasised about it, so have they, and reality hasn't got a hope in hell of matching expectations.
- **Admit you are nervous.** If the thought of them gazing at your flesh makes you faint, leave your underwear on and slip under the sheets. Say, 'I haven't had sex with anyone but Martha/Martin for years. I feel like a teenager.' It'll ease the tension for both of you. You're not the only one who's under pressure. Your new lover feels they have to at least measure up to the standard set by your ex – and that's pretty difficult when your old lover's a few hundred practice runs ahead of them.
- **Stick to the basics.** If you're really nervous, this is one situation where I advocate just getting through. Kiss, have some foreplay, do the deed. Get it over with, let most of your anxieties evaporate, *then* you can concentrate on getting to know each other properly (and don't be surprised if, after all that fuss, you're actually keen for a repeat within the next half an hour).
- **If it's awful, admit it and laugh.** Say, 'That was *such* a disaster because we were so nervous. But now it's out of the way we can relax and really get to know each other sexually.' It's not a big deal if she didn't lubricate or orgasm or if he couldn't get an erection, lost it or came too quickly. It

doesn't mean you're not compatible in bed. It doesn't mean you should have stuck it out with your ex. It just means you don't know each other's bodies, desires or needs yet.

- **Accept that you may feel sad afterward.** For many people, especially women, sleeping with someone new marks the true ending of the previous relationship. It'll hit you like a lightning bolt: My God, it really is over. Even if you broke out the champagne when your ex left, don't be surprised if you have a post-coital grief attack. Cry, *sob* if you must, but don't shut your new lover out. If you're open and explain your emotions, they'll understand. Remember an ending is often the glorious beginning of something even better.

6

Contraception and STIs

Avoiding pregnancy and the lumps, bumps and things that itch in the night

Sex can give us the most pleasurable moments of our life – and the most painful. Falling pregnant to the waiter in Greece who did more than lay your table or discovering a T-shirt wasn't the only thing your ex left behind are both very real consequences of not treating sex with the respect it demands. Don't kid yourself: having sex can be dangerous. Terminating an unwanted pregnancy is not fun. Getting very, very sick from a sexually transmitted infection (STI) is not fun. Dying from AIDS isn't ever top of our 'Things I want to do this year' list. And if you're not careful, all can happen to *you*, no matter how 'nice' you are.

Have I put you off sex for life? If you're not prepared to take the associated risks seriously, I truly hope I have. But the fact is, most of the 'nasties' of sex can be avoided. With all the contraceptive choices available today, you'd have to be a complete fusspot not to find a method that suits both you and your partner. That removes the pregnancy risk immediately. Condoms (used properly and every single time) significantly reduce the risk of sexually transmitted infection. Add a good dollop of common sense and sex education and your chances of catching one drop to almost zero. At the risk of sounding like your mother, reading this chapter will not only save you heartache, it could save your life.

HOW NOT TO GET PREGNANT

The ideal contraceptive is 100 per cent effective, easy to use and economical with no known side effects. Unfortunately it hasn't been invented yet. But here's the good news: not only are traditional methods of contraception being constantly improved, there's some new kids on the contraceptive block that you may never have heard of. So while there's no such thing as a *perfect* contraceptive, for most women there's one that comes pretty damn close! I spoke to the experts at Family Planning to compile this list of the latest and greatest to help you find a hassle-free method for your personality, lifestyle and relationship. Since most women take responsibility for contraception, I've devoted this section to them. I've listed the prices for contraception as a comparative guide only. They were correct at the time of publication but may increase over time.

The symptothermal method

It sounds complicated and it is, but if you're the 'herbal' type – drink green tea, own CDs of whales singing and recycle *everything* (including what the cat threw up on the carpet) – this could be the method for you. It's totally natural and completely cost free but, alas, only for the truly dedicated: fiddly, messy and time-consuming are adjectives that immediately spring to mind.

How it works

The symptothermal technique aims to pinpoint ovulation (the most likely time to get pregnant) by reading the body's signals. You use a combination of the calendar, mucus and temperature methods to work out what days to avoid intercourse. By combining the three natural methods, you up the effectiveness rate considerably.

The calendar method: Ovulatory cycles are usually around 28 days. It is assumed that ovulation takes place mid-cycle, that the released egg will die after 24 hours and that sperm live for no longer than 3 to 5 days. Note I said *assume*. One of the problems with this method is that everyone's body behaves differently. To be totally accurate, you should write down when you start and finish your periods for at least 6 months (8 to 12 if possible) to work out your own personal menstrual cycle. It's then a matter of counting up the number of days between each period and doing some rather complicated sums. If you're truly keen, invest in a book detailing the Billings method (the name of the people who formulated it). It's far too complex to summarise here – and not terribly reliable even if you do master it.

The temperature method: There's a minute increase in our body temperature following ovulation (in the range of 0.2 to 0.6 degrees Celsius). The theory is that by taking your temperature daily with a thermometer (either in your mouth or vagina), you'll know when ovulation has occurred and shouldn't have sex for three days after your temperature has risen.

The mucus method: Around ovulation time, vaginal mucus (the clear or whitish discharge that comes out between periods) is clearer and thinner; after ovulation has occurred it becomes sticky and tacky and stretches like chewing gum. Recording changes in your mucus, again over a period of months, helps pinpoint when in your cycle you tend to ovulate. Some months, the mucus may change from clear to tacky on day 14 (day 1 is the first day of your period), others on day 18. If a pattern forms, you can get a rough idea of when ovulation usually occurs (and avoid sex around those days in the future). It's best to test mucus at night, just before you go to bed.

What's good about it

By combining three natural methods, you up the effectiveness rate considerably. It's natural and involves no chemicals or equipment.

The bad news

It requires a lot of effort and it's horrifyingly easy to miscalculate. The method relies rather optimistically on ovaries and sperm behaving in a predictable manner; infections, viruses and other health problems can cause false readings for both temperature and mucus.

Best suited to

Long-term couples trying to space a family.

Protection against HIV and STIs
None.

The failure rate
The theoretical failure rate is 2 to 5 per cent but the actual failure rate is more like 15 to 20 per cent.

Do I need to see a doctor?
No, but you might like to buy a few books on the subject so you know exactly what you're doing.

How easy is it to use?
It's complicated.

Is it expensive?
The price of a thermometer.

How enthusiastic will he be about it?
If you're long-term and it doesn't matter if you have 'an accident', very. Sex is totally natural and he doesn't have to do a thing.

The withdrawal method

How it works
You probably used this method when you were a teenager. He removes his penis from your vagina before ejaculation (coming), so there's no sperm inside you and little chance of you getting pregnant. Pre-ejaculatory fluid (the stuff that comes out before he orgasms) does contain some sperm but it's unlikely to cause pregnancy. This method requires strong self-control on his part and many couples find it emotionally and physically unsatisfying, for obvious reasons.

What's good about it
If he's practised, it can be quite a successful method of contraception. It's natural, has no side effects and costs nothing.

The bad news
You need to trust your partner implicitly to withdraw at the right time.

Best suited to...
Couples in long-term relationships who could cope with an unexpected pregnancy.

Protection against HIV and STIs
None.

The failure rate
It depends on whether he withdraws every single time. Family Planning put the failure figure at once every four years with experienced couples.

Do I need to see a doctor?
No.

How easy is it to use?
There's no effort required on your part.

Is it expensive?
It's free.

How enthusiastic will he be?
He may feel 'robbed' of the grand *finale* of orgasming inside you. Good self-discipline on his part is a must.

The condom

Condoms, as well as diaphragms and cervical caps, prevent pregnancy by providing a physical barrier between the sperm and egg. Each is an ideal alternative if you don't want to, or can't, take the Pill and are prepared to do a little pre-planning.

For maximum effectiveness when using a condom, use a spermicide as well – possibly one containing the purported AIDS-fighter, Nonoxynol-9. (In the laboratory, Nonoxynol-9 had some effect against the HIV virus but no-one knows if it's equally effective in the human body. Still, there's no harm in hedging your bets on the right side!) You can buy spermicides from any chemist.

How it works

The condom was virtually ignored when the Pill appeared on the scene; now it's back in vogue because of AIDS. A very thin but strong latex (rubber) sheath, it's designed to fit over his erect penis and catch the sperm in a pocket at the tip. The main complaint? Intercourse doesn't feel as pleasurable. For this reason, scientists are currently researching a plastic condom which conducts heat more efficiently and feels much more like the 'real thing'. A condom with a looser end (which apparently feels better for him) is also in the trial stages.

Number of condoms sold by a popular condom shop in Kings Cross, Sydney per month: approximately 4650. Number of different varieties of condoms stocked: 60. Number of singles worldwide who carry condoms: 77 per cent.

'It was the first guy I'd ever slept with purely for sex. We used a condom but he obviously didn't put it on properly because it kept sliding off. We put on a new one but when he withdrew, found it had a huge tear in it. I was scared stupid. It wouldn't have been so bad with a boyfriend but a guy I didn't know and sure as hell didn't want a baby with? I got the Morning After Pill and a check-up for STIs that week, then waited three months for an AIDS test. Now I provide the condom, I put it on and make sure we use lubricant.'

Jenny, 26, secretary

What's good about it

It's a great germ stopper. Not only does it stop sperm, it helps prevent you catching viruses like HIV (which can lead to AIDS) as well as blocking bacteria which carry other nasties like gonorrhoea.

The bad news

Condoms only protect you against pregnancy and diseases if they're used properly, each and every time you have sex, and if they don't break. Breakages and tears are usually your fault not 'the bloody manufacturer'. If you haven't put the condom on properly and squeezed the air out of the end bit, an air pocket can form which heats up (as you two do) and expands during intercourse causing the condom to burst. Use plenty of water-based lubricants like K-Y to prevent splitting but avoid oil-based lubricants like baby oil and Vaseline, which can weaken the rubber.

Best suited to

Couples prepared to wear a condom every single time they have intercourse and put up with a decrease of sensation; anyone who's single and planning on having more than one sexual partner.

Protection against HIV and STIs

Not so long ago, newspapers shouted the dire news that HIV molecules could penetrate condoms. Thankfully, it's not true. At this stage anyway, it's a myth that condoms don't protect you against HIV if you use them each and every time you have sex and they don't break. As HIV can be present in pre-ejaculatory fluid, you must put the condom on before any kind of penetration and before it even touches your genitals. Check that the condom conforms to British Standards (look for the words Certified to British Standards and the ♡ logo on the packet), especially if you got it from a vending machine.

> **'Condoms. I hate them. I can't stand them. I use them for safety but can't wait to get to the point where we're serious, can get tested and dispense with the bloody things.'**
>
> Phillip, 27, promotions manager

The failure rate

Somewhere between 2 per cent and 60 per cent because it all depends on how often they're used and how; 30 per cent is probably a realistic figure.

Do I need to see a doctor?

No.

How easy is it to use?

Some couples complain that condoms interrupt the 'flow' because they have to stop sex to put them on. But it can become part of foreplay if *you* put it on for him (go on, at least try to do it with your mouth); besides, a seasoned condom user needs only a few seconds to prepare.

Is it expensive?

Condoms are free from Family Planning or Genital Urinary Medicine Clinics. Opt for the chemist and you'll be up for around £8.50 for a pack of 12.

How enthusiastic will he be?

Probably not very. You've heard the jokes (it feels like having sex with a raincoat on).

HOW TO USE A CONDOM

1. Be careful when you're unwrapping it. Don't rip the packet open with abandon (and don't even think about doing it with your teeth). Rings and fingernails can snag and while condoms are tough, they're not *that* tough.
2. Wait until he's erect. Put the condom on *before* the penis touches the vagina but only when he's hard.
3. Leave the condom unrolled and squeeze the tip to get rid of any air. Hold it against the tip of the penis, then . . .
4. Gently unroll the condom, all the way down to the base of the penis. Smooth out any air bubbles once it's on.
5. Have fun – guilt-free!
6. Withdraw the penis *immediately* after ejaculation while it's still erect. One of you should hold the condom firm at the base of the penis while he withdraws, to stop it slipping off or any sperm leaking out.
7. Point the penis downward and slip the condom off carefully.
8. Remember you can only use a condom once. If you want to have sex again, get him to wash his penis and use a new one.

➢

9. Tie a knot in the used condom, wrap it in paper and put it in a bin. Don't flush it down the loo – it's not biodegradeable. Do you enjoy dragging used condoms along with your toes while walking on your local beach?
10. Score full marks for putting it on with your mouth. If you can cope with the taste, unwrap it and place it (unrolled) on the top of your tongue, the open end facing upward. The first time, cheat and use your fingers to position it over the penis head, then use your tongue and mouth to unroll it.

The diaphragm

How it works

The diaphragm is a shallow dome of thin rubber with a firm, flexible rim. It looks like a tiny alien spaceship and can seem just as mysterious, according to frustrated users. You put it inside your vagina so it covers the cervix and tucks in behind the pelvic bone, held in position by the pelvic muscles. There are three types available: flat-spring, coil-spring and arcing-spring with fit and ease of insertion the main differences. The diaphragm isn't a popular method of contraception – in our 'instant' era, no-one wants to prepare for sex. You need to be fitted for one by Family Planning, your doctor or gynaecologist and change sizes after a baby, pelvic surgery, a miscarriage or significant weight loss (7 lbs or more). You'll be shown how to insert it then left for a little while to 'practise' – and practise you will, because for some women insertion is difficult. Lots feel squeamish, others can't quite get the hang of it but once you do, it's a 10-second job. It's a good idea to buy two diaphragms and leave one in continuously.

***!** A recent survey found that 66 per cent of women let trust interfere with their decision on whether to use a condom. In other words, factors like 'But I love him' and 'He's a nice guy' stopped them pulling on protection. Romantic but hideously dangerous.*

'My girlfriend had a diaphragm fitted and we had no end of problems. I could feel it inside and while it didn't hurt, it was irritating. She got constant urinary infections and used to disappear for ages inserting it. It was a major disaster.'

David, 25, psychologist

so you're always prepared. (The best place to carry a diaphragm is in your vagina, not your handbag!) Swap over every day or, if you only have one, take it out (but not before six hours after intercourse!) and wash and dry it before reinsertion. If it starts to get smelly, wash in one part vinegar, four parts water.

How to use it

The diaphragm needs to be left in for six hours after intercourse to ensure all the sperm are dead. Some experts recommend using spermicide to kill any renegade sperm. (Avoid the rim if you choose to, otherwise it can cause the diaphragm to slide around). There's no need to reapply spermicide each time you have sex, just when you first insert it. Replace your diaphragm with a new one every 30 weeks, if you intend wearing it regularly.

What's good about it

The diaphragm is fairly free of side effects, it's cheap and relatively reliable in capable hands. When fitted properly and inserted correctly it usually can't be felt by either partner and if you leave it in permanently, there's no pre-planning required.

! The first condom was so thick, it was washable. In the 1930s, there was a unisex condom that could be rolled up and used as a diaphragm.

The bad news

Lots of women find insertion difficult; others find the whole thing messy. Some women with persistent urinary tract infections claim it makes them worse; others believe diaphragms are plain uncomfortable, though this is usually the result of being fitted with the wrong size or inserting it incorrectly. A very small amount of women are allergic to rubber and/or the spermicide.

Best suited to

Women with strong pelvic floor muscles to hold the diaphragm in place who are comfortable with their bodies.

Protection against HIV and STIs

No protection against HIV but it does help protect you against chlamydia and gonorrhoea.

The failure rate

Theoretically, the failure rate is 4 per cent but in practice it's much higher because, like the condom, people don't use it properly every single time they have sex.

HOW TO INSERT A DIAPHRAGM

1. First, rescue it from him – he'll think it's a scream and whiz it around the room like a frisbee. You'll be less enthusiastic when it twangs out of *your* hands while you're struggling to insert it and it flies across the bathroom (again). But persevere you must. Master the insertion part and the rest is simple.
2. Stand with one foot on a chair, sit on the toilet, squat or lie down with your knees bent for insertion. Experiment with each position until you find the one easiest for you.
3. Feel with your fingers where the diaphragm is to sit – locate your cervix and pubic bone, as shown by the doctor who fitted you.
4. Squeeze the edges of the diaphragm into a long, narrow shape between your thumb and first finger.
5. Hold the vaginal lips apart with one hand and use the other to insert the diaphragm into the vagina. Press down along the back wall of the vagina (the side nearest your bottom) until the far rim passes the cervix. Then, tuck the front rim up behind the pubic bone.
6. Check it's in place properly by feeling your cervix through the rubber. It should be completely covered.

Do I need to see a doctor?
Yes. You need to be professionally 'sized' initially.

How easy is it to use
It's complicated at first, but once you're in a routine, changing diaphragms becomes part of your daily toiletry routine.

Is it expensive?
Diaphragms are free on the NHS; the spermicide will set you back a tiny £3.50. Diaphragms usually last about two years unless you're wearing the same one continuously which will cause it to deteriorate more quickly.

How enthusiastic will he be?
Some men claim they can feel the diaphragm with the head of their penis; most don't notice.

The cervical cap

How it works
The cap works like a diaphragm but it's smaller. A firm cup-shaped or dome-shaped device, it sits snugly over the cervix and is held in place by suction. Some women find it more difficult to insert than the diaphragm – you need to have a reasonably long cervix and to be able to reach it easily. Caps are generally only available through Family Planning and selected doctors. There are three types available in the UK.

What's good about it
Because it's smaller than a diaphragm, some women find it more comfortable. If the diaphragm triggers urinary infections for you, the cap could be a better alternative.

The bad news
Its design is also a disadvantage because it can be knocked off during intercourse.

Best suited to
Women with weak pelvic floor muscles who can't, but would like to, use the diaphragm.

Protection against HIV and STIs
Same as the diaphragm – no protection against HIV or vaginal infections but it protects you against chlamydia, gonorrhoea and cervical infections.

The failure rate
A US study put the figure at around 8 per cent.

Do I need to see a doctor?
Yes, for the initial fitting.

How easy is it to use?
Some women find it harder to insert and remove than the diaphragm.

Is it expensive?
Hardly – it's free on the NHS.

How enthusiastic will he be?
Very. He's unlikely to feel it.

> 'The Pill made me sick and bad-tempered. The diaphragm gave me cystitis. Condoms made me sore. I'd heard horror stories about the IUD but when my gyno suggested I try it, I did. It's brilliant. I've had no problems with contraception since.'
>
> Sally, 36, health worker

The intrauterine device (IUD)

How it works
The IUD has suffered some pretty bad press over the years – quite unfairly so, according to Family Planning. They say it's a fantastic method for the right person: once it's in, you can leave it there for years and it's extremely effective. There are two copper IUDs, both about 2 cm long, available. It's actually the copper that's the contraceptive not the IUD device (though a foreign body in the uterus also stops fertilisation): copper changes the environment in the uterus, preventing the transport of both sperm and ovum thus blocking fertilisation as well as implantation. Most gynaecologists and some GPs will insert an IUD in their consulting rooms. First, they'll do a pelvic examination and take swabs to check you're infection-free, then insert it on a subsequent

visit. Once it's inside, neither you nor your partner is aware of it. You can check it's still in place, however, by feeling for the nylon strings which are left on the device for checking purposes. Depending on which IUD you choose, it can stay there for five to eight years before being removed by your doctor.

What's good about it

It's cheap, long-term, totally maintenance free once inserted and highly effective because you don't need to remember to do or take anything before having intercourse.

The bad news

You may get heavier, more painful periods and could also get a slight infection on insertion (usually quickly cured by antibiotics). The IUD isn't recommended for young women who change partners frequently because you may be more susceptible to tubal infections if you're exposed to chlamydia or the like (this has never been proven but it's a risk all the same). Why the bad image? IUDs were commonly used by young women at the height of the sexual revolution and were blamed for all the STIs women picked up. In reality, we simply slept around more and didn't use condoms. Sometimes, IUDs come out, usually with the first few periods, so it's imperative that you check the strings each month after your period.

Best suited to

Women who don't have heavy or painful periods, do not have any vaginal or pelvic infections, have only one partner and have previously had children.

Effect on future fertility

A rare complication is the possibility of ectopic pregnancy (pregnancy in the tubes not the uterus) which can risk future fertility. If you fall pregnant with an IUD inserted there's a chance that you'll spontaneously miscarry. If you don't, the IUD can be removed during the early stages of pregnancy but there is a risk of inducing miscarriage. If the IUD is left in and the pregnancy progresses there's an increased chance of premature labour or early rupture of the membranes.

Protection against HIV and STIs
None.

The failure rate
1 per cent.

Do I need to see a doctor?
Yes, for insertion.

How easy is it to use?
After insertion, you simply need to check it's in place after each period.

Is it expensive?
It is free on the NHS. You'll need to replace them five to eight years after insertion.

How enthusiastic will he be?
The IUD is inserted deep inside so he won't feel a thing.

The combined oral contraceptive (the Pill)

How it works
The Pill has been around for more than 20 years and is the contraception chosen by most young women. The Pill gives a daily dose of synthetic hormones, oestrogen and progestogen, which act like the natural hormones in the body. When there's a certain level of these hormones acting on the brain, the ovary does not get stimulated to produce an egg – and if there's no egg, there's no pregnancy. There are lots of different Pills on the market, each containing various combinations of progestogen and oestrogen. They come in 21-day or 28-day packs; the latter includes sugar pills which you take during your period so you don't get out of the habit of taking a pill every day. Usually, you'll be started on a low dose Pill or a triphasic Pill (one which varies the amount of hormone taken throughout the month) but if breakthrough bleeding occurs and doesn't settle down within three months, a different dose is prescribed. It's quite normal to try a few Pill brands before settling on one that suits you.

The Pill is almost 100 per cent effective if you take it at around the same time every day and don't have any health problems which may affect its absorption. If you miss a tablet or are late by more than 12 hours, take it as soon as you remember, take the next Pill at the usual time and you'll still be protected. If you miss more than one tablet, use other contraception for seven days while continuing to take the Pill. Because it's designed to be swallowed and absorbed at a certain rate, vomiting and diarrhoea, some medication (including some antibiotics) and extraordinarily high doses of Vitamin C can interfere with its effectiveness.

The good news

It's easy to use and highly effective, and there's another great spin-off for women who hate having their periods – there's really no need to have one. Manufacturers believed women wanted periods (and some do like the reassurance that they're not pregnant) so they included the sugar pills to allow a break from the hormones, which brings on a 'period'. But lots take the Pill continuously (just skip the sugar ones and continue to the next packet), or break for a period every three to six months or so. If you do choose to still have periods, chances are they'll be lighter, less painful and nearly always on time. The Pill may also help cure acne and reduce PMS and there's scientific evidence that it may have other benefits: there's less chance of getting serious pelvic infection, cancer of the ovary, cancer of the endometrium (the lining of the womb), anaemia, non-cancerous breast lumps and cysts on the ovary.

The bad news

Some women shouldn't even consider taking the Pill. If you're over 35 and smoke, steer clear – the Pill makes smoking even more dangerous. The hormones in the Pill slightly increase the blood's natural tendency to form clots; combine this with an unhealthy diet, excessive drinking and smoking and you're asking for trouble. Before it's prescribed, your doctor will go through a long list of health problems and your family health history to check you're a suitable candidate. Women who have had liver problems or breast cancer, for instance, will probably be advised to use another method. Minor side effects may include chloeasma (a slight pigmentation of the skin which makes it look brown and blotchy) and some minor fluid retention (though it's a fallacy that the Pill makes you fat). Some women complain of mood changes and depression but changing to a lower dose or a different brand often solves the problem. Years ago, women were advised to take breaks from the Pill because they were high-dose formulas; today's newer, low-dose Pills are fine to take continuously.

Best suited to

Women who don't smoke and have no serious health problems or a family history of health problems.

Effect on future fertility

Contrary to common perceptions, the Pill doesn't 'build up' in your body and there's no need to wait a few cycles to get it out of your system before trying to get pregnant. Usually, you'll revert to a normal cycle within a month or two, with most women falling pregnant within 6 months after they've stopped taking it – about the same fertility rate as women who've never taken the Pill.

! Feeling sexy? It could be your Pill, not him! Women who take triphasic Pills, with varying levels of hormones, appear to be more interested in and enjoy sex more than women on fixed-dose Pills.

Protection against HIV and STIs

None.

The failure rate

When used properly the Pill has a tiny failure rate – only 5 pregnancies per 1000 women per year. Forgetting to take it every day is the most common cause of failure.

Do I need to see a doctor?

Yes, for the initial prescription and for subsequent health checks when you renew it.

How easy is it to use?
Simply swallow a tablet daily. If you're the forgetful type, work it into a routine (maybe keep the packet on your bedside table so it's the first thing you see when you open your eyes in the morning).

Is it expensive?
It is free on the NHS.

How enthusiastic will he be?
Over the moon. There's practically no chance of pregnancy if you take it every day.

The progestogen only pill (the Mini Pill)

How it works
The Mini Pill contains about one-third to one-fifth of the dose of progestogen that's in the combined oral contraceptive and it doesn't contain any oestrogen. It's slightly less reliable than the regular Pill but useful if you can't take oestrogen because it makes you feel sick or for medical reasons. The Pill works by delivering a daily dose of synthetic hormones which act on the brain and stop the ovary being stimulated to produce an egg. The Mini Pill works differently: its dosage of progestogen increases the mucus plug at the cervix, making it thick, tacky and difficult for sperm to penetrate. It also changes the lining of the uterus (the endometrium), making it less 'friendly' to fertilisation and it can have an effect on ovulation. It's taken every day without a break so it comes in a 28-day pack and it's essential that it's taken at around the same time every day. (Its contraceptive effect is greatest three to 21 hours after each tablet is taken so if you have sex at night and/or in the early morning, ideally you should take your tablet between midday and the early evening.)

What's good about it
Unlike the combined Pill, the Mini Pill can be taken by women who have a history of blood clotting, stroke, heart attack or smoke heavily.

The bad news

It's imperative that you take it at the same time every day and do not miss any pills. As for the combined Pill, if you're vomiting, or have diarrhoea, take extra precautions. A few medications may also affect its effectiveness. Unfortunately, the Mini Pill doesn't have the advantage of cycle control so you can't skip periods or manipulate your cycle to have a period at a certain time. You may experience spotting (bleeding in between periods) or mood changes like PMS. Depression is rare.

Best suited to

Organised women who can't take the combined oral contraceptive Pill, who are breast-feeding or can't take oestrogen.

Protection against HIV and STIs

None.

The failure rate

The failure rate is around 2 to 3 per cent.

Do I need to see a doctor?

Yes, for the same reasons as the Pill.

How easy is it to use?

You take one tablet daily but it must be at the same time.

Is it expensive?

It is free on the NHS.

How enthusiastic will he be?

Extremely if you're sensible and can be relied upon to remember to take it, nervous if you're not.

Depo Provera, injectable hormonal contraceptive

How it works

Depo Provera works just like the Pill by stopping the release of an egg from your ovaries. The difference is that it's injected once every twelve weeks rather than being taken orally every day –

which means a much lower failure rate because you can't forget to take it! The first injection of a progestogen preparation is given into the muscle of your upper arm, bottom or upper thigh during the first seven days of your period. You need a top up once every 12 weeks. Despite its obvious benefits, Depo Provera isn't a common method of contraception probably because it can cause havoc with your periods and can delay fertility for between 7 to 18 months.

What's good about it

It's effective immediately, has an extremely low failure rate and you can forget about contraception for three months at a time. Depo Provera is also used to treat endometrial cancers.

The bad news

You can't predict the effect it has on a period. Most women after two or three injections have no period at all, but you could experience erratic, unpredictable bleeding. You might get no period for two months, then bleed for eight to ten days. Depo Provera has also been associated with weight gain, headaches and depression.

Best suited to

Like the Pill, there are women who shouldn't use Depo Provera: those with a history of depression and cancer of the breast, for instance, but your doctor will discuss this with you. Otherwise, if you're constantly forgetting to take the Pill, this is a great alternative.

Effect on future fertility

This isn't the method to choose if you're planning on getting pregnant sometime soon. Depo Provera takes a long time to wear off; most women will take 7 to 18 months from the last injection to ovulate and become fertile with the average time being about 10 months.

Protection against HIV and STIs

None.

The failure rate

Theoretically, it's the same as the combined oral contraceptive Pill; in practice it's more effective because you can't forget to take it.

Do I need to see a doctor?

Yes. You'll need to visit your doctor or a Family Planning clinic once every 12 weeks.

How easy is it to use?

It's just a case of writing your appointments in your diary and sticking to them.

Is it expensive?

It is free on the NHS.

How enthusiastic will he be?

Highly.

Norplant

Norplant involves inserting a series of six small, narrow rods into the upper arm under local anaesthetic through a small incision in the skin. You can't see the rods, which are about 3 cm long, though you can feel them if you touch them. They release progestogen and work in much the same way as Depo Provera but you only need to replace them with a new set once every five years! Unfortunately, like Depo Provera, there's a side effect of erratic bleeding but researchers are working on controlling it.

The Morning After Pill

How it works

Despite its name, you can take the Morning After Pill (MAP) up to 72 hours after unprotected sex. Most regular users, according to a Family Planning study of 400 women, are in their 20s and used condoms that broke or a rather ineffective withdrawal method (that is, their boyfriends forgot to). This method of contraception involves taking two doses of high dose combined oestrogen and progestogen twelve hours apart. It prevents pregnancy in one of two ways: if the pills are taken before you ovulate they can delay ovulation (which means you need to be particularly careful for the rest of the month because you may ovulate later than usual). If they're taken after you've ovulated and an egg has been fertilised, the MAP prevents the fertilised egg from implanting in the womb.

What's good about it

While it shouldn't be relied upon as permanent contraception, it's ideal as a back-up when condoms break or if you suspect your regular contraception has failed or if no contraception has been used. Some women, who have sex *very* infrequently, use the MAP instead of using regular contraception.

The bad news

The major side effect isn't pleasant – about 50 per cent of women feel sick and are. For this reason, you'll often be given anti-nausea pills to take as well. If you're sick within two hours of taking a dose, you may not have absorbed the hormones and need to start all over again. You may get other mild symptoms – breast tenderness, headache or light bleeding – but these usually disappear within 48 hours and require no treatment.

Best suited to

Women who need an emergency back-up.

Effect on future fertility

If you're already pregnant (if you conceived in a previous cycle or earlier in your present cycle), the MAP will not stop that pregnancy continuing or harm the fetus.

Protection against HIV and STIs

None.

The failure rate

Up to 5 per cent.

Do I need to see a doctor?

Yes, contact your GP, Family Planning Clinic or the Casualty Department of some hospitals.

How easy is it to use?

It usually requires a hastily scheduled doctor's appointment and 24 hours time out if you feel ill.

Is it expensive?

It is free on the NHS.

> ❗ *Number of women who've failed to use contraception at least once: 87.1 per cent.*

How enthusiastic will he be?

Relieved that there's no unwanted pregnancy and hopefully sympathetic if the pills make you sick.

Permanent contraception

Forgive me for stating the obvious, but permanent contraception usually means *permanent.* Though some operations can be successfully reversed to make you fertile again, don't count on it. Proceed with caution. Are you absolutely, totally sure you're *that* serious?

Tubal ligation (or sterilisation)

Commonly known as 'getting your tubes tied', the fallopian tubes are cut, clipped or tied to stop sperm going up the tubes and eggs going down. The egg is still released but it's harmlessly absorbed by the body. Usually done under general anaesthetic through a laparoscope, it only requires one day in hospital, though it will be a week before you'll feel 'normal'. *Permanent* is the key word here; reversal is tricky and it's successful only 30 to 60 per cent of the time, depending on the particular case.

Vasectomy

> ❗ *Vasectomy is so straightforward, surgeons admit to performing the operation on themselves.*

This is a simple 20-minute operation which stops sperm travelling out of the testes and into the semen; sperm is still produced, but it's reabsorbed. Done under local or general anaesthetic, the surgeon cuts the front of the scrotum, picks up the vas deferens (the tube that carries the sperm) on each side in turn and cuts and seals the ends. Though pretty hazard free, it's not effective immediately: it may take as many as 16 ejaculations to clear sperm that's still in the tubes. You must continue using contraception until he gets a negative sperm count. Having a vasectomy isn't a decision that should be made flippantly. Even if the reversal procedure goes smoothly, there's no guarantee he'll go on to father a child.

Coming attractions

There are many contraceptives used widely overseas but which are not available because no-one has bothered to market them yet. Others are still in the trial stages but could well be ***your*** contraception of choice in years to come. Watch out for . . .

RU486 – Mifepristone

Some say RU486 is a better emergency contraception than the Morning After Pill because it has fewer side effects: it doesn't make you sick like the MAP. It's available in the UK but research continues to find the lowest possible effective dose.

The female condom (Femidom)

It appeared amidst a fanfare of publicity and fans swear by it. A long, thin polyurethane tube with a firm ring at the end, it's designed to fit in the vagina with any excess latex folding back over the opening. Some women claim it feels 'like having sex in a plastic bag' but it has pluses: because the condom covers the labia as well as the vagina, it helps protect against herpes.

The vaginal ring

Dubbed 'the contraception of the future', vaginal rings are as effective as the combined oral contraceptive Pill without the failure risk. This is what most of us will dump our current method for. As yet, the rings aren't available in the UK but may be in the future. A ring, smaller than the average diaphragm, is inserted into the vagina where it releases the same hormones that are in the combined oral contraceptive Pill. Once inserted, the ring stays there for three weeks – you remove it for a week only if you want to have a period or you can leave it in permanently and enjoy a period-free life for up to a year at a time. The obvious benefit? You don't have to remember to take a pill every day. Family Planning are also trialling a gel containing progestogen, which is rubbed onto the skin of the abdomen each day where it's absorbed like the Mini Pill.

Male contraception

Despite the odd excited announcement that a male contraceptive pill is in the planning stages, effective male contraception (apart from the condom) is light years away. It's not a conspiracy to keep contraception our problem; it's simply much easier to control our fertility than a man's – one egg per month as opposed to 50,000 sperm per minute which have taken three months to mature. A method involving a weekly injection of testosterone is very much in the experimental stages. If successful, it'll take the form of three-monthly injections or an implant similiar to Norplant. Researchers are currently experimenting with implants using Depo Provera. If successful, they may be available within three years. The problem is lots of contraception methods work on the pituitary gland, and if you stop it functioning in men the result is often impotence – effective contraception all right, but not quite what he (or you) had in mind!

SEX ON HOLIDAY

The sun's shining, the waves are lapping and the hardest decision you've had to make all week is which way to point your deckchair. That wonderfully relaxed holiday mood can make it seem like the yukkies of life don't exist. Unfortunately AIDS, STIs and unwanted pregnancies don't disappear just because you're feeling blissfully brain-dead. Holidays are danger time for many people. Make sure *you* don't come home with more souvenirs than you'd bargained on.

- Pack condoms, lubricant and enough supplies of your chosen contraceptive to last the trip, plus 'spares'. (It's tough enough asking directions when you can't speak the language; try explaining what a flat-spring diaphragm is and why you need one *now!*)
- Don't rely on the calendar, mucus or withdrawal methods. Symptothermal methods are notoriously unreliable at the best of times, worse on holidays. Time differences and long

flights play havoc with your menstrual cycle and it's difficult to keep track of fertile days. Heat, lounging around in spas, a case of thrush brought on by pre-holiday panic, all can affect vaginal secretions. Use condoms and lubricant instead; they'll protect you against pregnancy, HIV and STIs. Don't use the withdrawal method with holiday romancers. It's easy enough for a boyfriend to get carried away – can you trust a stranger to keep his word?

- It's Tuesday there and Thursday in the UK, so when should you take the Pill? Keep your watch on 'home' time during the flight and take the tablets as usual. When you get to your destination, take a tablet in the morning or evening (whichever is usual for you), even if it means taking it early. Then take one tablet per day until the flight home. Keep your watch on 'holiday' time on the flight back and continue taking the tablets. When you get home, repeat the process: take a tablet that morning or evening, then settle back into your old routine. Remember that the Pill's effectiveness is hampered by holiday bugs which cause vomiting and diarrhoea. If you vomit within an hour of taking it, it's not been absorbed. Use condoms or a diaphragm as back-up.
- If you use a diaphragm, pack two and keep them in separate bags (in case you lose a suitcase). Flying, swimming in salt water, even scuba diving won't affect your diaphragm. Just remember it must stay in for six hours, so don't get confused with changing time zones. If you get a particularly bad bout of gastric (or anything else that causes you to drop 5 kg or more), your diaphragm may be the wrong size and ineffective. That new, flat tummy won't stay flat for long if you're pregnant!
- Practice safe sex in all senses. What might pass as flirting back home may be interpreted as a blatant invitation for sex somewhere else. Quiz your travel agent on the customs and morals of the country you're visiting. And don't assume any guy you invite in for coffee will behave like a gentleman – no matter what country you're in.

THE (DREADED) STIs

It's no wonder soapie scriptwriters never write Sexually Transmitted Infections (STIs) into the plot. Since the entire cast of 'Melrose Place' have all slept with each other – without so much as a *rustle* of a condom being unwrapped – 'infecting' one character would have the whole lot on antibiotics. Hollywood isn't too fond of nasty little bugs and viruses either. We don't see the Bond girls doubled up in agony, peeing razor blades, two weeks after James has swept suavely through, or Kim Basinger braving a whopping great penicillin injection nine-and-a-half weeks after having unprotected sex in sewers and kitchens.

Which leads some people to believe life really *is* like a glamorous, exciting action film where people dive under the covers looking fabulous, and emerge, make-up intact, wonderously infection-free and ready for the next love scene. If only it were true. In real life, orgasms aren't the only things you can get through sex, so arm yourself with the facts as well as the condoms. Read this section *now* rather than frantically flicking through the pages searching for a symptom you have just discovered.

A sexually transmitted infection (STI) is any infection which can be passed from one person to another through sex. Unfortunately there are rather a lot of them. Some are fairly harmless and are cured by a course of antibiotics, others can kill you. They're usually passed on at the beginning of a new relationship so every time you have unprotected sex (sex without a condom) with a new partner, you should have a check-up for STIs.

Now here's some *really* bad news if you're feeling smug about that half-empty family-sized pack of condoms in the bedroom drawer. While condoms *will* protect you against STIs spread by the exchange of bodily fluids (like sperm, blood and mucus), you can still catch herpes and warts because they can be spread simply by touching infected skin. And pubic lice or scabies won't care if he's wearing *six* condoms; they'll still merrily jump on the nearest strand of hair they can find. In fact, the only guaranteed defence against *all* STIs is not to have sex at all.

Right, now you've spent a millisecond considering that option, what now? The next best thing is a monogamous relationship with an uninfected person (where neither of you sleep with anyone else), the third is to only have casual sex in ways that are considered 'safe' (like kissing, touching and mutual masturbation) and the fourth is to sleep with whoever you like but to use condoms (and common sense) every single time.

Like most diseases, STIs aren't fussy and you can't pick the people who have one. Avoid 'dirty', 'promiscuous' or 'bad boy' types all you like but if you think you're safe having sex only with 'sweet', 'nice', 'clean' or 'innocent' people, you're being unbelievably naive. Ditto those who think they're okay because they have asked their partner if they have any symptoms. Let's face it, they're hardly going to look up and say, 'Well, now you mention it, I had these Godawful blisters on my penis yesterday and now they've turned into pus-infested ulcers.' Besides, they may not have noticed anything unusual because some STIs are alarmingly symptom-free.

If *you* notice any change in the discharge from your penis or vagina, pain or irritation during intercourse or when you pee, any blisters, ulcers, warts, lumps or rashes anywhere on or around your genitals or bottom, or any itching or irritation there, put this book down and go see a doctor or a sexual health clinician NOW. If you find you are infected, it's not only polite but essential that you pick up the phone and tell anyone else you've slept with. No, they're not going to be thrilled by the news but they should be grateful. Left unchecked, many STIs can affect our ability to have children later in life. Others, like AIDS, are fatal.

Following, in no particular order, is a rundown of some of the most common STIs. I sincerely hope you never become intimately acquainted with any of them.

AIDS

What is it?

This gets top billing for obvious reasons – it's lethal. AIDS stands for acquired immune deficiency syndrome and HIV (human immunodeficiency virus) is the virus that causes the disease. It was first noticed in the early 1980s and it predominantly affected homosexual and bisexual men and people who injected drugs. They still make up the two biggest groups affected by AIDS. HIV is spread by sex (oral, anal and vaginal through semen and vaginal secretions), by needles (sharing a needle which is contaminated) and can be passed on during pregnancy and childbirth. It's not spread by saliva (except in one or two rare and extraordinary circumstances), touching, kissing, drinking out of the same cup as an HIV-infected person, toilet seats, shaking hands, mosquitoes, sneezing or swimming pools. HIV attacks the body's immune system which is our natural defence against disease. Eventually, it becomes so weak the body can't fight against any infections or diseases and you can die.

How do I know I've got it?

There's no immediate sign. A few weeks after exposure about *half* of its victims get a glandular fever type sickness (fevers, tiredness, swollen glands), which passes. At this stage you're 'healthy' but carrying the virus – known as 'HIV positive'. Months or years later, if you get really sick, you then 'have AIDS' or an 'AIDS-related illness'. Persistently swollen lymph glands is a typical symptom of the later stage and you may experience fevers, night sweats and a cough, lose weight, have chronic diarrhoea, develop skin lesions (sores or raised red marks) and be constantly tired and weak.

What now?

A blood test around three months after the initial infection can identify if you're carrying the HIV virus. If you tested negative it's wise to get re-tested three to six months later. Obviously, count the three months from when you last had sex without a condom or shared needles.

Can it be cured and will it come back?

At the moment, AIDS is incurable. Researchers the world over are working on a cure but, at the time of publication, none had proven to be effective though several are looking promising. Usually, the inevitable bugs and diseases you pick up are treated as they arise, until late in the disease when the body has so few defence cells, it can't respond to antibiotics.

Have I infected my partner?

Quite possibly. If your result is positive, the news will usually be delivered by a crisis counsellor who'll help you work through the pain, grief and anger you'll feel. They'll also advise you on how to tell your current partner (and any past partners) you may have infected. It goes without saying that not telling them is tantamount to sponsoring your own personal killing campaign, especially if the person that infected you doesn't know they're a carrier.

Your best defence against the virus?

Take it seriously, use condoms and lubricant (unless both of you have tested negative and you're 100 per cent certain there's no chance of unprotected infidelity), and don't share needles. Oral sex is considered low-risk.

Will it affect my chances of having children?

AIDS can be passed from mother to child, an important factor to consider if you're planning a pregnancy.

Gonorrhoea

What is it?

It sounds dreadful and it can be. Caused by bacteria passed on by an infected partner, it turns into an infection that sometimes spreads via the blood stream. Gonorrhoea isn't common among heterosexuals but it's still out there.

How do I know I've got it?

The incubation period (the time it takes to develop symptoms or show signs of exposure) is anywhere from 2 to 10 days and first symptoms are often so minor, you may not notice. Men may find peeing painful or notice a white or yellow discharge from their penis. Women may also find urination most unpleasant and/or that their vaginal discharge is heavier than usual. You can catch gonorrhoea in the anus or throat as well.

What now?

Your doctor will take a swab (a sample) from the pus discharge and test it. Gonorrhoea is usually sensitive to penicillin and you may be given a single, high dose by tablet or injection. Sometimes, it's resistant to penicillin and you'll need other antibiotics. You'll probably also be treated for chlamydia, since the two often go (miserably) hand in hand.

Can it be cured and will it come back?

That's usually the end of it, though repeat tests will be ordered to make sure it's totally gone.

Have I infected my partner?

Gonorrhoea is spread through vaginal, anal or oral sex. If you've done all or any of those and not used a condom, it is possible they've got it too (or gave it to you in the first place).

Will it affect my chances of having children?

Not if it's treated promptly.

Genital herpes

What is it?

Pre-AIDS, it was the Most Feared of all the STIs. Post-AIDS, coping with a little cold sore suddenly seems bearable. Herpes sounds bad, but it's not serious and just means you get cold sores on the genitals rather than on the mouth. It's an infection caused by the herpes simplex virus and it comes in two types, 1 and 2. It's the same virus that causes cold sores on your lips, so if your partner has one and gives you oral sex, he may leave more than just a nice memory.

How do I know I've got it?

Your first warning may be an odd, 'tingly' sensation on or around your genitals. Then – what a fabulous surprise! – one or several blisters form on or around the genitals around 2 to 20 days after exposure, rupturing to form ulcers. It's pretty hard to miss if you have a severe attack. In women, the sores or 'lesions' usually appear on the vulva or the entrance to the vagina, though you may develop some on your cervix. In men, they'll appear on the penis, sometimes on the testicles. The initial infection is often the worst and can last up to 20, horrible, sickly days. You may feel feverish and achy, your lymph nodes may swell and feel tender. The sores heal in about 12 days but – sorry – haven't disappeared forever. Further attacks usually occur in the same place but are less severe and heal quicker (around four to five days). You are more prone to attacks when you are run down, tired, stressed or have been drinking too much. The latest research has shown it's quite possible to pick up herpes and not get a lesion for several years afterward. Bear this in mind if your partner suddenly shows symptoms but swears they've been faithful – they might well have picked it up way before meeting you.

What's the single, most effective cancer screening tool in the history of modern medicine? The Pap smear test.

What now?

Your doctor will take a swab from one of the sores and analyse it. You may be given local anaesthetic jelly to apply and standard headache pills or codeine for the pain. Because herpes has been associated with cervical cancer, it's important you get an annual Pap smear.

Can it be cured and will it come back?

Herpes is manageable but not curable. The virus remains in the body, lurking in a nerve fibre, ready to come back out and party if *you* party too hard. Some people find taking relatively new anti-viral drugs, which shorten the length and severity of attacks, helpful (your doctor can give you a prescription), others simply treat each outbreak by bathing the area with salty water or antiseptics and taking painkillers. The better your general health is and the less stress you're under, the less prone you'll be to an attack.

Have I infected my partner?

Herpes is spread by vaginal, anal or oral sex or direct skin-to-skin contact with infected areas. As a general rule, you're unlikely to infect someone if you avoid sex from the moment you're warned of an attack (by the 'tingling' sensation) right through until the blisters have formed, dried up and the skin has returned to normal. However, some people have 'asymptomatic shedding' (the virus is present but there are no symptoms) or sores which are hidden from view and not noticed. It's rare but you can pass it on unawares during this time. Condoms help to stop transmission and, so long as the part that's infected is covered, provide 100 per cent protection if there's an active sore. Despite this, it's not recommended you have sex during an attack simply because it's painful.

> 'I've had herpes for years and I tell all my future sex partners. Some of them freak and assume I'm a male slut. It's so unfair since I caught it from a much-loved girlfriend, who'd been infected when she was really young.'
>
> Craig, 25, labourer

Will it affect my chances of having children?

If you have an attack at the time of birth, they'll deliver the baby by Caesarian to ensure you don't pass it on to the child.

Pubic lice (crabs) and scabies

What is it?

Pubic lice are tiny little crab-like insects that are spread through any intimate contact (in bedding, towels, etc.), not just intercourse. Scabies are a mite and spread the same way.

How do I know I've got it?

If you've got 'crabs', you'll be itching like mad on all your hairy bits (like your pubic hair or under your arms). Look closely and you'll discover it's not your imagination: there are tiny little insects scurrying around. Scabies cause red, itchy lumps in all the same places.

What now?

Race up to the nearest chemist, swallow your pride and ask for a lotion to kill pubic lice and/or scabies. They're sold over the counter and come with instructions.

Can it be cured and will it come back?

Simply apply a lotion to the affected areas (no, you don't have to shave your hair off) and that should be it.

Have I infected my partner?

If you've had close contact, yes. They should be treated as well.

Will it affect my chances of having children?

Not unless you're so put off by the experience, you never have sex again.

> 'I went to the toilet one day and felt this intense stinging sensation. When I had a look, I saw a tiny little blister inside my vagina and knew I had herpes. I just couldn't figure out how the hell it had happened since I'd been in a monogamous relationship for years. My boyfriend was as horrified as I was. We went along to an STI clinic, both eyeing each other very suspiciously, to find out he'd probably transmitted it to my genitals from a tiny cold sore on his mouth.'
>
> Trina, 20, student

Syphilis

What is it?

In the old days, anyone who was anyone had syphilis (artists, kings, queens, you name it); today it's very rare in the heterosexual population unless you've been travelling through Southeast Asia (and not used condoms) or your partner has (flashing red light alert if the unprotected sex he had was with a prostitute). Syphilis is spread through intercourse and goes through three stages.

How do I know if I've got it?

The first sign may be a painless sore on the penis, vagina, rectum or throat which sometimes develops during the *primary* stage, anywhere from three weeks to three months after exposure to the disease. The infection reaches the blood and spreads during the *secondary* stage, causing a fever, painful ulcers in the mouth or throat, rashes and sometimes warts on the genitals. Stupidly ignore the symptoms and you may think it was all a bad dream because all the body's defences now get to work and the symptoms fade away for anywhere from 2 to 50 years. Unfortunately, it's hidden, not eradicated. About one-third of sufferers go on to the *tertiary* stage, developing large ulcers which can damage the heart, major blood vessels, spinal cord and/or the brain or prove fatal.

What now?
If you've experienced any of the symptoms or fear you've been exposed, you'll need a blood test to identify the disease. If it's positive, you'll be given a course of high dose penicillin injections and carefully watched for several years to ensure it hasn't progressed.

Can it be cured and will it come back?
If it's treated before the tertiary stage, it's completely curable.

Have I infected my partner?
Syphilis is spread by vaginal, oral or anal sex. If you test positive, you must inform as many previous or current sexual partners as you possibly can.

Will it affect my chances of having children?
Not if it's treated promptly.

Trichomoniasis

What is it?
It's a common infection, caused by a one-celled organism of the same name, with ghastly symptoms. It incubates for between one and four weeks though some researchers claim women can carry the germ for years before showing symptoms. Trichomoniasis is usually passed on through intercourse.

How do I know if I've got it?
You'll know it if you're a woman and showing symptoms! A thin, revoltingly smelly, greenish-yellow and sometimes frothy discharge appears from your vagina. Most men have no symptoms though some notice a slight discharge and need to pee more often.

What now?
A smear (sample of the discharge) will be taken and analysed. If it's positive, you'll be put on a course of antibiotics – either one, strong single dose or a week's worth.

Can it be cured and will it come back?
Yes it's curable and, unless you're reinfected, it won't come back. A good home remedy to relieve symptoms until you can see your doctor is to soak a tampon in two tablespoons of white vinegar, one drop of baby shampoo and half a litre of warm water. Insert (which is easier said than done – tampons tend to explode to EXTRA-large size after being soaked) and leave in place for up to four hours. Don't do it immediatly before seeing a doctor because it can affect the swab results.

Have I infected my partner?
It's spread by vaginal sex so quite possibly. Both of you should be treated simultaneously.

Will it affect my chances of having children?
No.

Human papilloma virus (HPV) or warts

What is it?
In fairytales, the princess kisses the warty frog to turn him into a prince. In real life, having sex with a wart-infected person will simply get you warts. HPV is a virus that causes warts in the genital area.

How do I know if I've got it?
It's common – about 60 per cent of people carry the virus – but only a small percentage go on to develop warts on their genitals. They're small, painless lumps that look like tiny cauliflowers, and they appear on the vulva, vagina, penis or anus. They can take weeks or years to develop after exposure and you may not even notice very small lesions which, nonetheless, shed virus particles and make you infectious.

What now?
There are 52 different strains of the HPV virus. Numbers 6 and 11 cause genital warts, numbers 16 and 18 are the ones most likely to be associated with cervical cancer but they don't cause warts.

The reason I'm dazzling you with statistics is because lots of people think having genital warts puts them at risk of cervical cancer. It usually doesn't (though regular Pap smears are still a very good idea). If you have visible warts, a doctor will paint them with an acid solution, which causes them to dry up and fall off after a few treatments. Alternatively, you may need to have them removed in hospital through diathermy (burning), cryotherapy (freezing) or laser treatment.

> 'When I was 16, I was terrified of catching a disease but when I got to uni, everyone's attitude changed. It was like, "I've got a dose of the clap, I've got to see the doctor." You boasted about it. It was a bit of a hero thing; proof you'd been bonking girls.'
>
> Nathan, 21, student

Can it be cured and will it come back?

Recurrence is common, especially if you're stressed, smoke or use steroids. As with herpes, the better you look after yourself, the less likely you'll be plagued by attacks.

Have I infected my partner?

In adults, HPV is spread by having vaginal or anal intercourse with an infected partner. Condoms *help* prevent the spread but even they aren't 100 per cent protection against infection. Avoid having sex while one of you is having warts treated.

Will it affect my chances of having children?

No.

Hepatitis A, B and C

What is it?

Hepatitis is inflammation of the liver caused by a number of things including alcohol, chemicals, drugs and infections by viruses. Hep A is usually transmitted by contaminated food or drink and through anal sex if you're gay; it's not transmitted through intercourse but may be by oral sex. Hep B is passed on via semen, mucus or blood through intercourse (vaginal or anal) or needle-sharing. (In fact, you're more likely to pick up Hep B than you are

HIV through heterosexual sex because of the nature of the bug – it can survive for longer in less ideal environments.) Hep C is similar to Hep B but mainly blood borne and usually transmitted through sharing needles. Whether it's transmitted sexually or not is unclear at the moment. Both Hep B and C are associated with liver cancer.

How do I know if I've got it?

Hep A usually lasts a couple of weeks (causing vomiting and diarrhoea) then disappears spontaneously, leaving no lasting effects. The incubation period for Hep B and C is anywhere from six weeks to six months and you may show no symptoms or very serious ones. Yellowing of the skin and eyes (jaundice), unusual tiredness, darker than usual urine and paler than usual stools are some symptoms.

What now?

If you suspect you've been exposed to any of the three types, get a blood test (even if you aren't showing symptoms). As with AIDS, there's a 'window period' – which means you should be retested several months later. Unfortunately, there is no effective cure. Because it's a virus, it doesn't respond to antibiotics though some drug treatments have proved helpful.

Can it be cured and will it come back?

Hep B and C sufferers can be lucky – your body fights the bug, it goes away and you're no longer infected or infectious. Other times (for reasons unknown), the Hep B or C bug hangs around in the bloodstream and you're a carrier. Even if it doesn't make *you* sick (though it usually does cause problems like liver disease later in life), you can still pass it on to others. Hep B can be prevented with a vaccine which involves a course of three injections. If you inject drugs or have unprotected sex, it's worth getting vaccinated, (and therapy while you're at it, to stop you doing either).

Have I infected my partner?

Quite probably. It's safest to have all sexual partners tested.

Will it affect my chances of having children?
No.

Chlamydia

What is it?
It's common – in cities, one person in 50 has it, one in 10 in rural populations – but it's a shy little bug and few sufferers realise they have it. Nicknamed 'the silent STI' because it causes mild or no symptoms, chlamydia can make a woman infertile very rapidly indeed. It's picked up through intercourse with a person who's already infected and the ramifications are serious.

Chlamydia can cause permanent damage to the tubes vital for reproduction in both sexes, making you infertile. It's one of the major causes of pelvic inflammatory disease in women and ups the chances of ectopic pregnancy (where the baby grows in the tubes instead of the womb).

How do I know if I've got it?
It's silent, remember, which means it's often symptom-free. If symptoms do occur in women, they're likely to be a thick, sometimes blood-stained discharge, pain when you pee (or needing to go more often) or pain during intercourse. Men may also have a discharge, pain on urination, swelling of the testicles or diarrhoea.

What now?
It's tested by a swab taken from the cervix or inside the tip of the penis, or (more recently) by a urine test. Luckily, chlamydia is relatively easy to treat through antibiotics: either one high-dose pill or a 10-day course. You'll be re-tested after the course to make sure the disease is cleared.

'He was the first guy I'd ever slept with, a doctor and 12 years older than me. He gave me hepatitis and I was sick for months. I learned the hard way why condoms are a must.'
Flavia, 22, waitress

Can it be cured and will it come back?
If you test clear after treatment, you're cured.

Have I infected my partner?
It's spread through intercourse. Condoms help prevent passing it on but both of you should be treated simultaneously if you haven't used them *every* time, to avoid passing the disease back and forth. Avoid sex while you're taking the antibiotics and until you've both been given the all-clear.

Will it affect my chances of having children?
If it leads to pelvic inflammatory disease, yes.

Pelvic inflammatory disease (PID)
What is it?
It's something women should avoid like the plague if they plan on ever having babies. PID is an infection in the womb and tubes, often caused by bacteria passed on through sexual intercourse. As the name suggests, some or all of the organs and tissues in the pelvis become inflamed and sore. If you suspect you have it, see a doctor NOW. Left untreated, PID can permanently damage the tissue and affect fertility and/or increase your chances of ectopic pregnancy (pregnancy outside the womb). Chlamydia and gonorrhoea are common causes. A termination (abortion), childbirth and some gynaecological operations can also trigger PID.

How do I know if I've got it?
It can cause no symptoms or quite severe ones including stomach pain, vaginal discharge, pain on sexual intercourse, pain on passing stools or urine, bleeding between periods or heavy, painful periods, vomiting and fever.

What now?
Your doctor will give you a pelvic examination (feel your tummy and inside your vagina) and vaginal swabs (he or she will take samples of your discharge), particularly for chlamydia which is a common cause. PID can be 'acute' (you've noticed symptoms recently) or 'chronic' (it's been there a while but gone unnoticed).

Chronic PID can cause symptoms on and off over a period of months or years. Either way, once it's discovered, you'll probably be put on antibiotics, perhaps several types over a period of weeks. If it's a serious attack, you may need intravenous antibiotics in hospital (they'll put a drip in). It's important to rest and drink fluids during treatment and you must avoid having intercourse until two weeks after the treatment has ended. Follow-up examinations and tests will give you the all-clear.

Can it be cured and will it come back?

It won't recur if it's treated properly but if you're severely infected, you might well be in for bouts of chronic pain and general ill health before full recovery.

Have I infected my partner?

Condoms help prevent infection but usually your partner is treated as well, just in case, to stop passing the infection to and fro.

Will it affect my chances of having children?

Sadly, yes. Many women with PID have major difficulties falling pregnant. After one episode of PID, 10 per cent of women have damaged tubes. If untreated or reinfected, two episodes leaves 25 per cent of women infertile, and after three episodes the figure jumps to 50 per cent.

'FESSING UP – HOW TO TELL A LOVER YOU HAVE AN STI

Sarah got herpes when she was 17. At 27, she still had mild attacks about once every two years but avoided sex at those times and figured the chances of infecting her fiancé were pretty slim. Five years later, her now-husband found out – as she was about to give birth to their first child. The stress of pregnancy brought on a massive herpes attack and the child was at risk of being infected.

'We have to do a Caesarian,' the obstetrician explained to the anxious father, 'because Sarah's infected right now.'

'With *what?*' he answered. What should have been a gloriously happy event was marred by angry arguments about why he hadn't been told.

Lots of people don't tell their partner they've got an STI because they're worried they'll be branded 'cheap', 'slutty' or 'dirty'. And sometimes they're right – some sexually naive, uneducated or extremely narrow-minded people *will* judge you. But the way I figure it, if you explain the facts and your lover still thinks you're trash, surely it's better to find out early on in the piece that he/she's a righteous bigot? *Anyone* who's sexually active is at risk of getting an STI. If you've used condoms with the person you're about to tell, the most they can justifiably accuse you of is having unprotected sex in the past, though even *that* isn't true in some cases.

Here's some pointers to help guide you through a tricky discussion. (If you're carrying HIV, see 'Should I have an AIDS test' on page 187.)

- If you've just found out you've got an STI, had unprotected sex recently and think you may have infected your partner, there's nothing for it but to tell them immediately. (I'm taking it for granted no-one in their right mind would *knowingly* have sex without a condom if they knew they were infectious.) Say you had no idea you were carrying anything but are worried sick you may have inadvertently passed it on. If they're angry and accuse you of all sorts of irresponsible behaviour, calmly point out that the decision not to use a condom was made by both of you. You both took risks and who knows who gave it to who, anyway?
- If you have herpes or an STI, other than HIV or AIDS, that can't be cured, you don't need to tell every person you sleep with. If transmission of the STI is prevented by condoms, you use one and you aren't currently having an attack, it's unnecessary to tell casual lovers. They're not at risk so it's none of their business.
- Pick the moment carefully to tell long-term partners if you have herpes or an STI that can't be cured. The time to confess a long-standing STI is when you decide the relationship is serious, or has the potential to be. A good relationship is based on trust and if you leave it too long your partner will feel understandably 'had'. Pick a time and a place where you're both relaxed and won't be disturbed but . . .

- Prepare first. If you don't already have books or leaflets explaining the STI you have, get some (Family Planning clinics usually have great info you can take with you). Your partner can then read the facts for themselves. Rehearse what you're going to say so it doesn't get all mixed up on the way from your brain to your mouth. Imagine how you'd like to be told if the roles were reversed.
- Speak calmly. Say you have something to say and would appreciate it if they don't interrupt until you're finished. Then simply tell your story – how you got the disease, how upset you were when you found out, how you deal with it now. It's a very good idea to explain early in the piece that because you've been using condoms, there's no chance you've infected *them*. That way, they'll listen to what you're saying rather than sit there thinking, 'Oh my God, now I've got it too.' Tell them you're confessing because you trust them not to judge you, can see a future together and want to be completely honest. Now's the time to bring out the literature to back up the facts you're presenting.
- Refuse to be judged. Unless you got it from bonking their best friend behind their back, it's nothing to be ashamed of. Expect a little uncomfortableness (if they like you, they don't even want to *think* about you having sex with someone else, let alone what you got from it), but don't let anyone put you down. Once you've told them and worked out any effect the news will have on your sex life, drop the subject.
- Ask that they keep it confidential. It should go without saying but protect yourself anyway. Even if you are healthily undisturbed by others knowing you've got an STI, it's for you to tell people, not them. If they breach the agreement and blab to all and sundry, send him or her back to the nursery and get them out of your life.
- If they can't accept it, reconsider the relationship. If your partner has read all the facts and can't deal with the news, tell them they've got two choices: either talk to a counsellor (try an STI clinic) to get over any issues it's thrown up or leave. Do you want to be with someone who constantly

reminds you of how 'bad' you are or makes hurtful jokes at your expense?

- If someone's given you an STI, treat them with the respect you'd hope they'd show you. It's rarely deliberate, so don't point the finger and blame them; just get the facts and get on with your life – with or without them.

SHOULD I HAVE AN AIDS TEST?

Anyone who's ever had unprotected sex (in other words, pretty well all of us over the age of 25) has had those terrifying moments when we're convinced we've got AIDS. Even if it was one, stupid encounter, we huddle under the bedcovers, stare into the darkness and think, 'I bet I've got it, I know I've got it.' Health workers call us 'the worried well' – usually infection-free people in a low-risk category who take the test more for peace of mind than anything else. (That's not to say we *haven't* been infected, it's just pretty unlikely.) Others have been infected or are in a high-risk group. They've injected drugs, are homosexual men, have had sex with bisexual men who haven't used condoms or they've had lots of heterosexual unprotected sex with a number of people. Whichever category you fall into, having an AIDS test is well worth considering. It's not scary, no-one will look at you 'funny' or think you're promiscuous and they don't allow Big Brother cameras in clinic waiting rooms, honest.

> ***!*** ***Number of women globally infected with HIV: 5 million. The major mode of HIV transmission to women: heterosexual sex.***

Where do I go?

First wait three months from the last time you had unprotected sex or shared a needle, then head for a sexual health clinic (most major hospitals have them), Family Planning clinic or your GP. You can then be tested for *all* STIs, many of which have no obvious symptoms. The clinics are legally bound to ensure confidentiality, so they can't tell your parents, your partner or your boss (though they may suggest *you* tell them if you do test positive).

What will happen?

You'll be counselled first and asked about your sexual history, drug use and general health. The counsellor will ask why you want the test, how much you know about the disease and how you would react if you tested positive (they need to be satisfied you won't throw yourself off the nearest cliff immediately). Then, you'll be taken to an examining room and a doctor will take some blood (and swabs if you're getting a thorough check-up). The blood test will detect the antibodies produced by your body when it encounters HIV. Few clinics give results over the phone so you'll need a second appointment to find out the verdict.

What happens if it's negative?

Say a 'thank you God' prayer. Now's the time to make a personal pact to practise safer sex always.

What happens if it's positive?

Some people don't go further than pre-test counselling because they aren't prepared to deal with a positive result. Others take the plunge. Remember that if the news is bad it still doesn't mean you have AIDS – it could be 10 years before you experience symptoms. A counsellor will tell you the result and help you decide if or how you'll tell family, lover/s, friends and your employer. It's advisable to get regular counselling for at least a few months after; as you can imagine, being HIV positive isn't something that's easy to deal with. Your reaction to the news will vary over the next few months and years and it helps to know people in the same situation. The clinic will give you phone numbers of the many support groups available as well as explicit instructions on how not to pass it on.

! *Number of women who say they've changed their sexual behaviour because of AIDS: 53.6 per cent.*

OTHER THINGS THAT CAN HAPPEN 'DOWN THERE'

The human body is an amazing thing and awfully clever and efficient when it's well oiled and whirring along happily. But let's face it: if we were a car or a CD player, we'd have been recalled by now due to machinery faults. One microscopic, *teensy-weensy* bacteria or bug and the whole thing can muck up. Even if you're one of those sickeningly health-conscious, never-do-a-thing-wrong types, you'll still get sick occasionally. And while we'll all happily trot along to the chemist or doctor for help getting over the flu, we're not so quick to find out what's causing problems 'down there'. Many people, particularly women, get embarrassed – which is a bit silly when you think about it. Your doctor or gynaecologist has seen vaginas, penises and breasts before. Granted, maybe not yours, but they're all pretty similiar, don't you think? Then you have to admit you have – *What? SEX!* – to explain your symptoms or worries? I suspect this won't come as a horrible shock to your doctor either – she might even have it herself on the odd occasion.

In other words, there's no need to be shy, red-faced or self-conscious. If you suspect you have any of the following common infections, get professional help. Unless you're a seasoned sufferer (and your doctor's given you the go-ahead), don't attempt to cure yourself. I've listed some home-relief remedies to tide you over until you get to see your doctor and things you can do to avoid future attacks, but they're not substitutes for medical attention.

Cystitis and other urinary tract infections (UTIs)

Inflammation of the bladder can affect men, women and children. In adults, cystitis is the most common complaint (one in every two women will get it at some point). It's caused by germs entering the urethra and – guess what? – one of the most effective ways to get it is to have lots and lots of great sex, hence the nickname 'honeymoon disease'. (If you've had a big session, pee immediately after intercourse to flush out any germs; using lubricant during sex helps.) Classic symptoms for both sexes include an urgent need to pee (then nothing comes out when you get there), intense pain on urination or blood in your urine. Given that the symptoms are truly miserable, most people are begging their doctors for the first available appointment, which is just as well because it can lead to more serious things if left to fester. Once you start treatment – usually a course of high-dose antibiotics – it is wonderfully, immediately effective. The problem doesn't disappear that quickly (you need to take a full course), but the symptoms do.

DIY relief until you can see a doctor

Drink a solution of 1/4 teaspoon of baking soda in a cup of water once every eight hours and a glass of plain water once every two hours. Over the counter UTI remedies are also useful for mild attacks. To prevent future infections, drink cranberry juice (it helps stop bacteria latching onto the bladder walls), shower regularly, use mild soap, dry thoroughly and wipe front-to-back when you go to the toilet. Drink lots of water regularly to flush out germs and pee immediately after sex.

Thrush (candida)

This is a relatively harmless fungal infection. Why then, do some women run screaming from the room at the mere mention of it? Because it can be a living hell if it won't go away. As persistently annoying and as stubborn as a two-year-old, recurrent thrush is single-handedly capable of ruining sex lives, good moods and underwear without very much effort at all. In short, it can leave you feeling as hot for sex as a tub of ice-cream.

Candida is a yeast that most of us have growing in our vagina all the time. It's generally kept under control by the natural acidity of the vagina but things like the Pill, antibiotics, heavily perfumed soaps and bubble baths, vaginal deodorants, sex, pregnancy, diabetes, stress and general ill-health can cause an imbalance. It's not new – candida was found in the tombs of Ancient Egypt – and men get it too, but to a lesser extent (even so, he needs to be treated as well).

Symptoms include itchiness, a white, cheesy-looking discharge, vaginal swelling or redness, and pain during sex or peeing (usually caused by urine or sperm stinging the tiny cuts you've made by itching madly in your sleep). Your doctor will prescribe anti-fungal vaginal pessaries (you insert them and they 'melt' inside your vagina) or cream (with an applicator to insert inside). There's also a new, single-dose, oral anti-fungal tablet. He can use the cream or the tablet.

DIY relief

To prevent further infections, up the 'good' bacteria in your body by eating yoghurt with live lactobacillus cultures daily or go on a course of acidophilus tablets (available from chemists and health food shops). Eat less sugar, yeast products and alcohol. If you're plagued by it, pick up one of the many books on the subject which list umpteen theories on getting rid of it for good.

Gardnerella vaginalis

More common than thrush, it's something that normally lives in your vagina, keeping to itself until you do something to upset its home environment – like take the Pill. The first symptom may be a fishy smell (especially after intercourse) or a discharge, either thin and watery or frothy. It's cured with antibiotics and not passed on sexually, so he doesn't need to be treated.

DIY relief

Alter the pH of the vagina using a gel or vinegar douche (one-third vinegar to two-thirds warm water).

Endometriosis

This is a condition where the endometrial (lining) cells of the uterus grow in places outside the uterus like the ovaries, fallopian tubes, bladder or large bowel. It's not understood why but it affects women in their reproductive years (most commonly women in their 30s and 40s). Endometriosis doesn't always cause symptoms but it can stop you from falling pregnant easily, or at all. If you do get symptoms, they may include pain in your abdomen or while going to the toilet, during sex or during abnormally heavy periods. The most common symptom is severe pain just before or during your period that feels like a dull, dragging ache rather than the usual period cramps. It's diagnosed through an operation called a laparoscopy, where the surgeon looks for evidence inside. Treatment depends on how severe it is and whether or not you've had, or would like to have, children. You may be given medicine to relieve painful symptoms or hormonal drug therapy, which is designed to cause the tissue to disappear. In some cases, the tissue needs to be removed surgically. In severe cases, the surgeon will remove your uterus, tubes and/or ovaries as well.

EVEN IF EVERYTHING'S WORKING JUST FINE . . .

Look after your body and watch for changes

Get some info on how to examine your breasts for lumps. (He should examine his testicles for lumps on a regular basis also.) Wash regularly, using mild unscented soap, try really, really hard to wear cotton knickers most of the time and if you notice any abnormal lumps, discharge or redness, see a doctor.

Don't use feminine hygiene sprays or 'freshening' douches

For a start you don't need them, and secondly they alter the delicate pH (acidity) balance of the vagina and can lead to infections like thrush. If you're worried about being 'smelly', get a check-up to rule out infections, then shower regularly, use mild unscented soap, and wear cotton underwear. It's that simple.

Get regular check-ups and Pap smears with a gynaecologist or your GP

If you're sexually active, go every time you notice something unusual (or visit an STI clinic instead) or once every six months to a year. You'll probably be advised to get a Pap smear yearly or twice-yearly. They don't hurt and the payoff is enormous: a Pap smear not only can detect cervical cancer in its earliest stages, it picks up any cell changes that may be caused by infections you don't know you have.

First, your doctor will visually inspect your genitals and may do an 'internal' (put his or her fingers inside to check for swelling or pain). Then they'll use a speculum to look at your cervix and a cotton swab or cervical brush to scrape off a few cells. The sample is then sent to pathology to check for abnormalities.

Performance Problems

Some of the reasons sex goes wrong and how to get it lustily back on track

As a writer who specialises in sex, I discuss penises, clitorises and the pros and cons of G-spot orgasms as often as other people talk about where to go for lunch. I've done stories on dominatrixes and drag queens, prostitutes and premature ejaculators; I've visited bondage and discipline parlours, a sex addicts' club and sat around with a group of naked women armed with vibrators big enough to build houses with. All that experience makes me a popular dinner party guest – but it freaks penises out big time (not to mention the men they're attached to).

Add a tendency to forget not everyone's as open about sex as I am, and you can see why some men find me too hot to even think about handling. 'So, you can help me out with a story I'm doing,' I said to one guy on a first (never to be repeated) dinner date. 'Oh really?' he said nervously, Adam's apple doing an Irish jig. 'It's an easy one,' I continued chattily. 'All I need to know is this. When you're giving a girl oral sex, have you ever noticed if any fluid comes out? See, this story's on female ejaculation.' I scooped up a mouthful of pasta and beamed an encouraging, cheerful smile. 'Ummm . . . how's your meal?' he answered. Later, he told a mutual friend the only guy who'd be confident enough to sleep with me answered to the name of Bond.

No matter how much I tell men the pressure's on *me* to perform in bed, some still give me this watery, wan smile and continue to think, *Oh God, she knows so much, I'm bound to do something wrong*. And, of course, they do. Which probably explains why I can't really understand all the fuss over genital malfunctions. So our body bits don't behave as we want them to occasionally. So what? Genitals are like expensive electrical equipment – they play up now and again. Leave it until the next day and the problem often magically cures itself. Penises, vaginas and clitorises might be part of your body but they're not always within your control. Accept this one simple fact and you'll avoid the psychological head games that turn a lot of isolated technical hiccups into chronic sex problems.

As for other sex or relationship related trouble zones, again you'll notice the same advice given over and over. Talk to your partner. Discuss the problem. Tell him or her you're not happy. Your mouth is great for a lot of things to do with sex but its most important function in the bedroom is for talking. Good communication can solve lots of problems and make them *all* easier to cope with. Talk is cheap, cheaper than sex therapy.

This chapter looks at the common physical and emotional reasons why sex goes wrong and suggests practical solutions to the problem.

PENIS PROBLEMS

Personally, I'd hate to have a penis – it's so humiliatingly obvious when things go wrong! Because female bits are hidden, we get away with all sorts of things. We're *dying* to have sex but our vagina's as dry as a piece of unbuttered toast? No problem. A quick trip to the bathroom, a scoop of K-Y and our lover's none the wiser. Not so for men. A limp penis stands out like . . . well, it *doesn't* and that's pretty obvious to both of you. As for coming too soon, I'm yet to

> 'You never, ever talk about penis problems to other guys. It's almost like your penis is you. Guys are so ego-orientated and sex-orientated. If I confessed to a mate, he'd have one up on me. I actually find it easier to talk to women about it than men – women you're not sleeping with, that is.'
>
> Christopher, 23, music rep

hear a man complain if his girlfriend hits the target within three minutes (more like *hallelujah!*). The pressure on men to perform is enormous, even if nothing else is.

If you're a guy, chances are at some point in your life you'll find yourself in one of the following situations. If you're a woman, it's pretty obvious you could be the one he's with at the time. Men take their penises very, very seriously, so it pays for both of you to be prepared. How you react to the problem initially very often dictates how long it remains one.

He can't get it up (impotence)

Sometimes, penises and brains have different ideas of what's fun. You want to ravish her, but your penis wants to snuggle up into your Calvin's and have a kip. Nearly every man will have had problems getting an erection by the time he reaches 40. It's ***normal*** and usually explicable. Maybe you drank too much, work pressures are stressing you out or you're simply tired. Dismiss it as a one-off and chances are that's what it will be. Worry yourself sick about it and it may well happen again. The more wound-up and anxious you are the next time, the more nervous poor old Willy's going to be and the less likely he'll be to rise to the occasion. Your worst nightmare will be confirmed and you will be officially (if only temporarily) impotent.

! Only one-third of impotency cases are due to physical problems, and 90 per cent are treatable.

Why did it happen in the first place? Too much booze can do it, so can party drugs, physical exhaustion, pressure, stress and guilt (your penis may try to be faithful, even if you don't). Usually, it's psychological but there may be a medical reason. It's easy to figure out which category you slot into: if you have an erection when you wake up in the morning or during masturbation, it's probably psychological. You're not getting one

'The first thing that women do is grab your penis, and when they're used to grabbing firm erections not limp ones, they often visibly flinch. That makes me shrivel even further.'

Ethan, 35, mechanic

with your partner because you feel anxious, embarrassed or ashamed – maybe she's made you feel that way by being critical.

 FOR HIM

Real men don't always get erections whenever they want to. I'm not being kind, it's true. I asked every female who called the day I was writing this and out of 10 only one had never encountered the problem (my niece, who's five years old). Accepting that you're not the only one is often the solution to the problem. Many of you get horribly upset because you think of sex as intercourse – which needs an erect penis. Illogically, you'll think you're a dud in bed even if she's had 10 orgasms through oral sex. That's really silly. Take it from me, women don't think like you do. We'll go for the guy who gives us great head over an erect penis every time. So first up, change your mindset.

> 'It first happened when I was 19. I'd just met a girl and couldn't get it up. I thought it was a bit strange but put it down to the fact that I was really keen on her and wanted things to go really well. The second time it happened, I became obsessive – wound myself up into a complete state. The girl kept saying, "It must be me," and that made it worse. After her, I bonked a few girls casually with no problem, then I met my next long-term girlfriend and was back to square one. I finally figured it only ever happens with women that matter so I warn them and once I'm relaxed it goes away.'
>
> Tony, 28, teacher

Talk to your girlfriend and confess that you're going through a weird time. Don't avoid sex, just have it without penetration; use your tongue, hands and mouth to pleasure her instead. (She'll be praying you stay impotent forever.) Rule out any medical reasons for the condition. Give drugs, alcohol and cigarettes the big swerve and rethink your health and lifestyle generally. If you're on any prescribed medication, ask your doctor about possible side effects. If it's happening a lot, ask your GP for a referral to a urologist for a physical examination or book in to see a sex therapist. Think about why it's happening. Is it with all women or just this one? If it's just her, maybe you're mistaking friendship for lust or love. Sometimes, if you fancy her like mad, you're scared limp because you're so desperate to please her. Relax a little. If she's going to leave you because you can't get an erection, she wasn't worth the effort in the first place.

F FOR HER

- **Don't take it personally.** It doesn't mean your tummy is too big, he doesn't like your underwear or he fancies the blonde in accounts.
- **Don't pretend you don't notice.** Talk to him about it. Say, 'I know how that feels. Sometimes I want sex but I don't get wet.' Ask him if he'd like you to try to arouse him or whether he'd prefer to get some rest. Talk to his penis as well. Say, 'Poor thing, you're tired' or 'Too much beer, eh?' – anything to lighten the situation. The worst thing you can do is ignore it. Gently stroke it from base to tip or give him oral sex but don't labour the point. If he doesn't become hard in a few minutes, shift to another area – his nipples, his mouth, his testicles.
- **Turn it around. Say, 'Fantastic! This means I get you all to myself.'** Let him use his hands and tongue to bring you to orgasm. Masturbate for him. Relax and enjoy yourself – an orgasm each doesn't necessarily have to be the goal of lovemaking.
- **Have intercourse anyway.** If you can push it in (with his or your fingers), he'll often become erect inside you.

> 'The relationship was great, except we still hadn't had intercourse and it'd been six weeks! He'd give me these amazing passionate kisses out in public but while I couldn't wait to get home and rip our clothes off, he'd avoid it. Then I found out why: he'd been impotent for months. Of course, I was convinced I could solve it. When I couldn't, I thought, "Bloody hell, this guy really does have problems." I'm a really sexual person and I need to have sex and orgasms. If he'd taken the time to satisfy me with his hands and mouth, it wouldn't have been such a problem but he seemed so caught up with it, he forgot about me.'
>
> Carla, 24, secretary

He can't come

What's going on? You've been at it for so long she's not only planned the menu for tomorrow night's dinner party but the shopping list and what to wear as well. Rapid thrusting usually does the trick but this time, though you're close to orgasm, you can't quite get there. Usually it's because sensation in your penis is deadened by too much alcohol, drugs (especially speed) or (half your luck!) she's worn you out from too many previous climaxes. Women are used to having sex without the ultimate reward of orgasm – you're used to quite the opposite.

If it's not the result of overdoing it, it could be psychological. Have you just swapped girlfriends and are too shy to tell your new lover what you need to tip over the edge? Some men can only orgasm if their partner squeezes their testicles; others want her to insert a finger into their anus. If you've just split with someone and always orgasmed the same way, your body and brain may be waiting for the signal to let go. Alternatively, you might be feeling emotionally upset. Are you worried about losing her, having work hassles, or generally going through a stressful time? You're having trouble because your mind's not on the job.

Ⓜ FOR HIM

A good night's sleep is an instant fix-up if the problem's related to drugs or alcohol. Telling her what you need to orgasm is another. Communication is nearly always the key. Unload those problems by talking to her, or another sympathetic friend, and ask her if she ever has trouble coming (she does, believe me). A problem shared is a problem halved and all that. Are you spending too much time giving her foreplay and not enough on yourself? Encourage her to pull out all the stops, pull on the sexy underwear, tell you a fantasy while you're making love or just to let you know how horny she's feeling. Also get her to stimulate your anal region, massaging the area between your testicles and your anus. A well-lubricated finger up your bottom can work wonders.

Ⓕ FOR HER

- **Get wet.** You're not the only one who's sore – he is too. Add some K-Y (not too much) and it'll instantly feel more delicious for both of you.

- **Let him know how much he's turning you on. Appeal to all his fantasies.** Dress up, masturbate for him, do a Kim Basinger style striptease. Get him to bring you to orgasm as many times as you can stand it (a bore, I know), turn up the volume on the groans and the *'Oh yes'*es. Seeing you come can have a domino effect.
- **Use your mouth.** If you've been having intercourse for ages, your vagina's as worn out as you are. It's overstimulated and probably not gripping his penis as hard as usual. Switch to oral sex or mutual masturbation, using firmer pressure than usual.

He comes too soon

Premature ejaculation is the most common sex problem of all – 38 per cent of men don't last as long as they or their partner wants them to when they're having intercourse (and that's just the ones who'll admit it). As a teenager, you probably didn't worry too much (if indeed, you knew there was anything to worry about). Even when you're older, there are some situations that seem excusable (like living out a highly erotic fantasy, first-time sex with the girl of your dreams or sex with anyone if you haven't had it for a while). But when it happens every single time? Let me put it this way: even if you don't notice, she does.

> ***!** Four out of 10 men suffer from impotence or premature ejaculation.*

Defining a premature ejaculator (the technical term for it) is difficult. There's no set time period that you can measure yourself against, no 'test' to pass. It's horses for courses. Some couples think premature ejaculation is him coming after an hour's bonking, others are quite happy with (or used to) three minutes of intercourse. But if you feel out of control when it comes to coming, it's worth looking at for both your sakes.

Some men ejaculate when they touch breasts. Others get a little further but blow it on the very first (and undeniably the best) thrust. It's got a lot to do with the lessons you learned when you were young. If, as a teenager, you rushed through sex because you were worried you'd get 'caught', you've conditioned your penis to rapid ejaculations. Usually, age and a regular lover solve the problem – if they haven't, there's still lots you can do to fix it.

Ⓜ FOR HIM

Most sex therapists boast they can solve the problem within six weeks. Therapy usually revolves around learning to relax and relieving the pressure of performance. 'Homework' includes sex without penetration (taking the focus off intercourse through oral sex, mutual masturbation and generally exploring each other's bodies) and continuing to have sex even if you do ejaculate. Masturbation is one of the most effective means of control. The more you masturbate the better (it desensitises your penis), especially if each time you do you 'hold off' (try counting backwards, starting from 500).

The stop/start technique is 90 per cent successful if followed for a few months. Either you or your partner stroke your penis until you get an erection, you start having intercourse, then stop and withdraw the minute you feel close to coming. Stimulation stops until you start to lose your erection, then the whole process is repeated three or four times before you're allowed to ejaculate.

The squeeze technique – you or she grasps the penis just below the head and presses hard when you're close to orgasm – is another alternative.

Generally, the aim is to stop feeling so turned on. The more 'unsexy' your thoughts, the more control you're liable to have. Using distraction techniques, like mentally composing your résumé, can help; so can keeping your eyes closed so you can't see how sexy she looks. If the problem's really bad, zero foreplay for you and minimum for her; if necessary, don't touch her genitals at all. Use lubricant, put the penis in the vagina very carefully, avoiding too much stimulation and keep thrusting to a minimum. Stop and hold perfectly still or withdraw if you're losing control.

Ⓕ FOR HER

- **Get him to give you an orgasm first.** It takes the pressure off. Initiate non-penetrative sex like massage, oral and masturbation as well as intercourse.
- **Keep still.** This is one time he'll thank you for lying back and thinking of England. No groaning, moaning or raking your fingers down his back. Remain as passive as possible – don't contract your vaginal muscles or move your pelvis at all.

- **Keep going.** The more often he comes, the longer he'll last the next time. Try not to lose your temper or act bored (yawning is a no-no). Sure, it's frustrating not being able to touch him and lying there like a stuffed dummy isn't anyone's idea of hot sex, but (hopefully!) it's not forever. The more you have sex, the better it will get.

He doesn't feel like it

The honey-I've-got-a-headache line sounds awfully odd coming out of *his* mouth. Blame it on society (Hollywood or the soaps), but a *man* knocking back sex? Gosh, something must *really* be wrong. Not true, of course. These days, it's just as likely to be her ripping off your suit and you complaining you're too tired. And as women become more comfortable with sex, men are becoming less secure. Sex is demanded of you more often – and it's a massive blow to your ego if she wants it more than you do. The sheer pressure of trying to be the perfect 90s man can make sex seem more of a chore than a pleasure.

Men the world over are becoming less and less fertile. The average 90s man's sperm count is 50 per cent lower than his grandfather's was in the 40s.

Your desire could also be dampened by outside pressures. Men aren't sex robots; they're human and affected by stress and feelings just as much as women are. You're also individuals. Which means some of you have high sex drives (or libido) and somc don't. In an ideal world, we'd all find our libido equivalents. If you only want to have sex every two months and that suits her, it's not a problem. Hook a horny hedonist and it's a huge one.

Are you simply bored by sex and happy to let other things in life take precedence? Most of us move out of the can't-get-enough stage after those first few, fervent months. Unfortunately, it's often replaced by lovemaking that's as predictable as Grandpa's war stories. Physical tiredness is often to blame for temporary lack of interest. Are you trying desperately hard to establish a career, with not much energy left over for anything else? Working long hours (or partying too hard with too many drinks and ciggies) can mean sex is the last thing you feel like when your head hits the pillow.

Ⓜ FOR HIM

Holidays can do amazing things for a lagging libido, which means reducing stress is an obvious place to start. Sexual desire appears to originate in the brain. If you're juggling so much your brain feels like an amusement park, there aren't many cells free for fantasy. Make time for sex. Deliberately focus on it; read erotic books or watch some films. Get back to basics and spend more time on foreplay than intercourse. Let her massage you, rediscover sensuality and the simple delight of kissing and touching each other.

Ⓕ FOR HER

- **Help de-stress his life.** Schedule in 'pamper time' – an hour or two per week when you massage and stroke all his stress away. Don't panic and think that it's your fault (that you're obviously not sexy enough) and resist the urge to jolt him out of it by tying yourself naked to the bonnet of his car. He'll feel like a complete failure if you have to go to those extremes.
- **Have lots of 'quick' sex sessions.** If he's tired, he'll be much more interested in a quickie than in marathon sex. Get him to give you oral if he's not interested (you'll feel satisfied, he may find it the turn-on he needs), and return the favour on other occasions. Every sex session doesn't have to last an hour.

HOW TO GET YOUR LOVER TO SEE A SEX THERAPIST

Telling anyone it's time to seek professional help is tricky; getting your lover to see a sex therapist is even more delicate. Resist the temptation to blurt out 'You really should get help' immediately after (yet another) failed lovemaking session. Best to have this conversation outside the bedroom. Wait until you're both relaxed, then gently explain that although you love them and your sex life, you think a third party could help solve the problems you're both having. Use words like 'both' rather than 'you' when talking about the problem – it'll seem less attacking and more like you're making the suggestion for the sake of the relationship rather than pointing the finger.

Many people still think that only 'mad' people see therapists, so have the old 'you see an expert for every other problem, why not this one' argument ready. Once they agree to see someone, choose a sex therapist/psychologist carefully. Your doctor can usually help with a referral or look up 'psychologists' in the telephone book. Call the British Psychological Society (BPS) for referrals (see the Yellow Pages). They'll be able to provide you with a list of professionally trained counsellors in your area who specialise in sexual problems. If someone recommends one or you get a name from an ad, call the BPS to check they're registered. If your partner refuses outright to see an expert, you might want to rethink the relationship as well as your sex life – if they're not willing to compromise on this important issue, what about future problems?

FIVE WAYS TO HELP HIM THROUGH A ROUGH TIME

- **Don't overreact.** If he's having problems *most* of the time, he needs to see a doctor, possibly a sex therapist. But if it's only occasionally, what's the big deal?
- **Have orgasms from oral sex and masturbation.** Show him that an erect penis really isn't necessary.
- **Sympathise but don't lie.** Don't tell him he's hard if he isn't, don't tell him it was great if it wasn't. Pretending he doesn't have a problem will only make things worse.
- **Don't take it personally.** If he can't get an erection, it's not a personal indictment of your sexual attractiveness.
- **Talk to him about it.** Make it crystal clear you understand, don't blame him and are prepared to work *together* to solve the problem.

CAN'T, WON'T, SHOULDN'T: THE THREE MOST COMMON FEMALE SEX PROBLEMS

Psychologists recently did a word association test on a group of college students. They were given a subject (like 'family'), then asked to instantly list any other words they associated with it (children, mother, stroller, park, etc). Guess what happened when 'sex' came up? The male students smiled broadly, rubbed their hands over grubby Levi's and launched gleefully into a long list of adjectives like 'blonde, fun, legs, boobs, bed, orgasm, penis and sweat'. The girls paused, foreheads crinkled, put their hands between their knees and came up with 'guilty, wrong, bad, babies and tears'. To say they honed in on the negatives is an understatement. The study conclusion? Men focus on the in-out physical act of sex, women on the emotions associated with it. *Puhleeze!* They could have popped down to the nearest pub to find out that little gem of information.

Yet it's that fuzzy, emotional side that's at the root of most female sex problems. We worry too much about what people think. We won't let go in case he judges us, we don't tell a Godawful lover he's hopeless in case we scar him for life. Top of the class for being polite and caring, into the dunce corner for sexual enjoyment. We tend to take everything our mother, the church, our friends or ex-lovers have said in the past to bed with us. Even the neighbours get a look in – that planned Saturday afternoon orgy of lust turns into a reluctant rendezvous if they're home ('Shhhh! They'll hear you'). Hell, if the *dog* wanders in and looks at us the wrong way, it can put us off coming. All a bit ridiculous, don't you think? So stop worrying about everyone else during sex. The dog can't blab your secrets and Aunt Fanny's not peering in through the blinds.

She doesn't feel like it

It's easiest to divide sexual disinterest into *permanent* and *temporary*. At some point, all of us have found the thought of having sex about as appealing as cleaning the loo. The lifestyle of a typical 90s woman isn't conducive to great sex, for starters. Overloaded schedules leave us feeling stressed, unhealthy and unattractive. We don't feel sexy so we don't want sex. Stress and tiredness affect our hormones, blocking those that give a lovely libido lift, increasing others that make us anxious. Taking time out, making priorities and planning time for sex can solve the problem in a flash. Medication can also affect your sex drive. Anti-depressants like Prozac can make you feel great from the waist up, dead from the waist down.

Relationships are a common culprit – like being in the wrong one. Hooked up with a nice guy who does little for you sexually or hanging on to one who treats you badly? Sex slumps aren't usually just about sex; they're a sign that your relationship's gone awry. If you have problems outside the bedroom they'll filter through eventually. A bad lover is a common cause of sexual disinterest, particularly a selfish, inexperienced or incompetent one who's only interested in his own orgasm. If he's a bore in bed, why *would* you be champing at the bit to hop in?

If you've *never* enjoyed sex, have it only because 'you have to' and it rarely satisfies or arouses you, there are deeper psychological factors at play. If intercourse feels like being 'speared' or you divorce yourself from the act (experiencing that weird, *this-is-happening-to someone-else* feeling), you could be reacting to an earlier traumatic experience or a strict religious upbringing. Possibly, you've decided not to bother with relationships at all. Read 'If you're hung up about it' on page 10 and 'If you've never had an orgasm' on page 113. Consider seeing a therapist. It can be a sign of childhood abuse combined with repressed memories (see Chapter 8, 'Serious sex-related issues').

Ⓕ FOR HER

If it's temporary, consciously concentrate on feelings and sensations when you are having sex, and don't get too hung up on having an orgasm. Reacquaint yourself with your own body, learn what it responds to. Talk to your lover; tell him what turns you on, what doesn't, ask for more foreplay and use extra lubrication if you're dry. Deliberately focus on your erotic self. Do you *feel* like a sexual person? One therapist I know claims she can pick people who enjoy sex by the way they dress, walk and behave. People who like sex take care over their appearance, walk with confidence and like touching. People who don't aren't as aware of their bodies. Have sex more – the more you have it, the more you'll usually want it so indulge whenever you feel remotely turned on.

If your problem's long-term, you may have grown up feeling guilty about sex and may never have been 'woken' erotically. In other words, you simply don't know how to respond to sexual sensations in your body. A *sensate focus program* is what sex therapists use to help you 'learn' how to give and receive pleasure. The idea is to reawaken your sexual feelings gradually by using sensual massage to explore firstly your own, then your partner's, body. Intercourse is banned – you give and get pleasure through touch alone. Start by exploring *your own* body through massage. Have a bubble bath, use soap in the shower or oil your body and lie on the bed. Experiment with different strokes (soft, firm, fast, slow) to find out what feels good and arouses you. Don't just concentrate on the genitals and breasts; explore all of your body. Stage two involves massaging each other with oil in much the same way, this time avoiding the sex organs. In stage three, you're officially 'allowed' to touch more sexually sensitive parts with one proviso: you must talk constantly, keeping up a running commentary of what stroke and pressure feels best. When you've explored each stage thoroughly, you have permission to have intercourse. It helps if you also reduce stress as much as possible, opt for less 'threatening' sex (like massages and oral) and make a 'date' for sex at least once a week if you both have busy schedules.

Ⓜ FOR HIM

- **Don't make her feel guilty.** Pressuring her into having sex when she doesn't want to will kill any desire she may have. Make it clear you won't get upset or offended if she says 'no' to sex. Remove the pressure.
- **Talk to her.** Say you've noticed she doesn't seem that keen (lately or always). Ask her why. Is she just tired or do your techniques need improving? Does she need more foreplay? Would she like a massage?
- **Support her if her disinterest is caused by a painful past.** Encourage her to get professional help if she needs it. Don't insist she tells you every sordid detail of what happened but let her know you're there if she wants to talk. Don't judge her and don't offer advice. Instead, listen and give her lots of (non-sexual) hugs.

She can't come

Hands up if you expect to have an orgasm every single time you make love. Great! An optimistic attitude alone will guarantee you more climaxes. But it's a tad unrealistic all the same. The mood you're in, what's happening in your life and relationship, the amount and type of foreplay – all these can affect whether we'll come or not and a lot are out of our control.

Inhibitions stop us feeling relaxed enough to orgasm with a partner. Inexperience – not knowing our own body – doesn't help either. But again, the biggest obstacle between us and the Big O is a partner who's just plain hopeless in bed. If his idea of foreplay is 'Are you awake?', the chances of orbiting into erotic ecstasy are pretty slim.

If you've never had an orgasm at all, there's a section devoted exclusively to you in Chapter 4, page 113. Here, we'll deal with women who have trouble coming with their lover.

Ⓕ FOR HER

First up, look at how you orgasm when you're on your own. Are you addicted to your vibrator? Learn a more couple-friendly technique by learning to climax with your fingers. It's then simply a matter of showing him the right buttons to push by doing some serious communication, both in and out of bed. Use a bridge technique if you have no trouble coming while masturbating. While he's inside you, get him to stimulate your clitoris with his fingers; or bring you to the brink through oral sex, then use your own finger to continue stimulating your clitoris during intercourse. Try the 'fake it till you make it' technique (act as if it's happening and it might).

Some women subconsciously stop themselves going over the edge with a partner because they're worried they'll lose control or get too attached to him. If this rings true, ask yourself, 'What's the worst thing that could happen if I did come with him?' He'll think you enjoy sex? (How awful!) You might fall in love? (He might feel the same way and if he doesn't, you'll survive.)

About 80 to 90 per cent of women can be taught to orgasm with a partner through sex therapy. All it takes is time, patience, a relaxed and open attitude and (most importantly) a skilled, sensitive lover. (Remember, sex can be 'taught'.) If you need professional help, get it. Call the British Psychological Society (see the Yellow Pages) and ask for a referral to someone in your area. Why miss out on one of life's most pleasurable experiences?

Ⓜ FOR HIM

- **Stimulate her clitoris.** Add extra lubrication and use your fingers to stroke it gently throughout intercourse.

- **Become a better lover.** Read some good sex books, rent a few how-to-do-it videos (I don't mean porn – try Andrew Stanway's *The Lover's Guide* series), ask her for feedback.
- **Give her time.** Women take longer to reach orgasm than men do. If you only masturbate her or give her oral for a few minutes, you might as well not bother. Settle in and tell her to take as long as she likes.

> **'I can masturbate to orgasm within a minute. With my boyfriend, it takes at least 15 minutes of skilled stimulation. I don't know why but it's always been that way for me.'**
>
> Ellen, 27, advertising executive

Sex is painful

Almost all of us have occasionally let out a loud *'Ouch!'* at some stage during sex, particularly if we're trying a new position which goes too deep. But if it's hurting on a regular basis and you're mainlining martinis to cope with the pain, it's a warning something's wrong.

Painful intercourse is officially called *dyspareunia*. The pain may be deep and aching, sharp, a momentary twinge or intensely uncomfortable. It can be selective (it's only painful at certain times) or permanent (all the time) and the causes are diverse. It could be the result of an infection (even a flare-up of thrush can make us dry and sex painful), constipation, a sexually transmitted infection, a disorder of the reproductive system (like endometriosis), a urinary tract infection (like cystitis) or again (sorry guys!) clumsy or rough technique on the part of your partner. If he doesn't spend enough time on foreplay (or isn't very good at it), your vagina doesn't expand and lubricate in preparation for penetration. Instead, it stays tight and dry which makes intercourse uncomfortable or shoot-through-the-roof painful.

Not being wet is one of the most common causes of painful sex. Our natural lubrication is affected by the menstrual cycle, stress and tiredness, your age – a million things! The best way to increase lubrication is to have more (good) foreplay, the second best way is to add some K-Y or another water-based lubricant at the beginning of making love. It'll make sex more pleasurable, encouraging your natural secretions to kick in. The Pill can cause vaginal mucosa, a thinning of your natural lubrication; fix it by switching to a Pill higher in oestrogen or change contraception. Hot spas, vaginal deodorants and scented soap all also rob moisture.

If the pain is severe, you may have *vaginismus* which causes the vaginal muscles to go into spasm, stopping penetration entirely. It may start from the first time you have sex or occur later, usually after a painful infection or unexpected pain from a deep thrust. (It's a little like impotence: dismiss it as a one-off and you may be okay, worry about it and you'll get tense and start to associate intercourse with pain.) The causes are usually psychological and it's not something you can control because it's a reflex.

In almost all extreme, chronic cases of vaginismus, the woman has had a frightening early experience with intercourse – been raped, sexually abused or always suffered pain. (If you suspect or know this has happened to you, get professional help. At the very least, read Chapter 8, 'Serious sex-related issues'.) If your parents saw sex as 'wicked', the mere mention of the word can leave you feeling terrified and tense.

> 'Guys seem to think if they can hump away for hours, it makes them a stud. The fact is, after five or 10 minutes, I'm bored. If he's still thrusting after 20 minutes, I'm sore and also thinking, "He can't be that turned on by me or he'd have come by now".'
>
> Robyn, 24, dental assistant

Ⓕ FOR HER

Your first point of call is the gynaecologist or your doctor. If a chronic infection or urinary tract disorder is responsible, a course of antibiotics may be all you need. Your vagina tenses up on the odd occasion? It could be to do with relationship fears. Are you frightened of getting pregnant or an STI? Don't trust your partner? Maybe you're just not in the mood for sex and your vagina is telling you so. If you've ruled out medical reasons and it's a major problem, consider therapy.

A sex therapist will concentrate on two areas to solve your problem: how you feel about sex generally and your lover's sexual technique (or lack of it). In the meantime have more foreplay to make sure you're lubricated, add extra lubricant, spread your thighs wide and bend your knees to aid penetration, bearing down (pushing out) as your partner enters you to relax the muscles of the vagina.

If you have vaginismus, try these self-help exercises. Do them daily for several weeks and avoid intercourse until you're ready.

1. Start by having a bath or simply lying quietly for a little while. Then look at your genitals in a hand mirror. Touch the entrance with a lubricated finger, then try inserting it when you feel relaxed, bearing down slightly.
2. Leave the finger in place for a few minutes, then push it in a bit further. If you start to tighten up, stop, then *deliberately* tighten the muscles around your finger, to a count of three then release. Repeat until you feel in control; aim for at least 20 contractions. These are called Kegel exercises. Keep practising until you can push a finger all the way in without spasming.
3. Try the same thing with two fingers, using lots of lubrication. Then . . .
4. Repeat the exercise with a trusted partner. You set the pace. When you feel ready for intercourse, try a woman-on-top position. Get him to lie still, lower yourself on and let him penetrate when you feel ready. Deliberately tighten and relax your vaginal muscles as he penetrates.

Ⓜ FOR HIM

- **Encourage her to get a check-up.** Make sure she rules out medical reasons, then suggest she sees a therapist if you think it's psychological.
- **Triple the foreplay.** The more relaxed and aroused she is, the less likely it is to hurt. Don't attempt intercourse if she feels dry and/or tight.
- **Always use lubricant.** It's the single most effective way to reduce pain.

'My ex-boyfriend was totally hung up on the fact that his penis was slightly smaller than normal. Every time I touched it or looked at it, he'd say, "You're disappointed aren't you?" I wasn't, but I was sick of having to give constant reassurance. I mean, get over it!'

Carla, 20, nurse

FIVE WAYS TO HELP HER THROUGH A ROUGH TIME

- **Vary your lovemaking as much as possible.** The more effort you put into making sex fun and erotic, the more likely she is to want it. Educate yourself. You can't be sexually experienced without being sexually educated.
- **Don't be negative.** Accuse her of being 'frigid' and she'll retreat even further. Do quite the opposite. Shower her with compliments (sexual and otherwise), lift her self-esteem to the clouds, spoil her with (non-sexual) massages, say you don't mind just cuddling if that's what makes her happy. If you feel frustrated, masturbate.
- **Talk to her about it.** Take on the problem as if it were your own. The more she opens up to you, the closer you'll both be at hitting on the cause.
- **Don't take it personally.** It doesn't mean you're not a 'man' if you can't satisfy her. Even if she blurts that you're not fab in bed, sex skills can be learned.
- **Tell her you love her.** A secure, loved woman drops inhibitions, relaxes and trusts enough to satisfy her deepest desires.

EMOTIONAL TIME BOMBS

Sex therapists estimate that for every 10 times a couple has sex, one or two sessions are fantastic, about five are mediocre and the remaining three are boring or disastrous. *No-one* has great sex all of the time and one reason is this: it's not just the two of you in the bed. Getting in beside you both are your ex-lovers, your mothers and fathers, sisters, brothers, the horrible teacher you had in year five, the man who 'flashed' at you when you were two, his grandmother and the girl in the corner shop he snogged when he was 10. In other words, by the time you're ready to settle down, both of you are products of numerous small and several significant life events. You can't turn him into a sexual or emotional version of you or vice versa. There will always be points of difference both in and out of the bedroom.

A lot of the way we relate to our partner is dependent on our parents. Psychologists believe most of our emotional programming happens when we are very young: 50 per cent between the ages of 0 to 5 years, 30 per cent between 5 to 8 years and 15 per cent between 8 and 18. So, by the time you're 18, you're 95 per cent programmed – which leaves 5 per cent to work with. Horrified? Don't be. That teensy 5 per cent can turn around most of your programming if you want it to.

! ***Take a good long look at your partner before waltzing down that wedding aisle: you could end up looking just like them! Just as pets often resemble their owners, evidence is now emerging that married couples look frighteningly similar after years together.***

The secret to a happy, successful, long-term sex life is compromise and communication. Here are some solutions to common couple sex problems.

What do I do if I'm bored with sex? I've been in the same relationship for years and we've done just about everything already. Is it inevitable that sex dies?

Nothing gets my blood boiling more than when people say to me, 'It's natural for sex to die. There's nothing you can do about it.' The sort of people who feed me that drivel take great offence at my standard reply of 'Actually there are lots of things you can do to keep sex hot, you just have to work at it' because they're lazy. The only advantage new lovers have over long-term ones is newness – the thrill of conquering unknown territory – pretty insignificant when weighed up against the positives: feeling comfortable with each other, talking openly and enjoying a total lack of inhibition because you trust each other implicitly. Believing sex always fizzles out eventually is like not applying for a job because you're convinced you won't get it. Who knows what might happen if you made the effort? It's the same with your sex life. It's *common* for couples to lose the sexual fizz but it's *preventable*. This whole book is devoted to suggesting ways to make sex varied and better. Forgive me for not believing you've done 'everything' already, but I don't.

Why do I find sex less exciting once I fall in love?

When we sleep with someone purely for sex, we can be as wanton and wicked as we like because we don't really care what they think of us. Once we decide we like them and do care, it's like a bucket of freezing water is poured over any and all sexual fantasies and desires that aren't considered 'normal'. Will he think I'm slutty? Will she think I'm weird? We switch from horny lover role to what we think is Husband or Wife material. Talk to your partner next time you feel like this, hopefully having a laugh about how silly your fears are. If they do expect you to act differently in bed now you're an item, I'd be considering whether I wanted to be.

I'm always the one to initiate sex and I hate the fact that she doesn't

When you initiate sex, does she enthusiastically respond or seem half-hearted? If it's the first scenario, she may feel she needs 'permission' (you suggesting it first) because good girls shouldn't really like it *that* much. Or perhaps you have a much higher libido than she does and simply want sex more often (she doesn't get a *chance* to get horny because you're always jumping in first). If she's lukewarm to your suggestions, she probably doesn't enjoy sex (with you or at all) and does it just because she has to. Ask her why. Maybe you're a bad lover and she's too shy to tell you. Ask her if there's anything you can do to make it more enjoyable. Wine and dine her, massage her, give her lots of foreplay and see if that makes a difference. If something feels good we *like* doing it often.

How come I always end up having sex his way?

I don't know. Presumably you can speak. Get a grip, girl! Tell him you want to try something new or just take control and jump on top of him. If you lie back like a receptacle, can you blame him for assuming you want him to call the shots?

My girlfriend loves sex but hates 'quickies'. Why?

It could be something as simple as this: it takes her a while to lubricate. Buy some lubricant and see if that helps. Lots of women get turned on rapidly mentally, but it takes a while for their body to follow (and 'dry' sex isn't fun). Ask *her* why she doesn't like them. Quickies are a great adjunct to leisurely sex but if you opt for one every second session, I don't blame her for not being thrilled.

Who sleeps in the wet spot?

One night you do, the next he does.

How do I say no to sex without upsetting him?

Here's a novel concept: don't worry if you do. Most men would prefer you say no than have sex when you don't want to. If he does want you to perform on demand, change partners. The fact is, you don't need his permission to refuse. If you're polite and he's a nice guy, he might well roll over huffily and sulk for a while but, hopefully, he'll be aware he's acting childishly. How best to say thanks but no thanks? That really depends on the guy. Try telling the truth. 'I'm exhausted and just feel like sleep' or 'I don't know why, I just don't feel like it. Let's have a cuddle instead'. Make it clear you're rejecting sex, not him and he should handle it okay.

Is it ever okay to fake it?

No (most of the time), maybe (sometimes). See 'Faking it' (page 96) for answers to these cryptic clues.

How do I tell a much-loved partner he's abysmal in bed without using words?

Try using body language to get the message across. When he does something you do like, exaggerate your response: moan loudly, move closer, kiss him harder so he can't help but get the message you like what he's doing. If you don't like something, make that abundantly clear as well: twist away, lift your body away from his touch or (better) redirect his hand/mouth or penis. Most people do to their partners what they'd like done to them. If you like having your ear licked and bitten, you'll lick and bite his. Slip this into a conversation as a bit of interesting trivia then give him the attention *you'd* like the next time you're in bed.

If he still doesn't get the hint, you've got no other option but to talk to him. You really are better off using words than actions anyway. Just about every woman has lain there thinking, 'If I just hang in there a bit longer, he's *bound* to hit the right spot sooner or later.' But squirm all you want, sometimes it just isn't going to happen unless you say something. Sadly, you're not alone in wanting to stay silent. A lot of people don't say anything in bed, let alone 'Let me have it harder and a little to the left.' But how's he to know you think he's boring unless you tell him?

> 'I was bonking a girl doggie-style once and really getting into it, but all she could talk about was how big her bum must look. It was a turn-off! We don't notice your flaws so there's no need to hide them. When we stare at you walking around naked, we're appreciating the good bits, not focusing on what you think are the bad.'
>
> Jeremy, 18, bartender

I like doing 'kinky' things but get the feeling my current lover would be horrified. How do I feel her out about this, without embarrassing myself or scaring her off?

It really depends on what you, and she, define as kinky. No matter how broad-minded your lover is, I wouldn't suggest striding into the bedroom, dressed in her underwear, without giving her a little warning first. But if 'kinky' simply means trying something new, try using the third-person perspective to introduce a tricky topic. Say 'I heard a story about a friend who' or 'I had a dream about' and see what reaction you get. Or say you've got a fantasy about such-and-such. That way, you're insinuating rather than directly propositioning which can be erotic anyway. If she nervously starts wringing her hands, there's your answer. If she looks interested, follow it up with 'Why don't we try it next time?'

Will he think I've 'been around' if I suggest something unusual?

Again, it depends on what it is but I'd imagine most guys would be ecstatic rather than horrified if you'd like to try something new. If he thinks you're not a 'nice girl' for wanting to experiment, you're probably mismatched anyway. Do you want to spend the rest of your life acting like a nun?

Often, I don't orgasm during intercourse even though my lover always does. I know I could come if he gave me oral sex afterward. Is it fair to ask?

'Women who can achieve that up-but-falling-down look with their hair or put on a show and parade their new underwear, you can't help but love them. The sight of her, lying deliberately arranged on the bed in my underwear gives me an erection so hard, I could carve my initials in it.'

Phillip, 23, photographer

Is it fair that he has an orgasm and you don't? Of course it's fair to expect to feel satisfied at the end of making love. Just bear in mind that men aren't as blasé about body secretions as women are (they've never had to cope with things like periods) but a quick one-minute wash in the bathroom is likely to change his mind until he loosens up a little. Alternatively, have an orgasm before intercourse through oral sex, or ask him to manually masturbate you with his fingers afterward. Better still, get him to stimulate your clitoris *during* intercourse.

If he/she gives me an orgasm through oral sex, do I have to give him/her one, too?

You probably are expected to reciprocate, but it doesn't have to be immediately. Take turns. Lots of couples plan sex sessions where one partner concentrates on the other. One day, he can massage you, finish with oral sex and let you drift straight off into a delicious sleep; the next time, you do the same for him.

'I always feel vulnerable after sex – I think all women do. I don't want poetry, just some sort of acknowledgement that you enjoyed it and I wasn't just a notch on the bedpost.'

Katherine, 25, chef

He wants me to try anal sex but I don't want to.

Many men and women find anal sex a turn-on; lots of others would rather have pins stuck in their eyes. It's a personal decision and while him suggesting it doesn't make him secretly gay or a pervert, he shouldn't pressure you if you don't want to. If you do decide to give it a try, let him insert a finger into your rectum to see if you like the sensation before inserting his penis. See 'Anal stimulation' (page 80) for more details.

My lover wants me to masturbate in front of him. Am I being a prude by not doing it? Is this now considered normal behaviour?

Ten to 15 years ago, women didn't even admit that they masturbated, let alone put on live floor shows. Men, on the other hand, have always masturbated – a lot – and this is why he thinks it's no big deal to ask. There's a very good reason to go along with the idea – he'll have a front row seat to watch how you give yourself pleasure. (See in Chapter 1 for hints on doing it in front of each other.) Don't let him pressure you, but consider trying it: we should always push ourselves a little sexually. Stay in the comfort zone all the time and you won't grow.

Should I share my fantasies with my partner?

It depends on how well you know and trust your partner. A friend of mine once confessed to a new lover that she'd always fantasised about sleeping with another woman. The next time she saw him, they had company: an escort girl he'd hired. Lizzie, understandably, wasn't as impressed with his 'little surprise' as he thought she'd be. Kept secret or told to the right partner, most fantasies are harmless, terrific sex-boosters. Told to the wrong person, they become revenge material for the dumped and bitter. Personally, I'd save them for a long-term, committed and sexually liberated partner. (See 'Lights, camera, erection', page 261, if you do decide to share.)

Why does she hate it if I look at porn mags? Do I give up now on her ever watching porn *with* me?

Ever since Hugh Hefner launched *Playboy* in 1954, women the world over have got their knickers in a knot over pictures of women not wearing any. The fact is, the *majority* of men don't watch porn for the sinister reasons women think they do. They do it because it's fun. Ninety per cent of men are turned on by mainstream porn (which doesn't include material involving children, animals or extreme violence). Because men are better at separating love from sex than women are, they consider porn films an innocent 'boy thing', and most can't understand why girlfriends take offence. Quite frankly, neither can I if we're talking about the odd copy of *Playboy* or *Penthouse* or an occasional X-rated video. Just don't *expect* her to watch or read it with you unless she wants to – and if she's extremely anti-porn, yes, give up now on ever sharing it with her.

'A bed is good for two things, and the other one is sleeping. Why do women turn it into a cross between an analyst's couch and a confessional by wanting to talk about "us" in those post-sex, pre-sleep moments? Where do you get the energy? If you want to talk about the relationship, save it for dinner. Even worse, is the guilt tripper. "I wish I hadn't done that," you'll say. What we really want to hear is "That was great. Let's do it again tomorrow night".'

Alex, 36, musician

It's a different story, however, if you're obsessed with porn. Do you subscribe to *all* the porn mags, including the hard core ones? Have you given up work to sit by the video? Do you use it as a substitute for sex with her or can't perform without it? Then you've got problems best dealt with by a sex therapist. But research shows that the infrequent porn user is your average guy. It doesn't mean you don't love your girlfriend or find her sexy if you look at girlie mags. It doesn't mean you're comparing her to the girl on the page or screen or that you particularly want her to act like that. Men are turned on by pictures, women by words. You don't get upset when she curls up with a steamy novel, do you?

Why don't women like giving oral sex?

Some women think penises are unclean, 'yukky' or 'disgusting' because that's the place you pee from. Others have had a bad experience: some guy forced their head down until they gagged or maybe he didn't wash his genitals properly (particularly nasty if he's not circumcised). Some women don't like giving fellatio simply because they're frightened they'll gag and be sick, others don't like swallowing the semen at the end. If you shower regularly and thoroughly, let her control the position and depth, don't put your hands on the back of her head and don't make a fuss if she doesn't swallow, a lot more women would be converts. Let her know this is how you'll behave. Also tell her even if she's a novice, you don't really care what she does, it'll feel great. Men love oral sex because their girlfriend appears to be worshipping what he's worshipped since he discovered it – his penis. Plus, he gets to do nothing, while she becomes the aggressor.

Must I swallow?

Most men are so happy to have their penis in your mouth, not swallowing at the crucial moment is a small part of the whole process (only a handful think it's like watching the Cup Final without a beer). So long as you don't abandon him completely as he's about to climax, chances are he won't really care. Some women don't swallow but simply hold the semen in their mouths for a minute until they can spit it out in a tissue or the sink. Others switch to using a hand or let him thrust between their breasts.

I'm more turned on during my period than at any other time of the month. Should I warn a new lover or just continue having sex?

Definitely warn him – looking down to see blood isn't pleasant even when you are expecting it; when you're not, it's run-out-of-the-room stuff. If you have your period and want to have intercourse, all you need to do is have an old towel handy (and hopefully a shower close by) and say something like, 'I've got my period but I don't want to wait. It doesn't worry me if it doesn't worry you.' Don't get too huffy if he baulks at the idea. Blood makes lots of us squeamish and remember, he's had a lifetime of women saying, 'I can't. I've got my

> **'Some men think if a woman's experienced and really gets into it, she must have slept with the Foreign Legion. I think there's nothing *worse* than a girl who lies there like a sack of potatoes. If she doesn't seem interested, I'm not either. Moan, move, sprout Russian – do *something* to let us know if you're enjoying it.'**
> Alex, 32, architect

period.' He may just need a little time to get used to it. For some women, the thought of having sex during their period is unthinkable; others can't see what all the fuss is about. It depends on your mood and the heaviness of your flow.

He wants to know how many lovers I've had. How many should I admit to? Must I tell the truth?

What you did before you met him is your business, what he did before meeting you is his. There's no obligation to tell him anything at all about your sexual past unless it could directly affect his health. If you do decide to bare all, be aware that you will be judged – and not necessarily by the same rules he judges himself on. If he confesses to 50 lovers, your 15 may still be five too many. The most commonly cited statistic is 10 lovers for the 'average' female. Just who she is, is anyone's guess. It also depends on your age – a 25-year-old would reasonably be expected to have had more lovers than an 18-year-old. Plenty of women sleep with just one or two people, others clock up more than 50 guilt-free and lots hover around the 20 to 30 mark. Instead of reducing your sexual history to a number, why not let the truth slowly emerge over the years? As the relationship deepens, you soon figure out each other's significant previous relationships. The rest don't count.

OTHER RELATIONSHIP WRECKERS

Unless that's *all* you're in it for, you can't separate sex from your relationship. Here are some common couple 'love' complaints and how to handle them.

My boyfriend cheated on me when we were going through a problem patch and I can't forget about it

Don't try because you won't. Some couples do survive infidelity, most don't. A lot depends on his reason. The fact that he was drunk and it just happened isn't acceptable to most people. Did he wear a condom? If he was together enough to get it out of the wrapper, he was lucid enough to spare you a thought. Could he get an erection? He wasn't that drunk. Saying sorry isn't enough. You need to find out why he did it and why he thinks he won't do it again. If he's remorseful for a few weeks then gets tired of discussing the subject, ditch him now. *He* screwed up, you're the one trying to live with *his* mistake, so it's up to *him* to make you feel better. If you've only just started going out and you still can't look at him months later without feeling angry, give it a miss. If you've been going out for years and intellectually understand why he did it (even if it still hurts like hell), hang in there for six months, maybe even get some counselling. But it's up to him to earn back your trust. Sometimes an affair can unearth problems and something good comes out of it. Most of the time it simply means he can't control himself and doesn't respect you.

> **'I appreciate that lots of women aren't obvious when they orgasm but does he have to ask if I've had one every five minutes? I'll just be starting to enjoy oral when his head pops up to ask the question. It puts me off and I feel like I have to hurry. I wish he'd shut-up and get on with it.'**
>
> Erica, 19, journalist

I love my fiancé but I can't honestly say I lust after him. Am I being too picky to want chemistry when everything else is so perfect?

No. A relationship without sexual attraction is friendship. If you don't lust after your boyfriend, he's your best friend, not a prospective husband. This is hard to accept and there are plenty of people out there who will tell you to ignore my advice and marry him anyway. If you do, I hope you have a happy, contented life together but I fear you'll spend most of it eyeing up waiters, flirting with the butcher and probably having a series of sex affairs. Living a sexless life isn't fair on you and it's not fair on him. He might do nothing for your libido but there's someone out there who thinks he's sex-on-legs. Let her find him. If you're lucky and treat the situation sensitively, your fiancé could well end up being what he should have always been: a very special friend.

My partner constantly eyes up other women. How do I stop him?

There's a difference between noticing and admiring good looking people and that creepy undressing-with-their-eyes lecherous leer some men have perfected. The first is normal, the second disrespectful. He'll probably say you're 'paranoid', 'jealous' or 'insecure' when you confront him. Some women *do* over-react, so do a reality check first. Ask a well-trusted friend (even better, a well-trusted ex) if they think you have a history of imagining things. If they don't, you're convinced you're viewing the situation objectively and you really like the guy, start by telling him calmly how much you dislike him looking at other women while you're with him. Ask him to stop it. If he denies he behaves that way in the first place, simply say, 'Great. But I just want you to know it upsets me.' Wait until you've been out a few times to see if there's an improvement. If there isn't, sit him down again and say that unless he stops now, you're not interested in being with him. If he changes his tune immediately, give him *one* more chance. If he doesn't and you find it intolerable, leave.

***!** Number of women who think men judge their sexual attractiveness by the size of their breasts: 25 per cent. Number of men who admit to it: 11 per cent.*

My partner is smothering me. She wants to be with me every second, calls (the few hours) when we aren't together and sucks every last drop of energy I have. I love her but when I ask her to give me space, she gets upset

Relationships guru Barbara De Angelis calls people like this 'emotional vampires' and that's exactly what they are: desperately needy, scared of being alone, feeding off your energy, your *life*. The constant attention is tremendously flattering to start with but quickly becomes tremendously irritating. The fact is, no matter how much time or love you give her, it will never be enough. Someone or something has hurt her in the past – and you're not her therapist. Don't hang around out of pity (or fear that she'll do something 'silly').

Do suggest she seeks professional help to unravel why she's so insecure. People who love themselves aren't leeches – they enjoy their own company and draw on their own resources rather than always relying on others.

My old boyfriend/ girlfriend hurt me badly. I'm taking it *very* slow with my new lover but am frightened I'll never love again

19 – 5 = happy: Count the number of times you and your partner had sex last month, then subtract the number of arguments you had over the same period. A positive number means your relationship is strong. A negative number means you've got a lot more to solve than just this sum!

Good for you. It's prudent and sensible to take it slowly. You really *shouldn't* wear your heart on your sleeve: it belongs where nature put it – protected inside. Keep your eyes wide open, look at your new partner objectively and don't rush things. Make sure you've learned from old mistakes. Why did the relationship break down? Did you pick the wrong person or were you also at fault? Work on your self-esteem. You deserve to be treated well – don't settle for anything less.

I've been seeing a girl for months but still never met her friends or family. What's the story?

Pretty much what you fear, I suspect. There are some situations which could explain it: like she's married (do you ever meet at her home?) or recently separated (she doesn't feel the people close to her are ready to be introduced to a new lover). Alternatively, maybe her friends and family have given her previous boyfriends a hard time and she's protecting you. But if she appears to adore them, refuses to discuss the problem and simply doesn't include you, she either doesn't think you're good enough to parade in public or can't see a future together. Ask her outright, don't be fobbed off and have pride.

THE THREESOME THAT WORKS: UNHAPPY COUPLE PLUS COUNSELLOR

Lucky I'm not in charge of granting wedding licenses – I'd refuse to hand one over until all in-love couples had counselling. Look at it this way: would you go and see a doctor if he didn't have qualifications? Then why commit to live with someone for the rest of your life if they don't have good relationship skills? Counselling isn't just a way to repair the past, it's great preparation for the future.

There's a psychological questionnaire now available called 'Prepare'. You can't pick one up at your local newsagent but most good psychologists have it. Based on 12 major areas (like communication, children, sex and conflict resolution), 'Prepare' can predict what bits of your relationship you both need to work on and which are coasting along nicely. Do it *before* you move in or get married and you'll know what you're up against. The counsellor will also give you practical tips on handling the problems before you hit them. Makes sense to me.

Already in a serious relationship which isn't too fab? You've got two options: walk out or work it out. If counselling can't save the relationship you're in, the next will benefit from it anyway!

Get help if you're:

- arguing about the same things, over and over.
- feeling irritable and moody, bored or frustrated.
- finding excuses not to be together and spending less time with each other.
- not having regular sex.
- feeling like you're 'beating your head against a brick wall' when you talk to each other.
- noticing (and fancying) others.
- feeling more like flatmates than lovers.
- considering ending it – or having an affair.

FOUR THINGS MEN WISH WOMEN KNEW ABOUT SEX

1. We hate pillow talk.
2. We love it when you're obviously sexy.
3. We hate it if you just lie there.
4. The only lumps we notice on your body are your breasts.

FOUR THINGS WOMEN WISH MEN KNEW ABOUT SEX

1. We don't want to sleep with King Dong.
2. We don't want you to go on all night.
3. Asking 'Have you come yet?' stops it happening.
4. Saying something nice afterward is a good idea.

What will happen if we go to a counsellor?

> **!** ***Researchers claim British men are more likely to ditch their wives or girlfriends than any other nationality!***

It depends on what state your relationship's in and how good your communication skills are. Most troubled couples have between six and 12 hour-long sessions, starting off once a week, then spreading them out over a longer period. During the first session, the counsellor will talk about your problems and get an idea of the relationship dynamics – your personalities and how you relate to each other. After that, they'll start problem solving, put some action plans in place and teach skills. Don't be surprised if the problem you went for doesn't turn out to be the real issue. While him not helping around the house is driving you nuts, it could be his refusal to even consider marriage that's *really* bothering you.

A good therapist will tailor a program to suit you both, but make no mistake, it will be incredibly demanding. For a start, you'll be given lots of 'homework' (no point learning skills unless you practise them) and it's hard to break old habits, even if you know they're getting you nowhere. (P.S. The counsellor won't tell you if it's best you split, but they will guide you in that direction if they honestly think you're beyond help.)

Counselling works for couples:

- who get help early. The sooner you go, the less damage the problems will cause long-term.
- who want the therapy to work. If one of you has fallen out of love or is going under sufferance, the odds aren't tipped in your favour.
- who have a sense of humour. If you can laugh together, you're off and running.

Counselling doesn't work for couples:

- in the middle of a crisis. By the time you've sorted out the mess, you're too exhausted to work on change and you settle back into your old habits.
- who use it as a last resort. If one of you has already decided to leave, counselling just softens the blow.

- if one (or both) of you is having an affair and has no intention of ending it. Do I really need to explain why?
- who think the therapist will solve all their problems. They can only help you help yourselves.
- who aren't prepared to change. If you're so addicted to work/your friends/Friday night football and refuse to put the relationship first, the prospects aren't great.

How to find one

Call the British Psychological Society (look up the number in the Yellow Pages) and ask for a list of recommended counsellors in your area. You might get one on the NHS and some private health funds cover it. Lifeline and community groups offer free counselling; some private psychologists will charge you pro-rata on what you earn.

THE EX-FACTOR

Sometimes, sex problems stem from an unhealthy obsession with an unfairly intoxicating ex who seemed to steal your libido along with that favourite CD. If you're still fantasising about an old lover months or years on (come on – no-one's that good!), try the following.

1. Write down why sex was so great with them: what you did (be as specific as possible), where you did it, why it felt sensational. It'll lean heavier on one of two sides: you'll discover the physical act was irrelevant and it was the person that turned you on *or* you did things with them you haven't done with others.
2. Can you recreate it? If it was the person, think about the circumstances of your life at the time. You can't compare dating Bill in humdrum, daily life to bonking Brad while holidaying in Bali. Put Brad in your *real* life and sex would seem just as mundane. Utterly convinced it was a case of chemistry? Fine. If it's that important to you, hang out until the sparks fly with someone else. If you're pining over what you did during sex, what's stopping you doing it with your new partner? Don't tell him ➢

how great it felt when Brad teased your clitoris with his tongue, tell him how great it would feel if *he* did it.

3. Do a reality check. Still convinced they're the only person who can ever make you feel like that again? You're not only being unrealistic, it's futile. For a start, you've idealised it: *no-one's* that good in the sack. Go back to the start of the exercise, work out what it was that made sex so earth-shattering, then find someone to recreate it with.
4. Look hard at the relationship you're in. Is it a bandaid? Are you having sex to dull the pain? Or are you so blinded by the past, you can't see that what you've got is actually better? Decide which category it falls into, then do something about it. Leave or give it 100 per cent. Get some therapy if you seriously can't let go on your own.

8

Serious Sex-related Issues

Coping with the aftermath of abortion, rape and incest

There are some sex-related problems that no-one likes to talk about; consequently information is scarce and myths abound. This chapter is for women and men who have suffered the devastation of sexual abuse, either as a child or an adult, and I've also included a section for women who are contemplating having, or have had, a pregnancy terminated.

I've only scratched the surface of the emotions you may be struggling with but hopefully you'll find helpful, practical information and answers to your most commonly asked questions.

HAVING A TERMINATION

About 65 million abortions are performed worldwide per year. Despite the fact that safe abortion is readily available, most women would probably prefer not to think about it, let alone have one. Unfortunately, you may need to at some stage in your life. This is what to expect if you do.

What should I do if I think I'm at risk of an unwanted pregnancy?

If you've had unprotected sex, go to a doctor and get the Morning After Pill. Taken within 72 hours, it will stop the pregnancy from happening. Having an IUD inserted within five days of conception is another option. If it's too late for either, pick up a home pregnancy test from a chemist (they're almost 100 per cent accurate) and test two days after your missed period. Family Planning clinics also offer on-the-spot pregnancy testing.

What are my options if I am pregnant?

You have three: have the baby and keep it, put it up for adoption or have an abortion. Deciding which is best for you isn't easy. For some women, falling accidentally pregnant is a blessing in disguise. For others, particularly young women or those not in a serious, long-term relationship, it's devastating.

Some of the questions you need to ask yourself include:

- Do I want to bring up a child with the father? Would I have stayed with him if I wasn't pregnant?
- If I go it alone, do I think the child will suffer from not having a father? How will I cope as a single parent?
- Am I emotionally mature and able to cope with a child and all the associated responsibilities?
- How would I cope with the emotional fallout of adopting out a child I've carried.
- Will having a child affect my earning capacity? Will I feel resentful later because it detrimentally affected my career and my lifestyle? Can I/we financially afford to support a child?
- Do I have a good support network – family and friends who will help out if I decide to have the baby?

You may also struggle with moral issues. For obvious reasons, abortion is a highly emotional subject. Some religions, cultures and anti-abortion campaigners (like the Right to Life organisation) believe it can't be justified under any circumstances (though some will make allowances for pregnancy resulting from rape). If you do decide to proceed with a termination, you may have to pass through protesters on the day of the procedure. If this concerns you, try to get it done during the week. (Most protests are scheduled for the weekends, particularly Saturdays.)

If adoption appeals, call the Social Services (look in the Yellow Pages, under 'Adoption'). Explain that you're considering adopting out your child and ask for counselling.

Should I tell the father?

Advice from the experts varies here. Some say, barring exceptional circumstances (you were sexually abused or fear the father may become violent), he should be told. If he has trouble fathering a child in the future, it's important for him to know he was fertile in the past. Others say, if it's a casual relationship, you'll gain little by confessing. But if the relationship is serious and you plan to continuing going out after the termination, it's probably advisable to share the burden. It takes two to get pregnant and telling him means you can support each other throughout the trauma. Despite the odd case in the United States, where fathers have taken women to court in a bid to stop them having an abortion, (at the time of publication) the father can't legally stop you having a termination.

Who do I call to arrange a termination?

There are specialist termination clinics in most cities, run privately or through public hospitals. Many private gynaecologists also perform abortions; simply get a referral from your doctor. Otherwise, call Family Planning, consult a friend who's had one or look up the Yellow Pages under 'abortion' or 'termination'. Be aware that some Right to Life groups list their numbers under these headings. How do you know you're not calling one? You don't, but it will become obvious. Explain that you want a termination, ask how much it costs and a few medical questions (about things like physical complications) and it will soon become clear whether the group performs abortions or wants to counsel you to change your mind.

You can make an appointment over the phone. Terminations are free on the NHS or you can choose to pay for one at a private clinic.

Is it legal?

Abortion is legal as long as it complies with the 1967 Abortion Act which in effect means that two doctors have to be satisfied that you need and can legally have an abortion. Both doctors have to be willing to sign the necessary legal papers.

When is it too late to have one?

The best time is between your sixth and twelfth week of pregnancy; they can't operate before the sixth week because the fetus is so small it's easily missed. Some clinics will operate up to 18 weeks, but the more advanced you are, the more it costs, the more complicated and unpleasant it is and the higher the risks. If you're 18 weeks or over, it's a two-day procedure. On the first, you have counselling, an ultrasound and dilators inserted into your cervix which stay in overnight; you come back the next morning for the actual operation. A few clinics will perform terminations on women who are 20 weeks pregnant, but that's usually the cut-off point.

What will happen to me on the day?

In most clinics, counselling and the procedure are done on the same day with the whole process taking between three and four hours. You'll fill out some paperwork on your arrival, then be taken in for a counselling session to ensure the decision to have a termination was yours and that you're happy to proceed.

The counsellor will ask questions like: Did someone else pressure you into having the abortion? Did you consider having the baby? How do you think you'll feel afterward? If the counsellor is not totally convinced it is your choice, they won't give permission for the operation. They'll also send you away to think things through if you're not certain you're doing the right thing. If you haven't told anyone about it (you're too embarrassed or worried people will judge you), the clinic may arrange for support through community or private counselling.

Counselling will also focus on the reason you're there in the first place: ineffective (or no) contraception. They'll help find a method of birth control that suits you, perhaps give you a Pill prescription or Depo Provera injection (which covers you for three months). They'll also go through your medical history, check you get regular Pap smears and talk about general sexual health (like the importance of wearing condoms).

If the decision is made to go ahead with the abortion, you'll be seen by two doctors: one who will sedate you and one who will perform the procedure. Then you'll be asked to change into a T-shirt or nightie (which you will have been told to bring with you) and taken into the operating theatre. Most clinics use intravenous sedation as well as injecting local anaesthetic into the cervix. The sedation ensures you won't feel pain during the operation and you may even not remember it.

There are various methods of performing an abortion but all involve removing the products of conception from the uterus: the placenta, the sac, an embryo (up to 8 weeks after conception) or fetus (after 8 weeks). The technique is called *suction curettage* and it's similar to the dilate and curette (D and C) procedure sometimes used to investigate abnormal bleeding. The cervix is numbed with a local anaesthetic and gently dilated, allowing a fine tube to be inserted into the uterus. The contents of the uterus are then suctioned out and the walls gently scraped with an instrument called a curette. The entire procedure takes between 5 and 10 minutes.

Afterward, you'll be taken to a recovery room to rest for an hour or so and given something to eat and drink. A nurse will check the bleeding, take your blood pressure and pulse and ensure you're coping emotionally. It's wise to rest when you get home and to take it easy for a few days since you'll feel physically tired and emotionally drained.

What if I change my mind?

Some women decide they've made the wrong decision as they're taken into the operating theatre. This is totally acceptable. You'll simply be sent home and told to come back if you decide to go ahead with the termination. (About 50 per cent of women return.)

How will I feel afterwards?

Physically

Many women experience a cramping pain on the first day, and most bleed. Some bleed heavily for a few days, then it lightens and should stop completely within 7 to 10 days. Intercourse, swimming and baths (though you can shower) are not allowed for at least two weeks until the cervix returns to normal. You're also not allowed to use tampons (use pads instead) for the same period. The clinic will give you a week's supply of antibiotics to avoid infection. After two weeks, you'll need a check-up either at the clinic, Family Planning or with your doctor to ensure there's no infection and the uterus has returned to its normal size.

> **'I got pregnant when I was 15 and my mother wouldn't let me have an abortion. I was forbidden to tell anyone and sent away to a home for unmarried, pregnant women when it started to show. My baby was taken from me and given to adoptive parents immediately after the birth. I didn't even get to hold her. It screwed me up for years and I've never forgiven my family. Why couldn't they have just organised an abortion rather than put me through all that pain?'**
>
> Wendy, 35, housewife

Complications are rare in the UK because most abortions are performed by experienced doctors. But there are two things that can go wrong: infection (make sure you take the full course of your antibiotics and alert the clinic of abnormal bleeding and/or pain) or 'retained product'. Retained product means they missed some of the fetus. Emotionally that can be hard to cope with, but physically it's easily fixed. Persistent bleeding, passing blood clots or cramping pain (similar to a really heavy period) are all warning signs. If this happens, you need to go back to the clinic for another curette.

One termination won't usually affect future pregnancies. Some doctors claim 10 won't either, as long as they're all performed by experienced doctors and you have no complications. Others say frequently dilating the cervix can make it 'incompetent' (unable to support a fetus) or cause scar tissue.

Emotionally

Judging by the latest research, the vast majority of women who've had an abortion don't suffer long-term emotional trauma. But the best clue to how you'll cope is your mental well-being before the termination. One recent US report, which focused on more than 5000 women who'd had an abortion in an ongoing study, found those with high self-esteem were able to put the event behind them and get on with their life. In other words, those who found the procedure traumatic were troubled long before they showed up at an abortion clinic.

Having said that, there is obviously some emotional fallout. Almost all women experience a bewildering mix of relief and grief afterward. Even if you know it was the correct decision for you, you may mourn the loss and need to work through feelings of sadness, anger or guilt. (Don't confuse regret with sadness – just because you feel sad, doesn't necessarily mean you've done the wrong thing.) It's important that you talk through any feelings you're experiencing, either with a counsellor or a non-judgemental friend or relative. Try keeping a diary for a few weeks or months afterward. Record how you feel about the loss of the baby as well as the man who fathered it. If he left you, it's a good way to vent anger; if you didn't tell him, write him a letter (even if you don't send it). You'll also experience hormonal changes (like depression) because you've gone from being pregnant to not pregnant. It can take up to a week to readjust hormonally.

How will the father feel?

You're not the only one who may struggle with guilt and grief and *both* of you may view sex differently. Some men are so fearful of it happening again, they'll avoid sex, have trouble getting an erection or not want to orgasm inside you. You may also lose enthusiasm for obvious reasons. Usually, time heals; if it doesn't, get professional counselling.

CHILDHOOD SEXUAL ABUSE

As a child, you were probably told not to talk to strangers. In reality, you're far more likely to be abused by someone who's a member of, or well-known by, your family. Usually it's a close relative. In the western world 17 per cent of men and 25 per cent of women are believed to have been sexually abused at some stage of their life. According to a study by the Australian Institute of Criminology, more than 42 per cent of sexual assault victims are under the age of 15. Most people are horrified by these statistics but it's a sad fact that abuse, particularly childhood sexual abuse (like incest), is common.

Unfortunately, that doesn't make it any less emotionally devastating for its victims. If you were abused as a child, or suspect you might have been, please seek professional help rather than simply reading this section of the book. It's designed as a starting point only. Obviously, this information is aimed at adults who've been abused in the past, not at the children tragically suffering now.

'My father sexually abused me from age 4 to 12 but refuses to acknowledge it because he didn't penetrate me with his penis. I confronted him when I turned 20, after confessing to a close girlfriend. I said I remembered him making me perform oral sex and him doing the same to me and all he said was, "Don't be silly. That was just a game we played." My mother doesn't believe me and the police said I didn't have a strong enough case to prosecute. But he knows I remember and I tell everyone what happened. I don't care if they don't believe me, at least I'm planting doubt in their mind.'

Shirley, 32, nurse

When is child abuse usually 'found out'?

In the vast majority of cases, abuse is not discovered at the time it is happening because incredible pressure is put on the child to keep quiet; usually, the abuser tells the child they'll harm them or someone they love if they tell. Occasionally, an astute teacher or parent will notice sexual knowledge that seems inappropriate for the child's age or unusual or sudden depression, aggression or even suicidal tendencies. Or the child gets pregnant or picks up a sexually transmitted disease. Sometimes, if the memory of abuse is buried, it can burst out later in life through some significant experience – perhaps when you have your own children or your kids reach the age when you were abused. Even watching a program or reading an article about abuse can trigger the memory and cause someone to seek help.

What emotions and feelings usually result from abuse?

At the time of the assault, regardless of your age and sex, you felt totally terrified or shocked, possibly disorientated. Immediately after, you were in crisis: you experienced anything from hysteria and tears to feeling cold and cut off from your emotions. You may have fluctuated between the two. Older girls may feel ashamed, disgusted and blame themselves. A few people are furious (this is a good sign as it shows your 'sense of self' is intact), lots of others kick into denial or ***minimisation***. They think, 'I can't deny it happened but it wasn't so bad. I'll put it behind me and won't let it drag me down.' This head-in-the-sand approach usually doesn't work because it's very difficult to work through the after effects of abuse without facing up to them.

Other people develop *post traumatic stress disorder* (PTSD), a condition where you're susceptible to reliving the event whenever a *trigger* sets off a memory (something reminds you of the event). War veterans who dive to the ground when they hear a car backfire like a bomb are suffering from PTSD. For you, it might be the bristles on a man's face, the smell of aftershave, the feel of a naked body or the act of penetration itself.

A common reaction is to feel responsible for the abuse, that somehow you 'asked for it'. Rape victims think, 'It was my fault for walking down that dark street.' Childhood abuse victims think, 'Maybe I acted like it was okay; maybe I didn't make it clear enough that I didn't want to do it.' Because of this, you keep your mouth shut and suffer guiltily and silently.

What about people who remember years later they've been abused? Can memories be put into people's heads by overenthusiastic psychologists?

Most therapists are adamant that at the age of 30 you can suddenly remember what happened to you when you were 12. This is because our psychological defences, through a process called *disassociation*, sometimes don't allow us to experience or remember 'bad' things. In extreme cases, particularly if you were very young, you may have felt like you left your body while you were being abused (as though it was happening to someone else, not you, and you were watching).

People can disassociate in four different ways: from the sensations (you can't remember the feeling of the person touching you), the behaviour (you don't register what the person actually did), the emotions (you take away your emotional reaction of fear, terror or sadness) or the knowledge (you deny the experience ever happened). You can disassociate from all four things or any combination of them. So it's quite possible that you have no conscious memory of what happened to you, particularly if the abuse was violent or ongoing or by someone very close to you. You may sense *something* bad happened – feel depressed and fearful your entire life – but not know why. Later, at a time when your brain decides you're strong enough to remember, something can happen to bring back the memories.

Needless to say, discovering you've been abused as a child is intensely shocking. Therapists who specialise in abuse say the emotional after-effects are something you wouldn't wish on your worst enemy. So it's unlikely they'll 'plant' memories in your head or encourage you to remember things that didn't actually happen.

How can I tell if I've been abused but 'forgotten' it?

Common signs of past abuse are often caused by events other than abuse, so don't jump to conclusions! But some things to look for are difficulties in forming and maintaining relationships and problems with sex. If you were repeatedly abused as a child, how you dealt with the abuse can be carried through to your adult life. Feeling like it's not really happening to you, feeling numb or weirdly uninvolved during sex could be a sign. You may also feel extremely vulnerable. Vaginismus (when the vaginal muscles spasm and prevent penetration) is a common reaction; so is pain on intercourse, and not being able to orgasm or get aroused at all. Alternatively, so is being overly promiscuous: you may be trying to 'prove' there's nothing wrong with you. High achievers, people who strive to be perfect, and 'good' people are also possible victims. Abuse often leaves you feeling like you're a 'bad' person, so you try, often unrealistically, to be as pure as the driven snow.

Childhood abuse is a gross betrayal of trust, and trust is central to almost all human interaction. Children don't just trust those who are close to them; we start out with an inherent belief that people in general won't hurt us. So feeling abnormally cautious and paranoid may also be a warning sign.

Where do I get help?

The surest route to ridding yourself of the effects of abuse is through counselling. Your doctor can refer you to a psychologist or you can call any major hospital – most have assault units. Alternatively, ring a helpline, such as the London Centre on 0171 837 1600. You could also call the British Psychological Society for recommendations of psychologists who specialise in that area. For therapy to work, it's imperative you feel you can trust your counsellor (check they're qualified and registered with the British Psychological Society for a start). Even if you haven't got a logical reason not to trust or like a particular therapist, keep searching until you find someone you do feel comfortable with.

What will happen if I accuse or charge the person?

Most people spend the first half of their life trying to deny they've been abused, and the second half acknowledging it happened and trying to get over it. Therapy drags up feelings you've buried for years and you may feel incredibly angry at the person who did it to you. It's often at this point that the truth finally comes out: you decide to accuse the person, perhaps take them to court, or confess to the rest of your family what happened.

In 1995, 2272 cases of sexual assault (child and adult) were reported to the NSW police. In the same year, 218 people charged with a sexual offence against a child were dealt with in local courts, 341 in higher courts. A lot of charges are withdrawn or there's insufficient evidence to proceed, though, according to most therapists, very rarely is an allegation made that isn't founded on truth.

One reason you may decide not to proceed is family pressure: other members may be terrified of the scandal it will cause. If you're accusing your father and he's still supporting your mother and other children, it could mean she and they will lose their income if he's convicted. In the vast majority of cases, however, victims are supported by their families. A child is easily silenced and often accused of 'telling tales'. An adult is more powerful, able to articulate what happened and a lot more likely to be believed. (Your therapist won't recommend you tell your family because it's *you* who has to wear the consequences. If you feel they are pushing you to do so against your will, report them to the British Psychological Society and change counsellors.)

Sadly, most perpetrators of sexual abuse aren't arrested or charged. Often, the person is dead or (thankfully) no longer in your life and you don't know how to find them. Of those that are charged, relatively few are found guilty. Your chances of winning the case are higher if you told people along the way: maybe a girlfriend, sister or your mother. Repressed memory – discovering later in life you were abused – is still a bit of a hot potato in the courts but a competent solicitor can advise you on the strength of your case.

What will a counsellor do?

The road to recovery is different for each person. It depends not only on the degree of damage done but also on practical things like your finances, how much time you have and how you're able to handle the emotions it unearths. Usually, you'll be counselled at least once a week for between two and five years, talking during these sessions about things you'd still rather avoid remembering. It's a painful and draining process and humans are oddly resistant to change: part of us is more comfortable with the way things are now, even though it's horrible. There's no short-term cure, though you'll progress faster if you're highly motivated and attend more than once a week. It's also acceptable to take breaks rather than do it all in one stint.

The counsellor will talk about your life, the abuse and how it's affecting you. It may take a long time before you're able to talk through a lot of what happened but that's normal – and far preferable to leaving the memories smouldering away inside. Some people aren't interested in counselling and find *doing* something helps restore their sense of power. Taking the person to court or helping someone else in the same situation by joining an action group are common reactions. At the end of the day, however, most victims find they need to sit down with another human being to work things through. And the best person for that job is a professional counsellor.

ADULT SEXUAL ASSAULT

Outdated, ridiculous and largely offensive myths still surround rape. Some of the more common ones include:

- Women attract rape by the way they dress and behave (only certain types of women get raped).
- Women secretly enjoy it.
- Men who rape are sick and can't help or control themselves.
- Rapists don't look like normal people.
- It's a woman's responsibility to control a man's behaviour.
- When a woman says 'no', she sometimes means 'yes'.
- Rape always involves violence or the use of a weapon.
- Unless you can show physical injury, don't bother reporting it.

All of the above are false. Rape or sexual assault is when a person is forced into any kind of sexual activity with someone, known or unknown to them, without their consent. In other words, *no-one has a legal right to touch any part of your body unless you want them to.* Let me reiterate two points because these are myths many women still believe. Rape doesn't always include physical force – verbal threats are just as (if not more) effective. Rape doesn't always include him putting his penis in your vagina. You can be raped with fingers or objects; you can be orally or anally raped. Don't believe anyone who tries to tell you this isn't true. Rape is now officially called 'sexual assault', though victims and workers in the field still usually refer to it as rape (which is why I have done so in this chapter).

As with childhood abuse, rapists usually know their victims in one way or another. We think they only hang around dark alleys, but they don't. Quite often they're someone we trust, even like. Family members, friends, acquaintances and colleagues count for about half of most offenders. A further one-fifth are people the victim met that day for the first time. More than half of all sexual assaults occur in the home – yours or his. In many cases, the victim let the rapist in – not surprising, given that she usually knows him. Outdoor areas like parks, the street and carparks are second favourites. Most assaults happen on Fridays and Saturdays between 6 pm and 6 am, rather than during the day with about 60 to 80 per cent of rapes happening at night.

'When I was in grade 10, a girl at my school pressed rape charges against another student. She was very academic and pretty, he was the quintessential good-looking school athlete. It divided the school: the girls believed her, the boys sided with him. But when he was found guilty, everything changed. We all knew how hard they'd been on the girl in court and we looked at her with a new respect. His reputation was shot. "Why did you do it? You could have any girl you wanted," I asked the guy. He answered with, "Mate, she asked for it and she wanted it." He had no guilt whatsoever.'

Tony, 26, electrician

Almost all the time, it's a man raping a woman. In the period 1989 to 1991 (the latest released figures), 90.2 per cent of the adult sexual assault victims reported to police in NSW were female. The average annual rate was about nine times higher than that for males (66.8 victims per 100,000 population, compared to 7.5 for men). Adult male rape isn't common, though it's becoming more so, particularly for gay men. If a man is sexually abused it's usually when he's a child or serving a gaol sentence and the abuser of a man is nearly always another man. For these reasons, I've slanted this section toward female rape victims though men will experience similiar feelings and (hopefully) receive the same treatment by police.

What should you do immediately after the attack?

Your first priority is safety: get yourself somewhere safe as fast as possible. If the rape happened in your home, lock all the doors and windows then ring a friend (or family) and the police on 999 or call your local police station. The police *prefer* you to call them first but totally understand that your first reaction is to call someone close to you. (Besides, they can be used later to testify if you take the matter to court.) If you don't want to call the police, contact a local sexual assault centre.

It's crucial that you don't wash your clothing. By all means change, but put the clothes straight into a bag to hand over to police. Don't wash yourself or treat any physical injuries and try not to smoke, eat or drink, particularly if you were orally raped (all could affect swabs that will be taken from your mouth, vagina and anus). Try not to go to the toilet until after your medical examination: that will also hinder the collection of forensic evidence. If it happened in your home, leave everything as it is – don't clean up. (If you're extremely distressed and do all of these things, don't panic – the police will be well aware you're not thinking straight.)

Emotionally, you'll react in a number of ways. You'll no doubt feel terrified the person will return, feel you've lost control and may go into shock. Some women feel (rightfully) furious; alternatively, you may feel guilty and blame yourself. You could be a confused, hysterical, blithering mess by the time the police arrive or feel strangely calm, unemotional and cold. Quite often, rape victims are rude to police (a male raped you, the police that attend are usually male). All reactions are common and normal; there's no 'expected' way for you to behave.

'I met this guy in a nightclub and he ended up coming back to my place for coffee. He'd spent the entire evening telling me how upset he was because his girlfriend had been raped recently and he didn't know how to handle it. I thought it was obvious we were just going to be friends and thought he'd be the last person to try anything. Wrong. The minute the door closed he pushed me back onto the couch, held me down with one hand and ripped my pants off with the other. I was terrified but kept my head. I told him I had to go to the bathroom to put my diaphragm in and when I came out, I walked straight to the phone and dialled 999 before he figured out what I was doing. The police answered immediately but he'd already bolted.'

Annette, 24, PR consultant

What will happen after you call the police?

If you live in a capital city, two of the closest available police officers will come out pretty well immediately, followed by an Initial Responses Officer and a detective. If you live in a country area, your local police officer will attend. They will question you and take a brief outline of what happened, examine and preserve the crime scene, and ask if you want (or will agree to) a medical examination, which needs to be done within 72 hours.

Even if you're not sure if you want to press charges, get the medical examination done. You'll also be asked if you want a sexual assault counsellor to come out immediately.

When you're up to it, they'll take you to a police station or hospital, where a doctor will do a medical examination (usually using a specially designed sexual assault investigation kit). The police will take a full statement and fill you in on what will happen if you press charges. The police won't push you to charge the rapist; it's up to you if you want to proceed formally. (If you don't, that'll be the end of it though they'll usually arrange some sort of follow-up counselling.) You're then allowed to go home and the police will start investigating the matter if you have chosen to press charges.

Usually, you're not needed again until your case is scheduled for court, though you might be asked to identify the attacker from pictures or a line-up if you didn't know them.

If your attacker threatened to return, the police can enforce strong bail conditions or take out apprehended violence orders with specified conditions (like not to assault, molest or harass you).

Unfortunately, you won't be assigned your very own police officer to protect you like they do in the movies, so you might consider moving in with your family or friends, or getting someone to live with you for a while if you live alone. It's a bit of a myth that attackers come back – they usually don't. Having said that, you'll understandably feel an intense need to be somewhere safe and it's wise to take precautions. Going straight home to an empty apartment isn't advisable.

What are the pros and cons of going through with the charge?

A very large number of sexual assaults are not reported to the police. According to the most recent victim study by the Australian Bureau of Statistics, only one-quarter of sexual assaults committed against women aged 18 and over are reported to police. Male victims are even less likely to report rape because of the stigma attached. So why don't we? Two common reasons are 'the police can't or won't do anything about it' or 'the incident is too "trivial" to make a fuss over' (especially if you're a date rape victim). Other reasons include feeling guilty or ashamed, worrying the police won't believe you or that the court case will be too stressful.

If you do report the crime, the majority of you do want to take it to court, especially if it's happened recently. (You can charge someone years later but lack of hard evidence, like a medical report, can decrease what could have been a strong case.)

Don't kid yourself if you do decide to press on: rape cases are very unpleasant for the victim. The rapist's defence team will use whatever they can dredge up to discredit you and paint a shining picture of their client. Technically, it's not legal to drag your past sexual history, what you were wearing or your character into the case, but that doesn't mean they won't try. All will be alluded to and used against you by a clever solicitor who's aware of the loopholes. You have to be pretty tough to get through. The police and a counsellor will support you but at the end of the day, the witness box is a pretty lonely place. You'll be asked to recount, in minute detail, the whole traumatic experience, possibly several times over. His lawyer will ask you questions which will make you feel that you're not believed, that you somehow 'asked' for it and that you said 'no' but your body language and behaviour screamed 'yes'. Stick to what happened and think before you answer seemingly innocent questions. I'm not telling you this to put you off, just so you know what you're in for.

A little over one-third of the sexual assault charges heard in the local and higher courts in NSW in 1991 were proven. If you win, it can be one of the most empowering moments of your life. If you lose, it's possibly the worst. You'll think people didn't believe you, but this often isn't the case. It simply means your attacker bought himself a good solicitor or, for some reason, your case was hard to prove. Some rape victims make better witnesses than others: they sound and look capable, are articulate and are very composed. Others are so traumatised they can do little more than cry.

How might people close to you react?

No two families are the same. Some will rally around and want to wrap you in cotton wool, others may not believe you or say things like 'I told you wearing mini-skirts will get you in trouble'. Friends are usually shocked, female friends frightened, both for you and themselves. Sometimes people won't want to believe that you're telling the truth because it means that they, too, are in danger. Because of this they may imply there was something you could have done to avoid it.

Your male friends, boyfriend, father and brother will probably experience feelings of intense anger and hatred for the rapist. Lots will plot revenge, though few follow through with it. This isn't your problem. Make it clear this won't help your case, then stay out of it. Sometimes family and friends will push you into pressing charges when you don't want to; other times the opposite occurs. It can depend on who the rapist was: a friend or neighbour or a stranger who grabbed you on a dark street. Regardless, make your own decision and don't be swayed by others.

According to the police I have spoken to, most boyfriends are supportive of their girlfriends (but that obviously depends on what sort of guy he was *before* the attack). If he loves you, he'll be angry at the rapist and tremendously concerned and supportive of you. He may also feel responsible, that it's his fault for not being there with you.

How might it affect you in the future?

Rape can (and usually does) have a profound effect on the lives of victims for many years after. It's a violating and traumatic experience. How *you* react depends on what sort of person you are, the seriousness of the attack, your feelings about yourself and your sexuality, your age, your cultural background, maybe your religion. Serious physical injury isn't typical (there's usually only minor cuts and bruising) but there are a wide range of psychological symptoms that just about all victims experience. Fear, anxiety, depression, anger, shame, sleep or eating disorders, and a feeling of powerlessness are all common. But by far the biggest effect will be on your sexual relationships. You may feel that you never want to have sex again. The thought of being touched, being naked, of someone just kissing you may make you feel physically sick. Again, this is normal and best solved by professional counselling.

You may feel a burning need to be believed and listened to. Psychologists call this 'validation' of the experience: you want others to appreciate how serious, horrible and terrifying the assault was and for it to be seen as significant. Long-term counselling is recommended for *all* rape victims; popping along for a few months after the attack usually isn't enough. Don't try to struggle alone with the issues. You might well come out the other side, but you'll do so a lot quicker if you talk to someone with experience in helping victims of sexual abuse. The police, any sexual assault service or centre, or the British Psychological Society can refer you to a qualified counsellor. You survived the attack – counselling can help you move on and get back to enjoying your life.

Who should I call if it happened a while ago?

Threats, feeling ashamed, not being able to talk about or face up to what happened – a lot of things can stop you seeking help immediately after an attack. Maybe you thought you could cope with it yourself but now find you need help. It doesn't matter if you were raped 1 month or 10 years ago, you can still file a complaint, press charges or seek counselling. Contact the police or a sexual assault service attached to a hospital or community health centre for referral to a counsellor. Many are open 24 hours a day. Alternatively, call the Social Services or the police or a helpline, such as the London Centre on 0171 837 1600, or find a rape crisis centre or support group. Many cities will have their own rape crisis helpline.

How can you lower the chances of being raped?

When you're out

- Don't overload yourself with parcels or wear clothes that will stop you running.
- Wait for public transport in well-lit areas. If possible, avoid catching buses and trains late at night or very early in the morning.

- Sit near the bus driver or in the guard carriage on trains.
- Leave your car in well-lit areas, not deserted back streets.
- Stick to main, well-lit roads at night and avoid walking through parks or other large, dark areas.

At home

- Install a peephole and deadlocks.
- If you have the cash, install an alarm and a panic button near your bed.
- Don't answer the door unless you're sure you know who's there, and it's someone you trust.

On dates

- Be assertive and clearly communicate what you do and don't want to happen sexually.
- Think twice before inviting him back for coffee or going to his house – especially if one, or both of you, is drunk.
- Some men think that if they pay for your meal you owe them sex. If you have doubts, consider paying for yourself until you know them better.
- Take your own car the first few times. It's not uncommon for 'dates' to drive their victims to an assault site on the way home.
- Trust your gut reaction. If you're out with someone who seems weird, go to the toilet and on the way tell the waiter or barman to call you a cab. Warn them that your date seems odd. Tell the guy you feel ill and have called a cab to take you home. Refuse his offer to drive you.

If you are attacked

- Running away is often the best solution. If you can, do it.
- If you can't run, make as much noise as possible. Carry an ear-piercing whistle and blow it; scream and shout. Use your legs to kick, your mouth to bite and hit him where it hurts (in the testicles, throat, stick two fingers in his eyes). Use your keys or handbag as a weapon.
- If you think you can carry it off, try talking your way out of it. Tell him you're pregnant and he'll kill the baby by raping you, say you're AIDS positive, have an attack of herpes – anything to dissuade him.

9

Fantasies

Drop the but-I-thought-you-loved-*me* stuff – steamy fantasies make for even steamier real-life romps

I had my first sexual fantasy when I was seven years old and I'm ashamed to say it was about Engelbert Humperdinck. My father was dead keen on this singer, who looked twice as daggy as he sounds and was at least 100 years old even back then. Brylcreamed hair styled into rippling, Bob Hawke-like waves, swarthy skin set off by shiny suits, eyebrows a girl could tangle her fingers in – I thought he was sex-on-legs. Trouble was, I really didn't know what sex *was*, a fact that becomes rather obvious from the fantasy. I used to imagine that I'd kidnap Engelbert and keep him around the side of our house. (For some reason, he was quite happy to do nothing but stand on a concrete path for days on end.) I'd sneak out to visit him and then he would – wait for it – *roll bacon rinds up my arms*. What a turn-on, eh! Why the thought of this produced such a pleasant, naughty shiver up my girly spine is utterly beyond me. I've examined those record covers a million times since but still can't figure the connection between Engelbert and bacon fat – except maybe that they're both slimy.

You'll be relieved to hear my subsequent fantasies haven't come close to matching the oddness of that little gem but, like millions of others, I still thoroughly enjoy letting my imagination run riot. Just about everyone fantasises: men, women and (obviously) children and there are lots of reasons why. In fantasy land, there are no rules. No-one can accuse us of being right or wrong, nice or nasty, perverted, dirty or plain revolting because (thank God) no-one's invented a device to read minds. So, we're free to invent idealised situations that are totally impractical or unattainable in real life. Pimples, cellulite, cramps, periods, pissed off girlfriends or boyfriends, smelly genitals and children wanting biscuits – they all magically disappear in fantasies. Our dream lovers know exactly when, how and what to do to make us giddy with desire because *we're* directing the show.

No two people conjure up exactly the same fantasy but there is a unifying thread to them all: a longing to escape from what's socially acceptable. In real life, ripping off your secretary's skirt and bending her over your desk will land you a sexual harassment charge. In your fantasy, it gets you the blow-job of your life. Fantasies are a welcome escape from the stress of day-to-day living. Daydreaming about some gorgeous Jamaican delivering more than a cocktail on a sun-drenched beach is infinitely more appealing than worrying where next week's rent is coming from.

Most of the time, our fantasies revolve around things we'd never want to try in reality – some would ***horrify*** us if they actually happened. (Arriving home to find your girlfriend in bed with six workmen is a hell of a lot different from aimlessly daydreaming about it.) But their effect on our libido and sex life is immense all the same and, in some instances, our fantasies ***would*** delight us by coming true. The more you fantasise, the higher your libido. What came first, the chicken or the egg, is anyone's guess but it's pretty well established that the more you think about sex, the more you want it. That makes fantasies the cheapest, most effective sex aid around. Even better, they're tailor-made to suit the user. We can turn them on or off at will and they introduce variety into our sex lives without the complications and devastation of real-life affairs. They add the spice of infidelity without a price to pay for it.

Fantasy and masturbation go together like bacon and eggs and lots of people have one favourite that always guarantees an orgasm. Studies show more than 50 per cent of us fantasise every time we make love with our partner. Sexperts estimate the *real* figure (that is, when our partners aren't watching over our shoulder to see what survey box we tick) to be much higher. Of those that do fantasise during sex, all report a much more satisfying love life than those who don't. And our fantasies aren't necessarily about other people or other situations. Often, we'll imagine how we look or picture what our partner is doing to us as they're doing it, because we can't 'see' with our eyes because of the position.

Whatever the motivation and whatever *your* brain conjures up, you'd be hard pressed finding a sex therapist who didn't include fantasy in a recipe for hot sex. Here are a rundown on our most common themes, some real-life confessions, and hints on how to use them to enhance your sex life, both in and out of bed.

IN HIS DREAMS: THE 10 MOST COMMON MALE SEX FANTASIES

'What are you thinking darling?' she asks, snuggled up romantically on the couch, one head on your shoulder. 'Er . . . um . . . how much I love you.' 'Oh, how sweet!' she gushes. What was really running through your head was any of the following . . .

1. Fantasies about your current partner

No kidding. This is the number one sex fantasy for most men: things you've done, or would like to do, to your girlfriend. (It's her top fantasy too, by the way). Forget big-breasted blonde Swedish women begging for more – scenarios featuring your girlfriend are far more frequent and likely. Why? Because available flesh-and-blood is sometimes more of a turn on than the unattainable – there's a good chance it could come true or has already.

2. Having sex with a woman other than your partner

Often, she's a past lover, a friend of your girlfriend, perhaps a celebrity. The psychology behind this one isn't too difficult to work out: lots of people long to have sex with someone new and fantasy is a great way of indulging this longing without losing your partner in the process. If the woman in the fantasy is a virgin, you've cast yourself in the teacher role, initiating her into hedonistic pleasures through your skilful lovemaking. If she's got big boobs, choose from a variety of psychological theories. Freudians would say you haven't cut the apron strings; breasts (ie., sucking on Mum's) are a symbol of your childhood. More sensible therapists would say you're one of those blokes who equate big breasts with the ultimate sexy women.

3. Giving or receiving oral sex

This is near the top of the list for both sexes. Fantasy fellatio has one vital ingredient: the woman doesn't do it to *give* pleasure. She does it to *get* pleasure – worshipping your mighty penis, slurping, gobbling, begging you to let her take it into her mouth, giving long, lascivious licks. She accompanies the head-job with comments like 'God, it's huge' and (of course) not only swallows every last drop of sperm but licks her lips afterward. This one's heaven for just about all men (and a very easy one for her to turn into reality).

Fantasies about giving her oral sex aren't surprising either. Many women are more obviously turned on by oral than intercourse and as the ultimate pleasure-giver, this is what you *know* will drive her *craaazzy*. Plus there's still a part of us that secretly thinks of oral sex as 'dirtier' than intercourse, hence the huge turn-on factor.

4. Sex with two or more women

This is the adult male equivalent of the childhood fantasy of being accidentally locked up in a sweet shop. If having sex with one woman feels good, having sex with two *must* be double the fun. Throw in some lesbian lovemaking and this one sends most of you drifting off into la-la land with an if-only expression on your face. In your fantasy, you're super-stud: capable of bringing both women to screaming orgasms, over and over. In reality, lots of you worry (consciously or unconsciously) whether you're truly satisfying just one, so it's not surprising this is dream-fodder. Studies show the vast majority of men don't want (and actually couldn't cope with) such sexual demands in real life.

! *Fifty-five per cent of men have fantasised about a threesome compared to 27 per cent of women.*

'Orgy' type fantasies not only remove real-life logistical problems ('Umm, would you mind moving your leg? Your toe's going right up my nose'), but you can magically orgasm time and time again. Watching two women make love (especially women you know – your partner is often one of them) is another common male fantasy. The classic version has you arriving home from work unexpectedly to find your partner, dressed in some wispy thing, curled up on the bed with a divine-looking 'friend/goddess'. Hands, handcuffs and definitely tongues feature, but the climax is always them begging you to join in, so they can experience 'the real thing'.

5. Watching others have sex and/or being watched

It's called voyeurism (watching) and exhibitionism (being watched). In reality, few people would be able to stop themselves looking at a couple having sex if they were guaranteed not to get caught, but voyeurism is a fantasy, of both sexes, because sex is private and mostly hidden. Sure, we watch couples do it on telly, but it's rare we get to see *the real thing,* and there's also a narcissistic appeal: we imagine we're one of the couple because we can't *see* ourselves when we have sex. Even if you do it in front of a mirror, all angles aren't covered and you tend to forget to watch the good bits because you're too carried away by the sensation. Some of you are turned on by the thought of watching other men make love to your partner – she's a creature of such savage sexual appetites, you alone can't satisfy them. Not surprisingly, few (brave or stupid) individuals actually take that one through to real life.

Exhibitionistic fantasies often revolve around others admiring you. You put on a fine show (of course) and the voyeur is usually envious of your sexual skills, desperately wishing they were the person you were making love to. It's an ego-boosting fantasy.

6. Having her masturbate for you (or watching her without her knowing)

Watching her 'play with herself' is up there on most men's wish list, possibly because it reassures you that we're as into sex as you are. Secretly spying appeals to your curious side: what does she really get up to when you're not around?

7. Anal sex

It doesn't mean you've got 'gay tendencies' because the anus is undeniably an erotic zone, especially for men. A lot of you would love her to penetrate you with a finger – or want to have anal intercourse – but worry she'll think you're gay if you suggest it. So you fantasise instead.

8. Bondage (tying up fantasies)

Being tied up is her favourite, tying someone up is usually yours – which works out rather nicely if you play this one out in real life! Bondage fantasies are usually about power – having it or relinquishing it, and both have their appeal. Sometimes, it can mean you want to tie her *down*, rather than up (you don't feel she's truly yours); most of the time bondage springs to mind because it's the subject of many scenes in erotic books or movies.

Sado-masochistic (S and M) fantasies are less common but certainly not rare. Sadism is getting off on inflicting pain on someone else; masochism is getting off on someone hurting you. Most mild S and M fantasies revolve around whipping and spanking. Pleasure and pain is inextricably linked in the minds of some people and, in reality, spanking increases blood flow to the genital area (and therefore turns us on biologically). Aggression is common in the animal world: some female animals only ovulate if the male bites them. Masochistic fantasies sometimes stem from subconsciously thinking sex is bad (you need to be punished for liking it).

! Sex line workers say these are the most popular fantasy requests from men who call them:

- ***37 per cent want domination fantasies***
- ***23 per cent sex with schoolgirls***
- ***15 per cent anal sex with a woman***
- ***9 per cent sex with two girls***
- ***5 per cent to dress up in women's clothes***
- ***4 per cent sex with an older woman (often their mother-in-law!)***
- ***3 per cent an orgy***
- ***2 per cent sex with lesbians.***

9. Pretend rape

Contrary to what most women believe, when you fantasise about forcing a woman to have sex with you it's more about overpowering her through your amazing sexual technique and charisma than violence. She starts off saying 'no', then can't help but say 'yes' given the super-hunk that's on offer. Often set in Disney dungeons, nobody really gets hurt and the victim enjoys it even more than you do. If she's forcing you to have sex, you're indulging in a submissive sexual role quite unlike the one you probably have in real life. Usually, it's just a release from the day-to-day responsibility of always having to be in charge.

10. Sex with another man

Same sex fantasies or threesome fantasies involving another man are extremely common and don't mean you've got a secret wish to be gay; it just means you're sexually curious (see 'Am I gay?' on page 288).

HER HEDONISTIC HEAD GAMES: THE TOP 10 FEMALE SEX FANTASIES

Thinking sexy thoughts makes our tummies ache, skin tingle and vaginas moisten. Women who rate themselves as good lovers fantasise more often. Not only that, those who prepare for future sex by fantasising are more easily aroused and enjoy sex more when it happens. While just about all of us use fantasy while masturbating, lots also do it during sex, particularly if we're having trouble tipping over the orgasm brink.

1. Fantasising about our current partner

It's up there for both sexes, for all the reasons I've listed above.

2. Sex with a man other than your partner

For women, this is most often a past lover. Some feel adulterous or guilty reliving a particularly hot session from the past: don't. It's normal. Research shows we tend not to marry the person we were most sexually passionate with (most prefer to play it safe and settle for what we think are more sensible attributes). So, while you love your current boyfriend, an old one may have turned you on more.

If it's someone *new* you're fantasising about, it's the old want-what-you-can't-have syndrome. Alas, morals and nasty things like AIDS stop us having sex with whoever we please. But being involved with a partner doesn't mean all other desirable men go away and so those adulterous feelings have to be dealt with in one way or another. The safest outlet of all is our imagination – and it's remarkably fertile. In it, we have sex – if we're white – with black men (he's got a prize penis and his different skin colour makes him seem terribly exotic); toy boys (he's seen as more sexually active, gets harder, plus you're the experienced one who's calling the shots); and celebrities. In reality, stars are usually nothing like the public persona their publicity machine pumps out but, hey, they *seem* a lot more interesting than the average person. An extension of this is how famous you'll be if you get them: walking in with a Hollywood hunk on your arm is the quintessential ego boost and affirmation of your attractiveness.

3. Sex with another woman

We're more likely to have same sex fantasies than he is, probably because it's seen as more acceptable. We're also far less likely to get hung up on homophobic fears that we're gay. The woman featured isn't usually one we know but she always knows exactly what to do to turn us on because she's got what we've got.

4. Something new you'd like to try

It's that dreadful 'nice girls don't' stuff at work again. While many women are outrageously experimental and imaginative in their fantasies, not so many admit a desire for anything 'kinky' to a partner for fear of being judged. Playing out the scenario in your head is the next best thing. For those who are open, fantasising is also a form of rehearsal, upping the anticipation of experiencing it in reality. Included in this type of fantasy is being tied up, naughty threesomes, group sex and watching others. Having sex in public is another popular dream: we're turning on more than just our lover and our exhibitionistic side loves it.

5. Being given oral sex

It's the quickest, most effective (sometimes the *only*) way we orgasm, so it's not surprising it features heavily in our fantasies.

The guy of our dreams doesn't just like giving oral sex, he's so enthusiastic, he'd actually like to climb inside and stay there for days. Often he's a sex slave: tall, drop-dead good-looking and muscle-bound. We order him to give us oral sex on demand (for hours on end) but he also feeds us, gives fab massages, does the dishes and makes the bed.

6. Fantasies involving romantic sex

This is the one most women readily admit to, probably because it's the most 'acceptable'. Somehow, it seems more ladylike to say 'My fantasy is making love on a tropical beach at sunset' than 'Being given oral sex by the Pope during high mass while the rest of the congregation masturbate'. Romantic fantasies are sex with emotional attachment and most read like a Mills & Boon plot: gorgeous man, incapable of loving one woman, meets us, is knocked over by our looks and headstrong personality *then* ravishes us on a moonlit beach. Personally, I don't know one woman who has romantic fantasies but sex therapists assure me most 'normal' woman do (which I guess makes my friends deviants).

7. Being forced to have sex against our will

The 'safe rape' is a very common female fantasy but it's such a far cry from the real thing it seems silly even calling it rape. Passionate and forceful but rarely violent and painful, the 'rapes' in our head differ dramatically because we're always in control. Again, it's the good-girl thing: we relinquish responsibility as the man of our dreams overpowers us and 'makes' us submit – we can relax as we are just a pawn in the sex game. At the opposite end of the spectrum are fantasies where we force him to have sex with us, often in male-dominated situations like a

! *Number of women who have sexual dreams: 76.9 per cent. Number of women who enjoy and are turned on by some porn magazines and videos: 71.8 per cent. Number of women who tell their partners about their fantasies: 60 per cent. Those who go on to act them out: 33.6 per cent.*

courtroom or a business meeting. Being the aggressor or having physical power over him appeal because in real life it's usually the opposite.

8. Being found irresistible by a man

If you're so gorgeous/sexy/long-legged/stunning he can't help himself, you're absolved of responsibility once more. This is a favourite with women who still feel they need 'permission' to let go but also a pleasant daydream for most of us. Who ***wouldn't*** want to be so beautiful they have men drooling at their feet!

9. Working as a prostitute

Again, this one's popular with women who may be inhibited sexually in real life. In the fantasy, they indulge their true sexual selves under the guise of being paid for it. It's sex for sale, free of commitment – and a marvellous chance to show off. Men paying to have sex with you is also reassurance that you're attractive: you have something men want so badly, they'll hand over cash for it. Stripping is a more common variation on the theme: you tease the men mercilessly, and they're popping flies they're so turned on by your body.

10. Sex with a stranger

In reality, this sort of sex works out rather badly. In our fantasies, it's tremendously rewarding. Gone are the practical (often boring) needs of a relationship – this is sex for sex sake and the reward is pure, unadulterated pleasure. You can be as wicked as you like because not only will you never see them again, they don't know who *you* are so can't spread any nasty rumours. Sex with a 'faceless' man is even more of a turn-on. He comes up behind you, you feel rather than see him and you can experience the sensations of sex without the intimacy of eye contact.

AM I WEIRD, GAY OR LIKELY TO END UP IN A RAINCOAT?

Relax! In pretty well all cases, strange but sexy daydreams are a sign of a vivid imagination, not deviant leanings. Here are answers to some common questions about fantasies.

Do men and women fantasise about the same things?

Yes, though there are differences. His fantasies are often more explicit and men tend to centre on things they've done rather than things they'd like to try, while we do quite the opposite. Men are also more active in their fantasies, focusing on the effect they're having on the imaginary partner. Women focus more on feelings and responses. While he often fantasises when his sex life isn't great, we have more fantasies when it is, and while women who fantasise a lot tend to put at least some of their daydreaming into practice, he's not quite as lucky.

No two people's fantasies are identical, even if they are of the same sex, but a quick scan of the top 10 favourites shows there are common themes. Why doesn't everyone fantasise about the same thing? It's all to do with individual taste. Some people kill for freshly shucked oysters, others vomit at the thought. Same deal with sex.

Often, when I have sex with my boyfriend, I fantasise about someone else, and I feel guilty

Fantasising isn't just healthy for relationships, it can save them. It's natural to get jaded when you're sleeping with the same person night after night and playing a steamy sex fantasy in your head jazzes things up nicely, without hurting anyone. Many sex therapists recommend it. Indulge your desires guilt-free – imagining isn't being unfaithful, living it out in real life is. I bet he's transformed *you* into someone else on more than one occasion, too. The only time you really need to worry is if you have to fantasise *every single time* and are never turned on just by him. If that's the case, your sex life's in dire need of rescuing, or you've fallen out of lust with your boyfriend.

What if my fantasies are weird or completely out of character? Does it mean I'm a closet nutcase?

Most therapists say there's no such thing as an abnormal fantasy, *as long as the person can distinguish between fantasy and reality.* There's a big difference between thinking loony thoughts and wanting and intending to act them out. Deviant fantasies can be an indicator of true sexual deviancy but for the vast majority of people they're not.

If there's a consistently violent theme, if all your fantasies centre on a peculiar scenario which worries you, or if you find you now can't climax without thinking about the scenario, it could be worth checking it out with a sex therapist. It's rare that a person becomes so fixated on one particular scenario that they can't become aroused without it, but you might be the one in a million that it does happen to (in other words, you're probably worrying about nothing). Otherwise, think of your brain as a bus. You're the driver: drive it wherever you want, pick up as many passengers as you like and tell them to hop off once you reach your destination. If a seemingly weird fantasy is arousing you but you've got no inclination to do it in real life and it's not a fixation, what's wrong with it?

Am I gay if I have same-sex fantasies?

In a word, no. Just about everyone has (or has had) erotic daydreams about sleeping with the same sex – it's always up there in the top five. But fantasy alone isn't usually an indicator that you really are gay. Have you ever met anyone of the same sex in real life who you've longed to go to bed with? Do you consistently lust over the same sex in real life? Do you often feel that you're trapped in the wrong body? Do you enjoy having sex with the opposite sex? These are far more pertinent questions. Even if you have had a homosexual encounter, it doesn't necessarily mean you're gay. Many teenagers experiment in real life with their own sex (boys because the opposite is unattainable, girls because they're not 'allowed to' sleep with boys). Even as adults, we may have one or two gay encounters, simply for 'the experience'. These one-off sessions are usually more to do with sexual curiosity than a desire to switch camps for good.

Should I tell my partner about my fantasies?

This is a tricky one. On one hand, airing fantasies can zap your sex life through the roof. On the downside, it can destroy it. You're definitely taking a risk, especially if you don't know your partner very well. What you think of as normal, they might consider 'perverted'; it very much depends on their individual views, upbringing and morals. Don't assume that because something turns you on, your partner will feel the same.

Men often have problems accepting their partner's fantasies because they take it as a criticism – that you're not happy with 'just them'. Women often feel jealous and insecure for the same reasons. I really wouldn't recommend sharing any fantasies about people you know (with the exception of a celebrity, who you're unlikely to meet) and I also wouldn't share any unusual fantasies unless I trusted and knew the person so well I was guaranteed a non-judgemental, positive reaction. Be especially careful to ensure that your partner knows why you're sharing the fantasy. Spell out whether you want to 'play-act' it in any sense or are simply revealing intimate thoughts. (If you're female and share a rape fantasy, for instance, make it very, very clear that you're not asking for violence in real life.)

If someone shares their fantasy with you, treat the knowledge with respect. Don't be too scathing about their secret dreams, especially if their fantasy isn't one you were hoping for. Don't even think about telling your best friend and don't immediately launch into your theories as to why they're having *that* particular fantasy. He doesn't really want you to wear red leather with strategic cut-outs next time you visit his parents. It's a fantasy, that's all. On the other hand, beware the date who reveals a weird or violent fantasy very early, particularly if you're female.

What if I don't have any?

You're not alone, though you do belong to a small sub-section of the population. Those who claim not to fantasise usually have unconscious reasons for repressing them (such as they're unacceptable because of rigid morals or a strict upbringing). A few therapy sessions can work wonders for unblocking and unlocking our imagination.

Some people don't have any qualms about having sexual daydreams, they're just unpractised at using their creative side. Maybe you aren't very creative generally, prefer working with facts and figures, or you think making up stories is a waste of time (something weirdos and children do). Loosen up a little and read other people's fantasies (start with the real life confessions in this chapter; invest in Nancy Friday's *Woman on Top* or *Men in Love* if you want more). That's usually enough to get the brain ticking and trigger some of your own.

LIGHTS, CAMERA, ERECTION!

That lurid reverie about your primary school teacher and raspberry jelly isn't first date material. But sharing and acting out some fantasies is an excellent idea if you've been together a while, talk openly about sex and, most importantly, know that your innermost thoughts won't be the subject of your partner's next boys' or girls' night out.

Literally thousands of us secretly use fantasies to orgasm during sex, so owning up and acting them out can be the lustiest sex game you've played in years. Provocative barmaids, nymphomaniac nurses, dominatrixes and bootlicking toy boys, sexy slave girls and sultans, muscle-bound bikies and straight-laced career women: find the role which appeals to you and make like you're in the movies – though I strongly advise *against* turning it into one. 'Of course it's for our eyes only,' you both purr in the lovey-dovey stage. It's a different story when you ditch him for his best friend and a copy 'accidentally' gets dropped in your mother's postbox.

How do you suggest acting out a fantasy or finding out about theirs? Wait until you're both feeling relaxed and intimate, then say you had an amazingly sexy dream last night. Tell your partner about it and see what reaction you get. If they seem nicely titillated, confess that it's actually been a fantasy of yours for ages, and ask what are some of theirs. Once you're both talking, it's relatively easy to move into a line like, 'Hey, I've just had a great idea. Why don't we act them out for a bit of fun?'

Try to choose fantasies that appeal to *both* of you, particularly the first time round, and work out the scenario together beforehand: what you'll each wear, how you want them to act and vice versa. Then use your own imagination to embellish the story, adding a few surprises to the screenplay, maybe taking it even further. You could also try each writing down three favourite fantasies along with instructions on how you'd like to act them out. Write them on separate pieces of paper and put them in a jar for either of you to fish out when you feel like playing. You won't know what fantasy it is until you open it, and neither will they.

Acting out fantasies doesn't have to be literal: symbolism is often all that's needed. Got an anal sex fantasy but don't want to actually do it? Pretend you are while having vaginal sex doggie style. Use stockings and ties not rough ropes for tying-up games; and there's no need to tie knots tight – the idea is to fake a struggle rather than to have a real one because your circulation's cut off. Lavishly expensive props aren't necessary (though they are worth thinking about for favourite fantasies): black stockings and high heels turn her into a prostitute; jeans, no shirt (and a suitably subserviant expression) turn him into a sex slave.

Remember to set the scene using music and different rooms of the house (take it outside if it would work better) but don't stress about it. You don't have to be too literal – it's the 'sense' of the fantasy that you're recreating. Similarly, don't be surprised if the first time you do it, either (or both) of you nearly explode from trying to stop the giggles. Laughing together is all part of it. Keep going and you'll feel less ridiculous once you start getting into it.

Only one word of caution: work out an agreed 'stop-now' signal before starting anything. This is particularly important if your sex games include bondage or spanking. Part of the fantasy may be the person begging for mercy, but how are you supposed to know whether it's real or feigned without a sign? Apart from that, the world is your stage and you're the superstars. Here is a fantasy each for inspiration.

F FOR HER

Playing the stern mistress

Reverse the traditional roles and become the master of his destiny (well, for about an hour anyway).

If you own anything in leather, put it on. Improvise – a leather jacket worn over black underwear (stocking, suspenders, push-up bra and no knickers) with knee-high boots will do the trick. Otherwise, anything tight, black and short – the tartier the better! If you've got something in PVC (that horribly uncomfortable shiny stuff), drag it out from the back of the closet. His outfit's easy: nothing. Him naked while you're clothed sets the scene and makes him feel suitably helpless and vulnerable.

If you can't manage a thunderously threatening expression go for no expression. Be as unflinchingly mercenary as you can. Show him who's boss by telling him he's misbehaved and you're going to punish him. *Order* him to sit or lie down, face turned away from you, blindfold him and tie his hands together behind his back (pushing him forward into a submissive pose).

He's now naked, blindfolded and bound – completely in your power! If he's really into this one, he may want you to hit him with a riding crop or wooden spoon. By all means make your strokes sting but you don't want to cause serious pain. (Now isn't the time to show the bastard how you really felt when he flirted with Rachel at that party.)

Him begging you to stop is all part of the game. Refuse until you're either (a) so turned on, you're frothing at the mouth for sex or (b) either of you are finding the late night movie playing in the lounge room more interesting than your own acting. Tell him you will show mercy but on one proviso – that he ravishes you NOW!

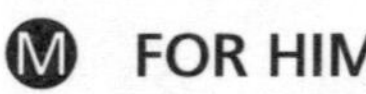

FOR HIM

'Forcibly' seducing an innocent

It's forbidden sex for both of you and an easy role-play to start with. Don't panic, there's absolutely no violence or pain involved. This is a very mild version of the common 'pretend rape' fantasy with a virgin element thrown in. Add more 'struggling' and 'force' to suit your taste!

She's naked, you're clothed (it doesn't usually matter what in but dressing formally can add to the older man, younger woman element). She pretends to be discovering her sexuality privately by standing in front of a mirror, running her hands over her body. You come up silently behind her and cover her eyes with your hand. The feel of her naked skin against your rough clothes feels exciting because it's a new sensation. Be suggestive, speaking in a low voice and tell her you've been watching and fantasising about her for weeks. If she likes you to talk dirty, here's your chance to let rip.

As you tell her what you intend to do with her and what she will have to do for you, begin to gently caress her body with your lips and hands. Just when she's starting to melt, turn on the tension and remind her she's in your power. You're still standing behind her, so pull her arms gently behind her back, hold them together at the wrists with one of your hands and use the other to continue exploring.

Now make good on your promises. She should resist any new advance initially, then be 'overcome' and let you continue (pretending all the time that she's not enjoying it). You take the lead, pretending each touch is her first.

'Come on, you want it,' you whisper finally. She half-heartedly protests, then surrenders and grants permission for you to penetrate her. Remember, she's inexperienced and this is her first time. Stop and ask if she's okay and once you're inside, thrust gently.

REAL PEOPLE REVEAL ALL

I asked four very different people to share their favourite fantasies and have faithfully recorded them in their own words. Be warned – there's a few nasty four-letter words!

Catherine, 24, nurse

'I have lots of fantasies but this one always gets me off. I'm walking past a building site and all these muscle-bound workmen start whistling at me. I'm so flustered I trip, fall over and sprain my ankle (though it never hurts, of course). Two of the men rush over to pick me up and ask if I want to sit down. They take me into their lunch room (the rest of the guys conveniently leave for a pub lunch), push beer cans, papers and over-flowing ashtrays out of the way and lay me down on a big table. One kneels to start massaging my ankle.

'"How does that feel?" he asks.

'"Great," I say enthusiastically.

'"You look a bit tense," says the other one. "Would you like me to massage your shoulders? You've had a real shock," and his big, powerful hands go to work.

'By this time, I'm horny, so say brazenly, "Seems a shame to stop there." They don't need any further encouragement and one guy runs his hand up my thigh and starts stroking my clit through my panties which are wet through. The other guy takes off my top and starts sucking and biting my nipples. My panties are off before I know it and hands plunge inside me and diddle my clit which feels like a marble in hot oil. The first guy is still licking my nipples and my neck, the second puts his head between my legs and gives me the best oral I've ever had. I come loudly and the first guy unzips and fucks me while his friend watches and masturbates.'

Karen, 21, student

'Every Tuesday night, me, my boyfriend and another couple go to see a movie. In my fantasy, I lock eyes with the cutest usher as we walk in: blue eyes, long hair, tall and well built. It's electric, that look, and we both know we're attracted to each other. Halfway through the film, I have to pee, and standing right outside is the usher. I stop, his eyes travel deliberately over my body. I'm instantly wet and start to throb. Without a word, he takes my hand and starts walking down a corridor. I follow like a lost little girl. He leads me into the projection room and I can see everyone in the theatre – including my boyfriend. Then he lays me down on a table and runs his hand up the inside of my thigh. His thumb massages my clitoris, then his tongue excites it and my whole body explodes in his mouth. It's incredibly erotic – this guy's a total stranger and I can see my boyfriend innocently watching the film. I'm so bad. I get off the table and stand against a wall, my ass in the air so he can take me from behind. Without warning, he's inside me and I groan so loud a few people in the back row turn to look. We fuck hard and fast while I watch my boyfriend polishing off the last of our popcorn.'

Jeff, 30, manufacturing manager

'In real life, I have to liaise with this fantastic looking woman who does our PR. In my fantasy, I arrive early for our weekly meeting. She walks ahead of me up the stairs and I watch her ass moving underneath her short business skirt. She's wearing a top I particularly like but this time it's open and she's got no bra on.

'"We never seem to have time together and that's a shame. I'd like to get to know you a lot better," she says, locking the office door and telling her secretary to hold all calls.

'I'm wondering why and hoping like hell it's what I think. She sits on the desk, motions me to a chair in front, then puts one high-heeled foot on either side of me. I can see she's not wearing knickers. She sits there, calmly talking about business and doesn't seem to mind me staring at her crotch which is wet and totally shaved. Eventually, she takes pity, stands up and unzips my fly. She takes out my prick then kneels down and sucks it expertly. I come a split second before her secretary knocks at the door saying the others have arrived. She straightens up, wipes her mouth with a tissue and waits for me to get myself together before letting the others in.'

Bruce, 26, electrician

'I've had the hard word put on me by bored housewives before but never the ones you want. In my fantasy, I'm asked to install a light fitting in a bathroom. I knock on the door and this total babe answers. She's obviously just about to have a shower because she's got a robe on and a towel over one arm. My cock stirs. She shows me into the bathroom and asks if I'd mind if she took a shower while I'm working because she's running late. Who am I to complain? I pretend to fix the light but she's so close and in full view, soaping her tits and slipping her fingers into her pussy. She turns the shower off and asks me to pass her a towel. I say, "No worries, let me dry you off."

'So I start drying her shoulders and then get down on the floor to dry her legs. She puts her hands on my head and stands with her legs apart so I nuzzle her sweet-smelling pussy and lick that little knob until she's clasping her thighs so hard around my head, I can't stand it. It's mushy and wet and her juices are dripping down her legs. She begs me to fuck her so I do. I bend her over the bath and fuck her from behind, thrusting so deep as I come, she has trouble keeping her balance.'

! Of all our sexual fantasies, bondage (tying each other up) is the one we're most likely to act out. Twenty-three per cent of men just fantasise about bondage, 27 per cent have done it. Twenty-five per cent of women just dream about it, 26 per cent take it through to real-life.

Sex Myths

Most couples do it 2.5 times a week, your best friend's bonking more than you are and other sex secrets and lies

It's funny the things we grow up believing about sex and our bodies. My friend Sarah was convinced for years that if men don't 'use' their erections their testicles hurt for hours afterward. Todd still refuses to budge from his theory that some girls are so fertile *nothing* will stop them getting pregnant. My grandmother claimed she could pick a good girl from a bad one by the way she threw her leg over a bicycle. I, of course, being sexually superior, was able to effortlessly separate fact from fantasy. Well, that's what I'd *like* to tell you. In reality, I was the biggest sucker of all – thanks to my best friend Jenny.

Jenny knew everything there was to know about sex, all of which she made up. Gullible old me, eyes like saucers, believed the lot. Penises have bones in them. You took the Pill vaginally. You could cut the finger off a rubber glove and use it as a condom. Men with big noses have big penises. Jenny was also the one who told me how to use tampons – you just lay them lengthways across the opening of your vagina. For weeks, I watched other girls lock themselves in the loo, armed with strange-looking cardboard cylinders, muttering about how they couldn't get the hang of tampons. I, on the other hand, was out and washing my hands before they'd even opened their instruction leaflets. Which is possibly what I should have done, since Jenny had no idea you were supposed to insert them *inside*. Those Carefree ads had me stumped. Girls swimming, surfing and bouncing around in aerobics classes? All I could manage was a painful hobble, legs tightly closed to keep the thing in place. Silly when you look back (thick, even) but also interesting how we cling to some sexual misconceptions for so long.

Some sex myths are simply outdated, reflecting different society values and morals. Times change, people change and even the facts change sometimes when new evidence comes to light. But what remains truly astonishing is this: for a subject that's the number one obsession of the western world, most of the general population still know little about sex. So, here's the truth, the whole truth, and nothing but the truth about all the things even the sexually educated have niggling doubts about. Jenny, this one's for you.

! Does love at first sight really happen? Instant desire certainly does but experts say 'knowing' right from the start is unlikely. That's merely knowledge after the event.

THE TOP 10 WHOPPERS

Our parents had them (you'll go blind if you masturbate, good girls don't) and we've invented a totally new set of sex myths. Most of us are surprisingly naive when it comes to sorting fact from fiction – so let's dispel the real biggies once and for all.

They're great looking so sex is going to be fantastic

Not only is this untrue (there is a God after all), but neither sex has the foggiest what the other truly finds attractive. While you're sweating it out at the gym in a desperate bid for a reed-thin body, the studies say he's eyeing up 'real women' – curvaceous, voluptuous creatures who probably qualify as 'plump' by today's standards. Ditto the muscle-man working out beside you: we consistently rate nice smiles and a sense of humour as far more appealing than abs-of-steel.

Even if you *do* get to bed the best-looking guy or girl on the block, sex rarely lives up to expectations. Because their whole self-image revolves around their looks (that's all they ever get

Money can't buy love, unless both of you are rich that is. The happiest matches are between partners whose assets balance in the categories of wealth, looks, status, knowledge, personality and temperament. If either of you far excels in any one area, the power is uneven. One of you thinks you could have 'done better', the other feels they're not good enough.

complimented on), the truly beautiful are often insecure, tense and inhibited in bed. If they're not admired for anything else, it's essential they keep up the beautiful look at *all* times – not great when sex is messy, sweaty and often unflattering at the best of times. A good lover doesn't notice sperm up their nose, pubic hairs in their teeth and a roll of fat squashed between you both because they're so immersed in the sensation, they've lost conscious thought. Call me cynical but if you're wondering if your Estée Lauder eyeshadow really has proved to be crease-free as he lines up for the final thrust, you're not into it. Ditto for men who worry about mussed-up hair.

Sex is the most important thing in a relationship

You can only spend so much time in the bedroom. So if it's a love (not a sex) affair, you're forced to relate on other levels at least some of the time. Most people's needs in life divide roughly equally into spiritual (connecting with others), mental (brain stimulation), emotional (loving and being loved) and sexual. You can't (and absolutely shouldn't) discount sex because it's definitely important; on the other hand, it's only 25 per cent of our lives. Surveys and studies on relationships reveal only 20 per cent of you consider earth-shattering sex 'crucial', the other 80 per cent consider it 'the icing on the cake' of a good relationship. According to the weighty Kinsey Institute 'New Report on Sex', bad sex isn't even a major cause of divorce (though it is certainly up there on the 'why I want to leave' list). The general consensus from the experts seems to be this: when sex is good, or even okay, it's afforded the same importance we place on things like shared goals, trust and love. It's when it's bad that it tends to become the focus of the relationship, insidiously destroying everything else.

Most couples have good sex most of the time

'If John doesn't do it at least once a day, he goes mad,' your best friend reveals after a bottle of wine. 'Oh, we haven't done it in bed for *years*,' boasts Jane. Why is it that everyone else's sex life seems better than our own? One reason could be that you're at different stages in your relationships. You can't compare new sex with a four-year-been-there-done-that relationship; the human nervous system is programmed to become desensitised the more of the same stimulation it gets. That's not to say long-term sex can't be as good; it's just different. If your partner knows all the right buttons to push (and they should after all that practice!) orgasm is often guaranteed for long-time lovers and, with effort, you can still be *very* passionate. But cut-your-arm-off-to-get-it, out-of-control, raging lust *every* night, after years of sharing the same bed? Possible, but you'd be flat out holding down a job with the amount of energy it would take to sustain it. Life and all its pressures get in the way and many couples are too tired to have sex at some stages in their life (kids, new job or skidding through a rough patch). So how come your sister still has mind-blowing sex after six years of marriage? She may think *you* have a fab sex life and doesn't want to admit she doesn't. Or she really does have terrific sex – once a month. It's all subjective.

Myth: Men always make the first move.
Reality: They think they do but in 70 per cent of cases women initiate the encounters by non-verbal come-ons like smiling or making eye contact.

The average couple make love 2.5 times a week

We forget that an average statistic is just that – an average. Researchers have lumped in the couple who *shred* the sheets three times a day with Bertha and George who manage it once a year and all those who fall somewhere inbetween, added up their weekly totals and averaged them all out. You could have sex every day for a month, then abstain totally for the next two and still make the average. Add to this that most women don't have sex during their period, most couples don't if they're sick, tired or arguing, *and* that on hols we make love three times more often, and you'd have a job trying to be Mr and Mrs Average. Besides, not everyone agrees on the old 2.5 figure. Last year's Australian stats put our national average at less than twice a week; a more recent survey claimed three out of five Aussies have sex less than once a week for a pathetic 10 to 15 minutes. Tragic but probably closer to the truth.

Australians have sex, on average, 116 times a year. The most sexually active people globally: couples who live together but aren't married (146 times a year). Number of times singles have sex: 69 times a year. Married couples: 118 times.

Men sleep around more than women do

A great deal of research has gone into solving the twentieth century mystery of why men consistently report having three times more sex partners than women do. (If it's true there's an awfully sore woman out there.) It could be that, generally, men overestimate and women do the opposite. What's more likely is this: a recent study by a British sexpert found women only tend to remember sex if it was part of a long-term relationship, 'forgetting' (somewhat conveniently) any one-night flings. He suggests the real partner total for women is three times more than they say or think. Funnily enough, that makes both sexes dead even.

It's men not women who are the real romantics. In one study of 700 lovers, 20 per cent of the men had fallen in love before the fourth date compared to 15 per cent of the women. By date 20, 45 per cent of the women were still unsure, compared to only 30 per cent of the men. Women usually initiate split-ups and men feel lonelier, more depressed and unloved afterward. They're also three times more prone to suicide after a break-up.

If they're having an affair, they don't love me

Wrong again. Affairs aren't about love, they're about sex, a certain *kind* of sex. It's the affair that's the turn-on, not the person. Sex on the sly, a bit on the side – even the expressions we use hint at the real reason people stray from home. It's the excitement of secrecy. One study found that not only were people more obsessed with past, secret relationships than those that were out in the open, but that the minute the forbidden relationship was revealed or (even worse) approved of, it fizzled out fast. The novelty of being with someone new is the other motivator. The thrill of the chase, the ego-boost – we're all suckers for a bit of attention. Having an affair doesn't mean your partner doesn't love you, but it *does* mean they don't respect you.

Most people now use condoms because of AIDS

I'd dearly love to tell you that this is so but although people are buying and carrying condoms, they aren't actually taking too many out of the packet. Youth, booze and hormones are proving a potentially lethal cocktail for teenagers the world over who regularly have unprotected sex. The newly single are another group who believe they're immune to AIDS: divorced, widowed or separated people have higher rates of unsafe sex than those who've never been married. It seems hard to believe intelligent people knowingly put their lives at risk. But they do. Often.

If you don't wake the neighbours, you're not enjoying yourself

Some people scream their heads off at the football, others just wave the odd flag – that doesn't mean one's enjoying it more than the other. While it's great if your partner does make noise (it's good feedback), it really depends on their personality. For many women, reaching orgasm is a long, private process which involves intense concentration. They're battling to stay focused on the sensation so, when they do climax, aren't likely to blow all that hard work by

! Opposites don't attract, similarity does. Couples who have the same values, attitudes, interests and ways of looking at the world are more likely to say they've found 'a soul mate' and more likely to stay together. On the other hand, hooking up with someone whose differences complement your own personality is a good idea. That's why worrier-relaxed and shy-outgoing combos work.

announcing the fact to the entire world. Some men are also quiet achievers. Horses for courses.

It's not what you've got, it's how you use it

Partly true, partly false. The saying should go, 'It's not what you've got, it's how you compensate for it.' If you're a centimetre or so under the average, chances are she hasn't noticed or cared. But if you're talking *really* little, you can 'use it' (that is, thrust) all you like and it probably won't be the best penetration she's experienced. The small guy who has extraordinary oral sex and foreplay skills, however, won't have too many problems; the guy hung like a horse *will* if he relies exclusively on his penis.

Women are turned off by porn

Both sexes are turned on by pornography and erotica, just different kinds. Generally, men go for more explicit, hard-core stuff; women usually prefer erotic, soft images (and a plot, if it's at all possible). Women also often need to look at the people on the screen and think 'I could/would like to do that' or they don't relate to it. But as for not enjoying it at all – bollocks. The recent boom in made-for-women-by-women flicks is evidence enough that if it's the right kind, we'll lap it up.

THE CUTTING EDGE: CIRCUMCISED VERSUS UNCIRCUMCISED

Circumcision – removing the foreskin of the penis – was commonly performed for 'hygienic' or religious reasons. These days, it's frowned upon by the general community and few Australian babies are circumcised despite theories that it reduces the risk of penile cancer and infections of the foreskin. Chances are, however, most women will encounter both 'cut' and 'uncut' penises so let's challenge a few misconceptions right here and now.

Circumcised penises are prettier

This is a matter of personal taste and what you're used to. Take a flip through some old photos and most of us will *cringe* at the ghastly get-ups we thought looked bloody marvellous ten years ago. The fact is, they did – at the time. Fashions change and so does our perception of what looks good. If you've only slept with circumcised guys, an uncircumcised penis looks different and our natural reaction is to go 'blah'. If everyone you've slept with is uncircumcised and you hit a circumcised one, it will look funny to you as well.

Uncircumcised men don't get as hard

Believe me, the blood pumps just as ferociously through an uncircumcised penis as it does a circumcised one. The reason it doesn't feel as hard around the glans (head), is that the extra skin 'cushions' it slightly. Ever so slightly.

Uncircumcised ones are smelly

The uncircumcised guy *does* need to be scrupulous about his personal hygiene to avoid odour problems. But if he showers regularly and washes properly – gently pulling the foreskin back from the penis and washing underneath with mild soap – he'll smell (and taste) just as sweet as the next guy.

Uncircumcised guys are more sensitive

Quite true. Because the head of his penis is covered by skin, it's not exposed to things like rubbing against clothing. But this doesn't mean he'll come more quickly. Inside the vagina, the sensation's essentially the same and it's what he's used to, so if he blames premature ejaculation problems on being uncircumcised, he's having you on. It's his brain, not his foreskin, that needs sorting.

Which feels best for him?

Adrian was circumcised at 24, so is in the unique position of having experienced both:

'I'm English and, as was the custom back then, not circumcised as a baby. A few girls commented that I was unusual, simply because most Aussie guys were, but I didn't think much about it until I was 23 and got a fibrous growth which caused thickening of the foreskin. It was incredibly painful. I couldn't pull the foreskin back to wash because it felt like my penis was being strangled. But I'd

! ***Not a myth after all: On average, an Asian man's penis is 2 cm smaller than a white man's, whose is 3 cm smaller than a black man's.***

force it, it would tear, scab over, then form scar tissue and make the whole problem worse. I was too embarrassed to see a doctor but when it got to the point that sex was agony, I went.

'I felt quite humiliated getting circumcised at such an old age and it hurt like hell afterward. It felt like someone had put a red hot poker up my penis and it stung for days. I had to wear sarongs around, much to the amusement of my girlfriend and her friends, and it took about two weeks to heal properly. Sex wasn't dramatically different – probably because I'd had a bit of a play and got used to it. I felt more sensitive the first few times we had intercourse but that quickly passed. As far as sensation and the time it took me to orgasm, there was no change whatsoever. But I'd probably say I prefer being circumcised. My penis is easier to look after (you don't have to fiddle about with the foreskin) and I think it looks cleaner and more attractive. If I had a child, I'd probably get him circumcised even though it's not politically correct, simply because I'd hate him to have to go through the pain I endured if he also had problems at a later age.'

ANSWERS TO SOME COMMON QUESTIONS

Am I normal (and is my partner)?

This is the most commonly asked question in sex therapy and the hardest to answer – 'normal' is virtually impossible to define because we're all individual. People ponder the question because they believe all the sex myths, know they don't apply to their own sex lives, don't realise they don't apply to other people's either and think everyone else is having a better time than they are. But not only is it unhealthy and inhibiting to aspire to be normal (not to mention boring – do you really want to be the quintessential Mr and Mrs Jones?), it's impossible. Read all the sex surveys you want but you still won't really know what other people do in bed because what people say and what people do are two totally different things.

Instead, steer toward another goal: developing a healthy, satisfying sex life where nothing is 'kinky' or wrong provided both of you agree. Don't fall for the 'but everyone else does ➢

it' argument and be pressured into doing things you don't want to, but consider trying things that sound reasonable at least once. If you're not sure if you're being narrow-minded, look up a few good sex books to get an impression of whether what your partner is suggesting is standard sexual practice or listed with more unusual things (like sexual deviance). That will give you a good idea of whether your attitude to sex is prudish – or prudent.

My vagina sometimes makes noises during sex and it sounds like I'm breaking wind. Help!

Some positions of intercourse – particularly him entering from behind – force air into the vagina which is expelled (usually in a most unelegant fashion) after he withdraws. It's a totally normal bodily function which most couples ignore or have a giggle over. Tongues licking, mouths kissing, bodies slapping together – sex is noisy and this should add to the excitement rather than detract from it. The only way to stop your body making noises is to stick exclusively to the missionary position and not get too carried away. Fun, eh?

My vagina's smelly – what should I do?

The French have a name for the smell of a woman's genitals – *cassolette* – which means perfume box. Most men are turned on by your natural scent (even if you aren't) and that slightly acidic smell is normal. If the smell has changed, become stronger or a discharge has appeared with it, see your doctor to make sure you don't have an infection. Otherwise, wash with unscented soap, wear cotton underwear and steer clear of too much garlic (your breath isn't the only place it turns up).

How much pubic hair is normal? I think I've got too much

Yikes! There's that awful 'normal' word again. Why is it some people have curly hair and others dead straight? It's called genes. If you feel Mum or Dad have been a little too generous in the pubic department, trim, wax, shave or have it removed by electrolysis. Bear in mind though, some men love it!

A HIGHER LOVE

We've all heard the hype about how great sex is meant to be if you've dropped an 'E' or are coked to the eyeballs. But what's the reality? According to one young women's magazine survey, 25 per cent of under 25-year-olds take 'party' drugs once a month or less, 23 per cent every weekend and 18 per cent every day (with the average starting age being 16). Faced with these stats, I figured I'd better find out. You can guess the conclusion by the fact that I've included it in this chapter – the one devoted to debunking myths. The fact is, most of the extravagant claims about the aphrodisiac effect of these drugs simply aren't true. And even if you have had an out-of-this-world sex session after taking them, there's a downside.

Some claims about drugs and sex *aren't* fiction. You *are* far more likely to have sex without a condom, for instance, so your chance of contracting an STI or the HIV virus rises sharply if you indulge. One-third of those surveyed in the magazine admitted they'd had unsafe sex while on drugs; others 'couldn't remember'. Other truisms: you're far more likely to end up in bed with someone you wouldn't have been remotely interested in sober or straight; you're more likely to put yourself in dangerous situations; you'll have sex sooner than you usually would with a new partner. Illicit drugs also up your chances of becoming intimate with someone you hadn't planned on – the police.

I haven't included the numerous general health risks associated with recreational drugs, just the effect they may have on your sex life. I can generalise though: all are bad for you, all can cause long-term, serious health problems, all are addictive and too much of some can kill you. All the information included here is provided by people who regularly use recreational drugs, as well as the health authorities who battle to clean up the not-so-fabulous side effects. I don't take illegal drugs. I hope you don't either. No-one's denying a few drinks can relax you and your inhibitions but *too* much alcohol and even teensy amounts of the other drugs I've covered here aren't safe and *won't improve your sex life long-term*. The best sex stimulants are your hands, your mouth, your genitals, your heart and, most importantly, a clear, active, imaginative brain. No chemicals necessary. If you need drugs to enhance your enjoyment of *anything*, you've got problems.

Alcohol

Users claim

In small or moderate amounts, alcohol has psychological effects which can help us feel and be more sexy. A few drinks reduce our inhibitions and lend 'Dutch courage' to those who are too shy to let loose sexually when sober. Alcohol makes us feel warm, fuzzy and affectionate, making us more approachable and open to sexual advances.

The downside

Too much can make us a little too uninhibited – we're far more likely to have unsafe sex when drunk as well as sleep with someone we wouldn't have otherwise.

Drunk, some people become aggressive and violent, others sink into morbid moods.

Booze is also notorious for stopping him getting an erection. In *Macbeth*, Shakespeare wrote that alcohol 'provokes the desire, but takes away the performance'. Clever bloke Shakespeare. Down more than the recommended two beers, spirits or wines in an hour and hello impotence!

! *Number of women who consider champagne the ultimate love drug: 81 per cent.*
Number of women who were drunk when they lost their virginity: 14 per cent.
Number of men: 10 per cent.
Number of women who think they had sex too young because of it: 25 per cent.
Number of men who agree: 12.5 per cent.

Because it's a depressant, alcohol chemically acts to slow down or stop the physical processes necessary for sexual arousal and orgasm. For men, this means either no erection or a semi-soft one – and he'll have trouble coming to orgasm. It also affects arousal, lubrication and ability to orgasm for women. Drink too much, and the only thing you'll do lying down is pass out.

! *Sobering news: The most popular aphrodisiac for men and women is alcohol.*

If you're having a ciggie along with that drink, your blood vessels will be narrowed. This reduces the blood flow into the penis (again, making for soft erections) and stops blood flow to the vaginal wall, decreasing lubrication. While 45 per cent of people say alcohol enhances sex, 42 per cent say it does quite the opposite.

Real life

'Booze has landed me in bed with ex's, married men and complete losers. They all look good when I've had a few too many and my morals go out the window. It's also made me sleep with guys I really do like way too early. They think I'm easy and I never see them again.' *Jamie, 21, secretary*

Dope (marijuana or cannabis)

Users claim

When the young readers of a UK magazine were surveyed, 56 per cent said they smoked it regularly and 63 per cent said it enhances sex.

Of all the party drugs, dope is the most sexually unpredictable of all. Some people swear it makes sex better, and chemically it just might. Dope increases blood levels of phenylethylamine, a neurotransmitter associated with love and lust.

Like alcohol, having a smoke can overcome inhibitions and make us feel more relaxed, so it can increase the chances of female orgasm in someone who's normally too uptight to let go. It also increases awareness and sensitivity of our skin and genitals. Sex is lazier and more leisurely; and it seems to last longer because marijuana affects our perception of time.

The downside

The effects vary dramatically from one user to the next, and there's no way of telling which way you, or your partner, will go. Lots of people withdraw or become anxious and irritable rather than snuggly or sexy. It's a bit of a lottery. Habitual users eventually lose desire: it's an effort to drum up the motivation to *think* about sex, let alone *do* it.

Real life

'I love having sex while I'm stoned but only with a long-term lover. I did it once with a guy I'd just met and felt like he was raping me.' *Tracey, 32, stylist*

'E' or ecstasy

Users claim

Eighty-three per cent of users say it enhances sex. Ecstasy is a chemical originally used as a diet pill. It was later rediscovered and flogged to party-goers as a drug that would boost desire and make sex better, along with feelings of intense happiness and affection (hence the name). Users say sex is 'full-on' on E: they feel loving, skin feels soft and wonderful to touch, their bodies feel sensitive all over and they spend longer on foreplay than usual.

***!** The best aphrodisiac for men over 40: sauerkraut. Tests on 500 men found 90 per cent were able to have sex daily for up to 30 minutes after eating the pickled cabbage three times a day.*

The downside

It's incredibly dangerous, especially in impure forms, and since it's illegal you have no idea what you're getting. Ecstasy alters our perceptions entirely: you 'love' everyone (and end up in bed with more than a few) and you are full of the joys of humankind (you can't imagine that anyone could cause you harm so put yourself in dangerous situations). While ecstasy can make us feel more like sex, it makes us take longer to reach orgasm – if you can manage one at all.

Real life

'Everyone looks good on E. You're up on the dance floor and you think you're with the most gorgeous guy in the club. So you take him home and sleep with him. Sometimes, if I do it when I'm coming down, I suddenly become really lucid and think, *Who is this guy? What am I doing?* Once, I tried to get the guy to stop but he was so off his face, he couldn't comprehend what I was saying. The next day, you wake up beside guys you'd cross the street to avoid when you're straight. I stopped doing Es for all those reasons.' *Annie, 26, hairstylist*

Coke (cocaine)

Users claim

Originally used as a local anaesthetic, coke has had a reputation as an aphrodisiac for centuries. Fifty-nine per cent of users agree it enhances their sex lives. Coke makes people feel confident and exhilarated and this increases their sense of desirability. In other words, they feel more attractive. Some people say it reduces their inhibitions while simultaneously increasing their libido and eroticism. The shy and insecure love coke because it helps them relate better to others and have more empathy. Advocates say it makes you 'go all night' and you feel strong and full of energy, making sex seem more animalistic. It's less 'touchy' than sex on an E and all your senses feel sharpened.

The most common side effects of party drugs:
Mood swings – 55 per cent of users have them
Depression – 46 per cent
Frightening flashbacks – 11 per cent
Bad skin – 26 per cent
Lack of concentration – 55 per cent
Memory loss – 44 per cent

The downside

It's so addictive, improving your sex life becomes the least of your problems – funding your expensive habit is what you have to worry about. Heavy users find the intense experiences produced by coke impossible to replicate without it, so lose interest in sex if there's no "Charlie" on offer as well. Coke can either boost erections or severely reduce the chances of getting one. It has similarly varied effects on women: some find their desire and capacity for orgasm enhanced, lots say regular use makes them feel dead from the waist down and they couldn't come if their life depended on it. Habitual users (those whose life does depend on it) lose sexual desire completely. Many coke users find orgasms elusive, hovering on the brink but not able to actually have one. Crack is a refined form of coke.

Real life

'It's fantastic, sex on coke. Everyone should try it. You feel so alive and buzzing. My girlfriend and I don't even bother to have sex if we don't have any or can't afford enough to last all week. I guess we're both addicts but hey, we're young. We're supposed to be having fun.' *Alan, 20, ad executive*

Speed (or uppers)

Users claim

Thirty-nine per cent of young people use amphetamines like speed regularly. It can stimulate sexual desire and lots take it to increase their stamina for sex because it gives an energy boost. Sex on it is 'a rush', your senses are heightened and your heart beats faster.

The downside

It's hard to orgasm, making sex decidedly frustrating. With regular use, desire fades completely. Speed can also make it difficult to get, and keep, an erection. Both sexes say they have trouble keeping their mind on the job, and they're eager to move onto something else.

Real life

'I'd been keen on this girl for ages and one night at a rave party, I took speed and she took an E. We went back to her place, had sex a few times and it felt fantastic but then she got dressed and said we had to go back to the party. She didn't want her boyfriend to catch us – I didn't even know she had one. I felt really let down and knew how girls felt when they've been used and abused. I haven't touched the stuff since.' *Mel, 23, psychology student*

THREE IN A BED: THREESOMES, SWAPPING AND GROUP SEX

'I must be the luckiest man alive,' confided my friend James, two sheets to the wind. 'My wife wants us to try a threesome with another woman.'

'So, are you going to?' I asked him.

'Of *course*!' he spluttered. 'God, what man in his right mind would knock back the chance to sleep with two women at once?' There was a telling pause. 'I mean, you'd have to be a real wimp to say no, wouldn't you . . . wouldn't you? It's every bloke's dream . . . isn't it?'

'But not yours,' I said, taking a risk.

'No,' he admitted, embarrassed as hell. 'Truth is, the idea frightens the hell out of me.'

James isn't alone. While just about all of us have fantasised about threesomes and group sex, taking that leap to reality is something else. James was terrified he wouldn't be able to satisfy both women, that they'd think he was hopeless, that he'd be left out and that his wife would turn gay and leave him.

'I'm also not entirely convinced I'll be able to handle watching someone I love getting it on with another person, male or female,' he confessed sadly.

I'm with him. I'm far too jealous to share but lots of people I know have had threesomes with varying results. Generalising outrageously, I'd say the ones that it worked for were couples who hadn't been together long and didn't really mind their partner being with someone else. They had a play, said it made great future fantasy material but wouldn't rush to repeat it. For older, long-term couples, it was an emotional disaster. Even if they enjoyed it at the time, most said the fallout afterward was incredibly destructive. Jealousy, 'broken' trust, paranoia that their partner secretly preferred the third person – three in a bed really is dicey stuff. Convinced your relationship could handle a *ménage à trois*? Read this first.

> 'I was 19 and had been going out with this guy for about a month. We had terrific sex but both of us knew that was all we had. We were mucking around with a girlfriend of mine who's really into sex as well and she French-kissed me as a joke, to see if he got jealous. He pretended to, so we hammed it up a bit and somewhere along the line, stopped laughing and started getting into it. It very naturally turned into a threesome and all of us enjoyed it but no-one instigated a repeat performance. My girlfriend and I haven't mentioned it since.'
>
> Debbie, 31, receptionist

Why we want to do it

Often, threesomes appeal because we're too lazy to put the work in to boost a flagging sex life. We think a quicker, easier way to add spice is to introduce a third party – let them do the work. On the other hand, lots of us are aroused by the sight and sounds of others having sex – that's why we watch erotic videos. It can be instructive to watch other people's sexual techniques, it can make us feel desirable if there's more than one person enjoying our body, it undoubtedly adds variety and, of course, it's taboo. The thrill of doing something both naughty and novel is often a turn-on in itself.

Some like the idea of being the centre of attention and the thought of all that pleasure – *two* tongues, *two* sets of hands, *two* penises or vaginas – sounds great. In our fantasy, many of us cast ourselves in the taking role. Generally, women are more aroused by the two women and a man combination than men are by two men and one woman.

Threesomes sometimes seem like a natural solution to couples who are bored with each other but don't want to leave or do something 'behind their back'. Doing it in front of their partner seems less of a betrayal and most imagine the third person as an enjoyable addition rather than a threat. The people I interviewed indulged with like-minded friends, placed or answered an ad in the personals, or went along to a massage parlour which catered for couples. Even if the experience was positive, in most cases, once was enough – they satisfied their curiosity but found one-on-one sex ultimately more fulfilling.

What can go wrong

Real life is very different to fantasy. Couples who love each other usually have a hard time seeing their partners with someone else and often the physical pleasure dulls because of the strong negative emotions threesomes throw up. Most of us are pretty territorial about relationships and our partners and not used to sharing them so there's often jealousy (of the third person's body, technique, how your partner related to them). Three people in one bed is, by virtue of the fact that it's an uneven number,

> **'My boyfriend called his flatmate in while we were having sex. I said nothing because I knew it was what my boyfriend wanted. When his friend said he was getting a hard-on, my boyfriend asked him to join us. They had a "sandwich": my boyfriend penetrated me anally, the other guy vaginally. They'd obviously discussed it before. I felt like a whore.'**
>
> Judith, 22, promotions manager

unequal – someone usually fancies someone else more and the attention seems to tilt that way.

After the thrill's worn off (and perhaps the alcohol – a few drinks can do wonders for turning us on physically and off mentally), lots of people feel guilty and resentful (particularly if they were talked into it), ashamed, 'cheap' or disgusted with themselves. But the most common negative of all is feeling betrayed and that trust has disappeared. 'I can't get the images out of my head' and 'I'm scared they'll see them without me' were common comments from the people I surveyed. If your partner wants a repeat and you don't, you feel threatened. Sometimes wanting group sex is a sign of immaturity. It's all about instant gratification and it's far less personal than the one-on-one variety. It can also mean one or both of you have intimacy problems.

> ***'If God had meant us to have group sex, I guess he'd have given us all more organs.' Malcolm Bradbury***

In a sense, going along to an arranged sex party is more honest and less tricky than a threesome with a friend. Everyone knows what they're there for, there's little chance of a relationship developing because people swap around a lot and you're not likely to see each other again. 'Swinging' or 'swapping' usually means your partner's not in the same room or doing it in front of you so there are no nasty images to replay in your head. Groups that organise swapping parties also usually enforce set rules about using condoms and stopping if one person isn't enjoying it.

If you are going to give it a whirl

If you decide to go ahead, here's what you should do:

- Have condoms ready.
- Talk through what will happen together: what's on, what isn't. Is kissing allowed? What if one person wants to stop and the other doesn't? Spell out who's having sex with who. Seeing your boyfriend take another guy's penis into his mouth can be pretty shocking if it didn't occur to you the two men would have sex as well.
- As a couple, ask yourselves: Are we good at communicating, problem-solving and negotiating? You need all three skills to get through this one.

- Ask yourself: *Do* I feel comfortable having three-way sex? Do I feel comfortable about *my partner* having sex with someone else? If you're not 100 per cent sure of either, don't do it.
- Examine your motives. Are you trying to hang onto someone by agreeing? Do you feel forced into it? Then don't do it.
- If you're intent on spicing up your sex life with other people, would you be better off agreeing on an open relationship, making a few rules like always using condoms, and then not talking about it? You don't have to have sex with someone new together.

Gay and Lesbian Sex

Am I? Is he? What now?

The hostess ushers me into the lounge room. 'This is Carrie and John,' she says. Smiles all round. 'And this is Peter and Mandy.' Ditto. ' . . . and Katie and Emma.'

It's pretty obvious from the body language that Emma and Katie aren't linked together because they're flatmates. Images whirl in my head: tongues plunging, mouths sucking, breasts colliding. I blink rapidly and wonder why the minute I clock a couple are gay or lesbian, I immediately imagine the two of them in bed. After all, the other couples also have sex – why don't I automatically think of them having 69ers? 'You focus on it because that's the point of difference,' a lesbian friend later explains patiently. 'But isn't that wrong?' I ask, nervous I'm guilty of some sort of subconscious homophobia. 'No,' she says, 'it's normal.' Fiona's incredibly tolerant of my many questions about her sexuality, as are all of my gay and lesbian friends. Pity some members of society aren't as tolerant of them.

It always strikes me as rather odd that anyone should take exception to what people do behind closed doors. In classical Rome, ancient China and pre-colonial America, homosexual sex was a part of everyday life. In Greece, it was common.

Unfortunately the liberal attitude disappeared in 1885 when homosexuality was criminalised in Great Britain and Australia. (Interestingly, lesbianism was never banned because Queen Victoria could not conceive of two women having sex!) The UK decriminalised homosexual activity in 1967.

Which is great – in theory. Unfortunately, laws can't stop whispering, ostracism and the many petty slights dealt out to gay and lesbian people daily throughout the UK. It's not easy being gay or lesbian. It's not easy being different from the majority in any sense. This chapter is not just for people who are confused about their sexuality or having difficulties coming to grips with being gay or lesbian, it's for 'straights' as well, most particularly those who find the topic slightly distasteful. Do yourself a favour if this is you: read it. You just might learn something.

AM I GAY?

As the agony aunt for *Cosmopolitan* magazine, I often receive letters from readers asking if they're gay. A simple enough question, they figure, but actually, it's not that easy to answer. As the psychologists, activists, counsellors and gay, lesbian and bi-sexual people I spoke to verified, *all* of us have a male and a female side. Which part of *you* is going to be dominant for life is anyone's guess.

What does 'gay' and 'lesbian' mean?

If someone says they're gay or lesbian it usually means they have sexual relationships with the same sex and have adapted their lifestyle to suit. Terms like 'gay' (men who have sexual relationships with men), 'lesbian' (women who have sexual relationships with women), 'straight' or 'heterosexual' (people who have sexual relationships with the opposite sex) or 'bi' (people who have same sex and opposite sex relationships) are society's way of simplifying sexuality. But while it's nice and easy to plonk people into simple categories, real life is a little different.

The fact is, our sexuality is fluid throughout our life. You may be 'gay' for a period of months or years, then straight for the rest of your life, or vice versa. In prison, with no access to the opposite sex, some inmates become attracted to, fall in love with or have sex with the same sex. Then, the minute they're out of gaol, turn straight again. They're not the only ones who experiment. Lots of straight people have one or two sexual encounters with the same sex before deciding which sex suits them best. So a more apt definition might be, 'I'm straight at the moment' or 'I'm gay right now'.

Some people identify with one group very early, are sure of their choice and that's the end of the story. Toward the end of adolescence or in our early adult years, most of us have figured out which group we 'belong' to, especially if we've decided we're straight. It's not quite so easy if we think we're gay. It may take a few more years before you accept that and you may struggle with all the issues it throws up. Bisexual people are those who are quite comfortable with and equally attracted to both males and females. Some people consider them the most confused of all the groups. Others think, 'How fabulous. They have the whole world to choose from!'

! Forty-eight per cent of gay or lesbian teenagers have run away from home. They're also more likely to drop out of school with 75 per cent reporting negative reactions from their peers and teachers.

What makes someone gay or lesbian?

Hundreds of thousands of studies have attempted to answer this question but, to date, there aren't any clear answers. Some tentative research points to a gay gene – that different structures of the brain may dictate our sexuality – but even that's not conclusive and there's no concrete proof. The only thing scientists *are* reasonably certain of is this: if there *is* a biological factor at play, it will only be one factor of the complex events which shape our sexuality.

How can I tell if I'm sexually curious or seriously gay or lesbian?

About 50 per cent of people experiment, to varying degrees, with the same sex during adolescence. That statistic includes everything from having a major crush on a same-sex teacher to actually having sex with the same sex. Of those who do experiment, the majority decide it's not for them after all. Others need to explore further before they decide. Some people stop having homosexual sex as they enjoy it with both sexes and it's less stressful and easier to be straight because that's what society accepts as normal. Others opt for casual sex with the same sex and relationships with the opposite for the same reason.

'I felt so isolated and didn't know any other lesbians. Eventually, I had to move to the city where I thought I'd be more accepted. I joined a support group immediately and was all set to attend my first meeting except I didn't go – I just couldn't walk in that front door. I rang the people who ran the group the next day and told them and they invited me to come into the office and have coffee. I did, got over my fears and my world changed from one of frustration and depression to feeling alive and good about myself.'

Fiona, 30,
personal assistant

It's probably best if you don't try to fit yourself neatly into one box. Some people have always known they're either exclusively homosexual or heterosexual and never, ever waver. Lots of others aren't sure where they fit in. How can *you* tell? The closest I can get to a definite answer seems to be this: you'll know you're gay if it feels right for you and if you're *consistently* and *repeatedly* drawn to the same sex and rarely or never to the opposite. Try to be honest with yourself. Are you fighting being gay because you're scared of rejection if people find out? Some people feel gay but when they look out at the visible, public face of the gay community, either feel they don't fit in there either or don't want to. Ask yourself, what sort of relationship would satisfy me most *at the moment*? You don't have to make a decision for life.

As for finding out 'for sure', start by working through your feelings and emotions. See a counsellor if you don't seem to be getting anywhere. Two or three sessions might make things crystal clear. The counsellor will focus on areas which may be holding you back from 'admitting' you're gay (like how your family will react, concerns about not having children, etc.). Once these concerns are addressed, you'll be less anxious about the consequences and more likely to unearth your real inclination.

You may decide you need to sleep with the same sex, the opposite sex or both before you can truly be sure. If you feel comfortable about that, go for it – just make sure you practise safe sex and don't get into dangerous situations. Know beforehand what you're prepared to do sexually and negotiate with your partner until you're sure they understand what you're hoping to get out of sex with them. Don't do it if it's going to get ugly with someone forcing you to continue if you don't want to. It's probably safer to meet someone through a support group and get to know them a little than it is to turn up at a gay or lesbian bar and take pot luck. One word of warning for guys who are thinking of sleeping with another man: it's not a myth that gay males are a high-risk group for HIV. You *must* wear a condom during anal penetration. Oral sex is low risk but if you've got cuts or ulcers in your mouth, or he does on his penis, use a condom.

! *Gay women have the best time in bed – at least that's the conclusion of a recent sex survey. Thirty-nine per cent of lesbians surveyed said their last sex session lasted more than one hour, with only 15 per cent of heterosexual women claiming the same. Only a fifth of the straight women had multiple orgasms compared to over a third of the lesbians. Gay men also clock up more orgasms per week than straight ones.*

! *Twenty-four per cent of men make homophobic statements compared to 3 per cent of females.*

If I sleep with the same sex once, does that make me gay, lesbian or bisexual? What about more than once?

In one study, psychologists found that half a random selection of men had had sex with another man to the point of ejaculation at least once in their life. For most, that was their only encounter and they were now straight. So an isolated encounter probably means you're curious, not gay. More than one probably doesn't mean you're gay or lesbian either. Again, it's only when you're *consistently* attracted to the same sex and have *lots* of sexual encounters with them that you probably are more gay or lesbian than straight.

Should I tell people if I'm convinced I'm gay or lesbian? How do I tell my parents?

This is called 'coming out' and whether it's wise to or not is something only you can decide. The upside: if everyone supports and accepts you, the relief is enormous. The downside: if they don't, your greatest fear is realised and you may be rejected, made fun of or ostracised, perhaps lose dearly loved friends or family.

There's no rule that says once you decide you're gay you have to come out of the closet with a brass band. Be selective with who you tell and your timing. Some people don't need to know and you'll gain nothing by telling them. Here are some questions and issues you might want to consider.

> 'I decided to finally tell my mother I was gay and she was terrific. The only thing she was concerned about was AIDS. Once I assured her I was up on the facts and only had safe sex, she said, "I'm honoured you've told me and my only regret is that you didn't tell me earlier. This must have been hard for you." It's no wonder I love her so much.'
>
> Tim, 25, student

- **How confident are you about your sexuality?** If you're confused or feel you might be passing through a phase, hold off.
- **Educate yourself about homosexuality.** Chances are, the people you tell will have some misconceptions about gays or lesbians. Prepare some answers to common questions like 'Aren't you scared of getting AIDS?' and 'It's Uncle John isn't it? He's turned you.'
- **Choose your time.** Are things okay at home? If your family is going through a stressful time – just moved, changed jobs or dealing with sickness or death – hang on. And try not to blurt it out in the middle of a fight.

- **What are your reasons for telling them?** If it's to build a more open, loving, trusting, respectful relationship, fine. If it's to deliberately hurt them, it's not very constructive for anyone.
- **Accept that people may say things they don't mean and will need time to get used to your news.** Think about it. It took you years to get used to the idea of being gay or lesbian; it will take them a little time to readjust as well. If the person is extremely conservative or very religious, it will be hard for them to accept your decision no matter how much time you give them. Are you sure they need to know? Can you keep this part of your life separate and still maintain a good relationship?
- **Are you financially dependent on them?** If they reject you, can you look after yourself?
- **Line up someone supportive to see afterward in case your friends or family react badly.** Call the lesbian and gay switchboard on 0171 837 7324 for help and advice.
- **Make sure the decision to 'come out' is *your* decision.** Ignore people who pressure you either way. Coming out will have a huge impact on your life – it could be positive, it could be negative. Make sure you've thought through the consequences before going ahead.

Twice as many career women as homemakers admit to having a homosexual experience.

The gay and lesbian bar scene doesn't appeal to me. Where else can I go to meet a partner?

Call the lesbian and gay switchboard for advice on what social groups operate in your area. There are gay and lesbian movie clubs, gay and lesbian basketball clubs; in other words, homosexual versions of lots of straight clubs. Some of them only mix within the gay community, others (like sport teams), play against straights. You could also try answering a personal ad but be careful. Arrange to meet in a public place and be aware that people often lie, not only about what they look like but what sort of relationship they're really after. Generally, the more gay people you know, the more gay people you'll meet. Cultivate friendships with people like you even if you don't fancy them. We all need friends as well as lovers!

The thought of being gay or lesbian frightens the hell out of me. I don't want to be different. How will I cope?

It's hard being different in anything. We all like being individuals but we also try to be like everyone else. It feels uncomfortable being singled out, especially if you live in a rural community and feel like you're the only one who is different. But the fact is, you're not. Numerous studies have tried to pinpoint the number of homosexuals and the verdict appears to be about 10 per cent of the population (people regularly having sex with the same sex). So, there are lots of people like you, in your situation.

Instead of focusing on how different you are and whether you're gay or straight, shift to what you could do to lead a fulfilling and happy life. You might need to make some changes to achieve this: maybe change jobs, friends or where you live. Moving to a city or neighbourhood where homosexuality is more accepted could be a good idea. For information ring the lesbian and gay switchboard on 0171 837 7324 which is open 24 hours. There are also a number of local services in many cities. Once you meet other gay people and realise they're not only 'normal' but everywhere, you'll feel more comfortable and be proud of who you are.

> **!** ***Twenty-five per cent of gay and lesbian Australians attempt suicide.***

Having said that, I'm not pretending for a moment that it's easy being in any minority group. Lots of people will judge you and many are prejudiced against homosexuals. The rewards for being 'normal' are so great that those who can pass for straight often will. But trying to deny who you are and pretending you're not gay or lesbian isn't a terribly good idea either. Those that do often suffer from low self-esteem, and tend to distance themselves from family and friends (can't let anyone get too close in case they 'find out'), thus feeling even more isolated and inferior. Their life is based on a lie so they never feel accepted.

It makes sense to surround yourself with people who accept you for who you are. If someone tells you you're sick, bad or wrong often enough, you'll start believing it and stop looking after yourself. Studies show the gay and lesbian population has more drug and alcohol problems and unsafe sex than the straight population. Suicide rates are also higher. Australia is in the unenviable position of having one of the highest suicide rates in the world; 80 per cent of suicides are males with rates peaking in the 16 to 25 age group. Causes include relationship issues – like realising you're gay.

! ***Of all the sex groups, gay and bi women:***

- ***have the most sex – 59 per cent have it two or three times a week***
- ***are most likely to have sex with someone they didn't like, 'just to be nice' – 27 per cent***
- ***masturbate the most – 38 per cent do it once a day or more***
- ***are most likely to have sex outdoors – 75 per cent***
- ***are most likely to use food to enhance masturbation – 22 per cent***
- ***are most likely to be involved in a relationship – 60 per cent***

How do I deal with homophobes (people who hate or fear homosexuals)?

It's an offence in a number of states to ridicule or harm gays and lesbians, so in these states you are protected by legislation. Most city police stations have gay and lesbian liaison officers who will help you make a complaint and all states have anti-violence laws.

If we're talking about a muttered 'poofter' or 'dyke' as you walk past some idiots in a bar, you're probably wise to ignore it (*especially* wise if you could end up hurt). Rise above the homophobes and recognise *they* are the ones with the problem. If you're the witty, articulate type, maybe you'll enjoy challenging them. Who knows, if you present an intelligent argument, you might even change their perception. On the other hand, if they're going to behave like that in the first place, it's not likely.

I think my boyfriend/girlfriend is gay. How do I tell?

Ask them. Say why you think they might be gay and try to be open to what they have to say rather than accusing. Of course it's upsetting if you love them and fear they'll leave you, but at least try to put yourself in their shoes. They've probably been struggling with the issue for years and your support could be a lifeline. If they agree they might be, you need to discuss the implications for the relationship. Maybe you could agree to be friends for a while until they decide for sure. If you think your guy is having unprotected sex with men (or other women, for that matter) behind your back, get an HIV test, use condoms and don't stop unless you're convinced you were just being paranoid.

I'm straight but my best friend's just told me they're gay/lesbian? What do I do now?

Nothing. Just because they're gay doesn't mean they fancy *you*. If you're worried about that, ask them. If they confess undying love, explain that you're straight and are sure of it. If they can accept a platonic relationship, the problem's solved; you might feel a bit funny for a little while but that will pass. If they can't, maybe see them less often until they find a partner.

! ***Bi-Bi BOYS . . . A large percentage of British women are giving the male population the flick and switching camps sexually. Only 14 per cent of readers of a British mainstream women's magazine considered themselves straight, with half describing themselves as bisexual. One quarter had had sex with another woman, 86 per cent fantasised about it.***

BUT I HEARD . . .

Lots of people, particularly straights, have certain misconceptions about gays and lesbians. Most aren't true and if there is a grain of truth under some piles of prejudice, the reasons for it aren't what you may assume.

Our new acceptance of gay and lesbian people will encourage confused teenagers to turn gay

There is absolutely no evidence to support the 'recruitment' theory which this thinking is based on. Equally as untrue is the fear that if someone hangs around gay people, they'll be taken advantage of or turn gay themselves even if they're straight. They won't. The only thing they may turn into is tolerant, accepting, non-judgemental people.

Lesbians all use dildos because they secretly miss the 'real thing'

Some straight couples use dildos, vibrators and other sex toys to add variety to their sex life, some don't. Lesbians are no different. Some like penetration and use dildos but I seriously doubt it's inspired by penis envy. Most are far too busy indulging in lots of mutual masturbation and oral sex to give it a thought. Lots of studies say gays and lesbians have more satisfying sex than straights. Certainly, they've got a distinct advantage: both partners have the same bits, so what usually feels good for them will feel good for their partner.

! ***Should gay people have the legal right to marry? Fifty-two per cent of straight men and 70 per cent of straight women say yes.***

All gay men have anal sex

Some gay men like being penetrated by a penis. Some gays only like doing it to their partner. Some gays don't like either doing it or receiving it, and some find it hurts. Like lesbians, gays usually have lots of oral sex, mutual masturbation or enjoy anal stimulation without penile penetration.

! ***Forget vampy, lipstick lesbian chic – the new lesbian is just as likely to be a blue-rinse bowls player. Psychologists now say women are increasingly likely to become lesbians in later life because of a shortage of men. There's already evidence of a radical change in the sexual habits of older women, revealing that many are turning to each other for love and sex.***

Gays are more promiscuous than straights

If you think of the gay community as being the few thousand people who go to gay venues and parade in the Gay and Lesbian Mardi Gras, studies show it's possible they are more promiscuous than the average heterosexual. But that's like judging all straight people on those who go to bars and nightclubs. Neither group is representative of the majority. (By all accounts, even those gays and lesbians who frequent the clubs tire of the scene after a couple of years anyway.) Once involved in relationships, they're as likely, or unlikely, as the rest of us to have a bit on the side.

> 'I was going out with this guy who had the most beautiful sister who was gay. I was fascinated by her and developed a massive crush. For a while there, I seriously toyed with the idea of switching camps – trouble was, I knew she wasn't interested in me. That was eight years ago. I've met a few women since who I've found attractive but know now I don't really want to act on it.'
>
> Zara, 27, dentist

As with all sex studies, it's difficult to find out exactly what Mr and Mr or Mrs and Mrs Average get up to in day-to-day life. Even harder to survey when it's a minority group used to being persecuted.

If gays do become promiscuous, researchers say it's often a reaction to the treatment dished out by society. Those who accept the negative images of gays are more likely to adopt the 'promiscuous' lifestyle society expects of them. Often, what seems like promiscuous behaviour – having sex in parks and public toilets – may not be a choice, but the only means they have of exploring homosexuality. Unfortunately, it still ups their chances of contracting an STI or HIV. As for gays not caring if they 'catch AIDS', that's not far off the mark in *some*, *isolated* instances. In one study, young gays who regularly practised unsafe sex weren't on drugs, drunk or particularly aroused, but were angry and depressed. Why should they care if they get AIDS, they figured, if no-one else does?

CHANGING CAMPS, SWITCHING BACK: REAL LIFE STORIES

Josh, 32, architect

Josh remained asexual for years until he came to terms with being gay.

'Looking back to primary school, I can make the connection that I've always been gay. I had a huge crush on a male teacher in Year six and always communicated better with girls than I did guys, which I think's pretty typical of gays. But it was when everyone started pairing off with girls and I didn't want to pair off with anyone that it hit. I went out with girls to prove to myself I couldn't be gay – I even slept with a few – but it was pretty sad. It felt weird; I was going against what I was. I decided that wasn't for me and gave up on sex, didn't do anything.

'My first reaction to thinking I was gay was, "Yuk! This can't be right. I don't want this." I'm very religious and homosexuality was contrary to the church's teachings. (Interestingly, it's not written in the Bible that it's wrong. It was Queen Victoria, the stupid cow, that made the church say it was wrong.) I was in my early 20s before I decided I had to become a sexual person. I'd had a lot to struggle through, particularly working out how my religious and sexual sides could ever mesh. Adrian, the guy I'm with now, was the first guy I slept with and it wasn't until him that I came to terms with it totally. I was scared shitless the first time I slept with Adrian. It felt right and very comfortable but all that "No, no, this is the wrong thing to do" stuff came up. Having sex with a man was the final thing: you're confronting it, you're doing it, you can't go back. The next morning I just got up and left. I was petrified! But the next day, there I was back and having lunch and I haven't looked back. Except then, of course, I had to decide whether to tell anyone or not.

'No-one knew I was gay and I briefly considered not telling anyone, thought maybe I could be celibate or get married and force myself to love a woman, but I'm so glad I didn't. I know so many people in that situation now and they've got kids but eventually it's going to come out and I think that's a horrible thing to do to the family. My boyfriend's sister has offered to have a baby for us but although Adrian would like kids, I'm not convinced it's fair on the child. It would have to be a girl. If it was a boy people would say, "There's two poofters who've got a little boy to play with." Politically, I think gay couples should have kids, but in reality it can be cruel.

'I've never actually told my parents I'm gay though I think they know. They're pretty sheltered people and deeply religious and I don't want to throw it in their face and say, "Deal with it." I'm breaking it to them by showing them. They know I live with Adrian and they know there's only one bed. They love me and they want whatever makes me happy and I'm demonstrating to them I'm not an Oxford queen but the son they know.

'I was never the sort of guy who wanted to bonk everything on Oxford Street [a 'gay' hangout in Sydney]. I think that's the way some guys come to terms with being gay. Sort of a "Shit! Okay, I'd better just go and do it" reaction, so they sleep with as many people as possible to comfort themselves. They're the ones that don't want to fit into straight society: they stick to their own small community because they don't want to face the big picture. When people think "gay", that's who they think of – the queens that parade in the Mardi Gras. I'm quite proud of the fact that I'm not like that. You don't have to throw your sexuality in people's faces all the time and people rarely pick me, or my partner, as being gay. Adrian and I have more straight friends than gay ones and are well integrated into "normal" society. A lot of gay guys are in touch with their feminine sides but scared of the masculine. We're in touch with both and that makes it easier for us to get on with straight guys as well.

'People who say you choose to be gay, well, that's bullshit. I didn't have a choice and I believe in the gay chromosome theory. If you're not gay there's no way you'd put yourself under all the emotional stress just to be fashionable. I mean, why would you do it? I know straight guys who've got pissed and ended up sleeping with another bloke and their reaction is to wake up the next day and vomit. I think the hardest thing for me is, because I appear straight, girls come onto me a lot. I don't want to go around saying, "Look honey, I'm gay" to everyone I meet, but there have been occasions where they find out and still persist. That annoys me. They're buying into that "all you need is a good woman" theory.

'My advice to other guys who think they might be gay is this: there's only one way to find out and that's to experiment. Sleep with the opposite sex first, then meet some gay people, talk to them and see if you connect. For God's sake, don't go to a gay bar if you're trying to find out: they're meat markets and you'll end up more screwed up than ever. The safest way is to contact a gay support group or gay counsellor. Also remember, you're a person first, gay second. Don't define yourself by who you sleep with.'

Amanda, 26, shop assistant

Amanda told her friends and family she was gay, then decided she wasn't.

'Sometimes I think my life sounds like a really bad script for a sit-com. Looking back, I actually think it's quite funny but it sure as hell wasn't at the time. I led a typical straight life up until I hit 22 – went out with guys, slept with them, the usual stuff. I'd had my share of bad boys but nothing none of my other girlfriends hadn't suffered through. I'd never thought much about being lesbian because it didn't seem relevant to me. I had a few girlfriends who were gay but what they did in bed was their business and I didn't think of them any differently from my straight girlfriends.

'Then I meet Darrell. She was introduced to me at a party, along with her boyfriend (who I thought was a complete jerk). She was amazing looking and reminded me of a young colt: all legs, a long neck and she held herself really proudly. I liked her and we chatted for ages when, much to my horror, I found myself flirting with her. I was a bit drunk but I couldn't stop looking at her lips and wondering what it would be like to kiss her. I felt strangely miffed when she left, arm-in-arm with her boyfriend, and thought, "Wow! I was attracted to another woman." That would have been that, except she got my phone number from the hostess and rang me. We went out for coffee and dinner a few times and I thought we were just going to be friends. Except a few weeks later, she turned up on my doorstep sobbing because her boyfriend had dumped her. She said she didn't know many people in our town because she'd just moved there. I let her in, cuddled her and said she could stay with me. That night, she slept in my bed and we became lovers. She'd slept with other women before and said she was bi.

'I should have recognised it for what it was: experimentation and a fling. But, oh no, I had to take it all seriously. I bought some books on lesbians and didn't identify with any of what was written but still I wasn't perturbed. I decided it wasn't fair on Darrell not to introduce her as my lover to my friends and family – so I did. I went around to my parents' house and made a dramatic announcement that I was a lesbian. They stared at me in absolute amazement and said, "Are you sure, darling?" To their credit, they were wonderful about it. My parents are pretty cool and they didn't overreact and welcomed Darrell into our home. My friends, on the other hand, were either horrified or thought it extremely amusing. My best friend, who'd always said her favourite fantasy was sleeping with another woman, was more perceptive than most. "Do you think you're lesbian or just have a thing about Darrell?" she said. "Because if it's Darrell, you're going to end up hurt." She was right, of course. I got up one morning and Darrell had split, leaving a beautiful letter saying she was a free spirit and thought I was getting in too deep, but it was a kiss-off all the same. The whole affair had lasted three months and I was devastated.

'I missed her heaps but, as the weeks went on, gradually started to accept what had happened to me. Then, I was sitting in a pub with a girlfriend and the most gorgeous guy walked in and I went to jelly. That was when I realised my best friend was right. I wasn't a lesbian, just attracted to one female. I now consider myself straight but it's taught me a lot about sexuality and I don't regret what happened for a minute. I don't even regret blabbing my business to everyone, even if my boss does think I'm a fruitcake now. Without exception, no-one ridiculed me or insulted me so I feel well and truly loved for whoever I am.'

Everyday Couples, Exceptional Sex

I'm sorry, did you say monogamy or monotony?

When I was 21, I got engaged to my childhood sweetheart. 'Do you know,' he said, gazing soulfully into my eyes, 'I'll be the last person you'll ever have sex with for the rest of your life'. It felt as though someone had kicked me in the stomach. I felt like a rabbit caught in the headlights of an approaching car. Like the gaoler had just turned the key on the lock to my prison cell. My vision of marriage transformed from trendy career couple swilling back wine while having wild sex on the back patio, to polyester dresses, aprons, floury fingers and twin single beds. The ring was off my finger within a week.

It wasn't that I hadn't thought about the sex side *or* that I wanted to do the entire male Olympic swim team (though I could think of worse ways to spend a week). It was the concept of one person being my first, my last and one and only. I just couldn't do it. The word 'monogamy' threw up frightening images of padded cells for years after that but somewhere along the line my attitude changed. I finally figured monogamy and monotony don't *have* to go together like peaches and cream. Here's how I look at it now . . .

Picture your favourite restaurant. Now imagine dining there *every single night for the rest of your life*. After a month, that greasy takeaway shop is looking appealing! Sex with the same person can be like that. Why would you fancy a hamburger when you could have prime rump? Simple. You're bloody sick of prime rump.

Okay. Now go back to the restaurant and imagine that each night you go there, something is different. One night, the music's soft and the lights are dimmed. The next, the stereo's blasting and they've cleared the tables to make a dance floor. One evening they serve French food, the next Italian, the following Thai. There's enough variety to order a different dish every night. The decor changes constantly: dark, gothic and moody one night, bright, light and stainless steel the next. In winter there's a fire, in summer the windows are flung open to catch the breeze and a view. Sometimes, you go alone and read a book. Other times, you and your lover solve the world's problems until the wee hours, or you're romantic and playful. The point is this: even if the place is the same, if you change the variables, it *seems* different. Ditto for monogamous sex.

You can make love to the same person for the rest of your life in a million different ways, places and situations. Naked, half-naked or clothed; clothes ripped off or stripped off. Sex can be slow and sensual, raw and wicked, intense and erotic; a two-hour marathon or a two-minute quickie up against the fridge. Dinner outside, dinner in – with dessert eaten off each other's bodies. Does monogamy *have* to be boring? In a word: no. Why then, do most people complain it is?

When pop gender-bender Boy George made headlines by admitting he'd prefer a cup of tea to sex most nights, thousands of couples secretly agreed with him. When Dr Patricia Love released a book called *Hot Monogamy*, hordes of desperate couples deviated from their sacred Saturday, Sainsburys/Ikea/Woolworths circuit to head for the local bookshop. Eavesdrop on any cappuccino-fuelled conversation between two females with kids and you'll hear, 'Sex? God! I couldn't care less if I never did it again.' Hell, neither would I if him on top, only on Sundays and always in bed sex was all that was on offer. If that's monogamy, no wonder it's very, very dull (if it was ever exciting in the first place). If slipping between the sheets and into the same sex ritual every time sums up *your* love life, full marks for even mustering up enough enthusiasm to open this book!

But here are the words you've been waiting to hear: sex can get *better* as the years roll on. Not only that, it can improve RIGHT NOW. There's just one catch: you have to be prepared to put creativity and effort into your sex life to introduce the variety that's lacking. At first, if you're mind-numbingly bored by each other's bits, this will be *a real slog*. One or two sessions later, it'll seem less like hard work. One month from that, you'll start grinning at each other whenever you think about last night. And two months on? Your friends will be calling to say, 'Where *were* you two last night? You never seem to go out much anymore . . . '

WHAT'S GREAT ABOUT MONOGAMY

- You can still have sex on 'fat-days' – you know he finds all of you sexy.
- You can relax a little – it doesn't matter if you don't get an erection, she knows it's a one-off.
- You don't have to use condoms – you've both had AIDS tests and don't want to have sex with other people.
- You can drop those inhibitions – you trust each other and know you won't be branded 'weird', 'slutty' or 'perverted' if you confide a fantasy.
- You're pretty well guaranteed an orgasm – if you've taught each other well, you each know the right buttons to push.
- You enjoy all different types of sex, not just the lusty sort. Sometimes it's romantic and lazy, and it's always loving and intimate.
- You smile when you wake up together the morning after – rather than wonder how the hell you got there.

WHAT ISN'T

There are two major complaints about monogamy: sex can become routine and boring (try everything in this chapter, then get back to me on that one!) and 'the newness' has gone. That's the number one beef of even happy couples. 'I love X, but you just can't recreate that fabulously erotic feeling you get when it's someone you've *never* done it with before.' Hmmm. I could lie and give you false hope. I could say, 'Don't be silly, of course it's possible.' But I honestly don't believe it is.

Playing games, acting out fantasies, introducing so much variety your head is spinning – all will help immeasurably. But it's still not the same as the very first time with someone new: that's the one downside of monogamy. But if it's the *only* bad thing, it's a small price to pay for all the pluses of being with someone you love. Cope with it by having sex with anyone you want – in your imagination. Fantasise madly that she's the girl in your office or he's your best friend's boyfriend but DON'T TAKE IT THROUGH TO REALITY even if you *can* get away with it.

! Number of women who say they wouldn't remarry if their current marriage failed: 80 per cent. The year of marriage you're most likely to have an affair: during the fourth or fifth.

Every time you're tempted, work through this exercise. Imagine your partner's face if they found out (and it's amazing how most people do). Picture how hurt they would be. Remember that they, too, feel the odd urge to roam but don't, out of respect for you. Even if they never find out, you know you've betrayed them. You've broken that special bond and can never, ever look them in the eye honestly again. Then imagine your partner being so hurt and angry, they leave you. You've broken their heart, you've lost everything, you feel like a complete scumbag. Was that thrill, that one blissful moment of experiencing a new body, worth it? If you run all this through your mind and still consider it would be, get out of the relationship NOW. You don't just want a bit on the side, you want to be single.

Some sex therapists say it's normal for each of you to have the odd sexual encounter during your lives together. What you don't know can't hurt you, etc. I don't agree. I've seen pointless they'll-*never*-find-out encounters destroy more than one otherwise blissfully happy couple. In all cases, the person who strayed counts it as the No. 1 Biggest Mistake of Their Life.

THEY'RE HOT, YOU'RE NOT

The third most common couple sex complaint is mismatched libidos: your partner wants sex more or less than you do. To a point, it's something you both have to learn to accept. Having said that, there's a hell of a lot you can do to even the scales.

Part of the turn-off of monogamous sex is that you've got sex on tap. It's *always* available. The single and sex-starved *crave* for someone to touch their naughty bits. Long-time lovers don't get a chance to build desire because it's always being satisfied. So, you start having sex when you don't really want to (because you feel you should), it becomes boring and your brain starts to associate the two. Part of the solution is obviously variety (see 'Foreplay for familiar lovers' on page 314), but you have to *want* to try the suggestions I've made – and if you don't feel like sex, why would you?

If your partner wants it more than you do

If you want sex less often than your partner, here are some tips from the experts for getting the urge back.

> ***More Please!***
> ***Number of men who want more sex: 60 per cent. Number of women who want more sex: 70 per cent. The most sexually active age for men and women: between 21 and 24.***

- **Put pen to paper.** Think back to the best sex you've had and work out what it was that made it so special. Who was your partner? Where were you? What led up to the experience? What did he do to you that made it so great? What did you do to him? Write down as many details as possible, then do the same for your worst sexual experiences, including the ho-hum ones. Compare the lists and use them to make another: list the significant things that make sex good for you and those that make it bad. Put them in order of importance and you should have a good idea of what you like, and what you don't. Regularly ask yourself: What would I like more of in bed? What would I like less of? What can I do to make it better?
- **Start keeping a diary.** Write down any sexy thoughts you have, any fantasies, how you felt when someone gave you a compliment. The aim is to remind yourself that you're a sexual person and find out what's stopping you feeling sexy all the time. If you don't think of anything at all even wildly related to sex and nothing happens, write that down too.

'Would rather have my fingernails pulled' is better than nothing. For every negative thought, try to write a reason why ('Because I'm so tired'). Keep the diary for at least three months. Re-reading it will provide valuable insights into what's stopping those juices flowing.

- **Buy some erotic books.** By that I mean whatever turns *you* on. It doesn't matter if it's *Gardening by the Stars*; if that causes a pleasant little ache down below, read it.
- **Start masturbating.** Contrary to popular myth, masturbating while you're living with someone doesn't stop you wanting 'real' sex. The more you masturbate, the more your body gets used to having orgasms and starts craving sex on a regular basis.
- **Now involve your partner.** The better sex is, the more you'll want it. Both of you write down, being as specific as possible, what you do and don't like about your sex lives. Things like: are you getting enough foreplay; what would you like more of, do the techniques suit you; are you happy with when, where, how often you have sex; what would you prefer; ideas on bringing back the 'newness'. Also include relationship issues: are you happy generally, what's upsetting you, what do and don't you like about the relationship. Be as honest as you can be.
- **Talk about it.** Don't just hand over your lists – you'll both end up huffy. Instead, flip a coin to decide who goes first. You won? Okay, now go through your list and explain, point by point, as clearly as possible what you mean. Get your partner to repeat back to you, in their own words, what they think you've just said. This way, there's no room for misinterpretation. Then, they get their turn and you summarise each of their points. When you've both said your piece, you can then move into thinking up ideas of how to overcome any of the issues thrown up.

White people are more likely to cheat on their partner than any other racial group.

- **Do something about it.** Each of you write down five things you could do to make sex better for your partner based on what they've just told you. Schedule one day per week or fortnight to do the things on the list (don't try to do them all at once). Make one small change each time you have sex. After a while, the new behaviour will become second nature.

- **Have sex even if the urge is tiny.** The more you do it, the more you'll want to. Stimulate yourself. Turn *yourself* on, don't expect your partner to do it and *make* time. If you're that busy, have a quickie.
- **Recharge your sex organs with the Sets of Nine.** This is a Taoist intercourse technique which 'massages' the vagina and penis. Basically, he thrusts in a carefully sequenced order. 1. Only the head of the penis is inserted and withdrawn, nine times, then he thrusts the entire length in once. 2. Eight shallow strokes (penis head only), two deep strokes (with the entire length). 3. Seven of the shallow strokes, three deep ones. 4. Six shallow, four deep. 5. Five shallow, five deep. 6. Four shallow, six deep. 7. Three shallow, seven deep. 8. Two shallow, eight deep. 9. One shallow, nine deep.

If you're the one who wants it more

- **Try masturbating every second time you feel like sex.** It takes the pressure off both of you.
- **Make it very clear when you want sex and stop hassling if they say no.** 'Tim *always* wants sex,' says Sarah. 'Every touch is sexual. Just once, I'd like him to touch me out of love and affection only.' 'I touch Sarah heaps and try to be as loving as possible,' says Tim. 'I make a real effort not to touch her only when I feel like a bit, but it's still not working.' Get the picture? If your partner's constantly feeling hassled, make it very clear when you are stroking them in an attempt to turn them on so that other times they'll interpret it as affection. Once they've said 'no', leave it alone. You'll put them off even more if they feel harassed.
- **Make sex enjoyable.** Know your partner and what turns them on. Ask them, talk it through, do whatever it takes to make sex fun and something they look forward to. The better lover you are, the more they'll want to sleep with you. A massage works wonders for changing minds.

WHY SHOULD I HAVE SEX WITH HIM?

Here's a fact: you can't have a great sex life if your relationship isn't good. If you've barely spoken all day, glared at each other over the (deliberately) burnt toast or are constantly flinging nasty, petty comments at each other, it's pretty unlikely you're going to turn into a sex kitten and Sensitive New Age Lover once you hop into bed. If you're not relating out of bed, you won't relate in it. This means (groan!) your sex life isn't the only thing you have to work at.

If the only time you touch each other sexually is under the blankets, I guarantee you'll be bored silly – with sex and each other – within a year. Treat each other as desirable creatures *all* the time and you'll be surprised how much you'll want to act on it. Sex can't provide the intimacy that's missing elsewhere in your relationship.

> ! ***Thirty-three per cent of men and 37 per cent of women feel unsure of how to satisfy their sex partner.***

- **Live life to the full.** People who love sex, love life and that attitude is attractive to everyone, not least of all their partners. Develop lots of passions, be energetic, get excited about new things and new people – don't just grab life with both hands, give it a big squeeze. Sexy is a state of mind. Hedonists are melt material.
- **Look sexy and keep fit.** Having dinner with a woman who only orders an entrée and mineral water isn't fun. One who orders up big, eats with gusto and appreciates a good wine is. The ability to let go, to stop counting kilojoules is a turn-on – but not if you let go completely. Taking care of your appearance should be a priority. Yeah, yeah, I know it's what's inside that should count but let's drop the politics and be realistic. Beer bellies, baggy tracksuits, greasy hair, bottoms straining to escape from too-tight jeans – they're not on *my* list of top turn-ons or yours. Exercise, eat well, get lots of sleep and don't hit the booze too heavily, too often. The better you look, the better you'll feel about yourself, and the sexier you'll be to your partner. You need energy to throw yourself around that bedroom.

- **Touch each other as much as possible.** Do it all the time, in public, at home, always. 'When I met Susan,' says my friend Kevin, 'the first thing I noticed was that she touched everyone. She couldn't help it. She hugged her best friend, smacked a huge kiss on her brother's cheek, threw her arms around the dog. I spent the whole night wishing she'd touch me and when she did, I was lost. Even now, three years on, I can't wait for her to make contact.'
- **Have confidence.** Don't get dragged into those, 'Oh, everyone plays around sooner or later' conversations. Ditto, any discussion which starts with, 'Of course, sex dies after a while . . . ' Refuse to believe your lover would want anyone else when he's already got you. Refuse to accept that sex isn't as good long-term – put the effort in and it'll get better and better and better and . . .
- **Respect each other. Be polite.** Say 'Thanks darling, that was great' for everything from a cup of coffee to a fab orgasm. Say 'You look sensational. Thanks for going to so much effort' if she looks stunning when you go out. Look after each other when you're sick; listen to each other's problems. Be *nice*.

! ***Always fighting and think the relationship is doomed? Not true if you're having good times too. Stormy twosomes clock up more bad times than their passive peers, but they have more highs as well. Of 73 married couples studied, the happiest were those who maintained a 5:1 ratio of good to bad times.***

- **Live your own life.** Spend too much time together, focus only on each other and you'll fast become bored – and boring. What are you going to talk about if you do everything as a twosome?
- **Fight fair.** Argue about one issue at a time. If you find yourself saying, 'And another thing . . . ', stop. Ditto 'This is just typical of you. It's like the time when you . . . '
- **Boost each other's egos.** 'Hi, handsome.' 'Here she is – isn't she gorgeous?' Silly little compliments feel good and reinforce those 'cosy couple' feelings.

- **Throw away your copy of *Mars and Venus*.** Forget all that men and women are aliens stuff and concentrate on the similarities. Men are taller, hairier, more oddly endowed versions of us. We're softer, curvier versions of them. He cries, you cry. He needs love, affection and sex; so do you. There are more points of similarity between the sexes than differences. Refuse to wage war. Make a deal to be more like each other. You'll try to be more upfront sexually if they'll promise to be more romantic.

Number of couples who say they're very satisfied with their sex life: 58 per cent. Twenty-seven per cent of couples say an unwilling partner is to blame for their dissatisfaction.

- **Let him be him, let her be her.** Remember what first attracted you to them? Why are you trying to change it?

FIVE THINGS BOTH OF YOU SHOULD KNOW ABOUT SEX BY NOW

There's been a trillion sex surveys done and certain themes emerge frequently. The sex lives of long-term couples who consistently rate theirs as 'excellent' all share the following characteristics.

1. You both know your way around your own and your partner's body. You know what you want in bed

It's surprising how often people say, 'I don't like my sex life but don't know what I need to make it better.' You have to know what you want in order to get it. You each should have read at least three good sex books, masturbate regularly and be able to bring yourself to orgasm without too much effort. If you don't know what your body requires to orgasm, how the hell is your partner expected to figure it out?

2. You talk about sex regularly to each other

Imagine if your lover chose what books you read and what programs you watched. You'd be incensed, right? I mean, how could he possibly know what you feel like *at that exact moment* without asking you? Most people have no problems agreeing with this statement. Apply the same logic to the bedroom, however, and they become quite indignant. Sex should be spontaneous, instinctual, something that 'just happens'. Sex should all come naturally. Nice thought. Pity it doesn't work like that in real life.

Will someone please tell me why people say, 'If you have to tell your lover what you want, it takes all the fun out of it'? Does sticky date pudding with caramel sauce taste awful because we had to order it? Would it taste better if the waitress plonked it down in front of us because she got a telepathic signal that it's what we wanted? I don't think so. Lots of people expect their partners to be sexual mind-readers. They think, 'If he or she *really* loved me, they'd know exactly what to do in bed to make me happy.' They don't. If there's one thing you can do to instantly improve your sex life, it's to talk to your lover about sex, as clearly and *specifically* as you can.

! *Sixty-two per cent of men and 73 per cent of women say they find their partners more sexually attractive now than when they first met.*

'I want you to kiss me more' isn't enough. Spell out where, how hard, what sort of kissing and when during sex you'd like it to happen: 'When we have intercourse, I'd love you to kiss me hard on the mouth just before I orgasm.' Use phrases like 'instead of' rather than 'I don't like it when' and don't forget to say what you like as well as what you don't. If you're embarrassed, do whatever it takes to get over it. If you don't open your mouth at some point, your sex life (and relationship) really is destined for failure.

3. You plan for good sex and put thought into it

These are the words just about all couples dread because they think it (a) means the lust has gone, (b) they must be *really* unhappy sexually to go to such extremes, and (c) it sounds like hard work. Wipe all three thoughts from your head. Accept that it's possible to put a little intellectual effort into your sex life without losing spontaneity.

Simmering is an American technique which therapists often find quite successful. Every time you have an erotic thought during the day, write it down then use it as a jumping-off point. Develop a fantasy around the thought and tell your partner what it is and what you'd like to do with it *before you see them*. By the time you see each other, you're 'simmering' with desire. Writing '10 pm Saturday' and sticking it on the fridge *won't* work. Simmering will. If you don't actively try to vary your sex life, you'll end up doing that fumbled first-thing-in-the-morning bleary stuff all the time. Hello monotonous monogamy.

Who has the best sex – stay-at-home-and-watch-television couples or those who party the night away? Studies prove those who stay in have better sex, more often.

4. You make your own rules and have stopped worrying about what other people are doing in bed

There are two types of sex: manufactured sex and real sex. Manufactured sex is the sex that's dished up on TV, in erotic movies and books. Women orgasm after three good thrusts; men never, ever lose their erection from too many beers. Real sex isn't like that. You are both individuals with your own sexual desires and preferences and your sex life isn't going to be like Jake and Amanda's on 'Melrose' - or the couple next door. There are no universal rules about what people should enjoy in bed and what they shouldn't. If she can only orgasm if you suck her right toe or he needs to wear a shower cap on his head, so what? Whatever makes both of you happy is fine. Don't be afraid to be different from the norm.

5. You're not embarrassed to let loose

If it's your long-term lover, what have you got to be shy about? Be willing to experiment and take a few chances. Loosen up a little, laugh a lot, drop the inhibitions and let your imagination run rampant.

FOREPLAY FOR FAMILIAR LOVERS (AND SOME GREAT IDEAS FOR JUST ABOUT ANYONE!)

Think back to when you met each other. The first few dates, particularly the ones before you've had intercourse – are one, long, deliciously exciting foreplay session. Remember getting an erection by simply watching her walk across a room? Being told off by your friends for snogging him in hallways at parties? People chastising you for not being able to keep your hands off each other? This is what we're aiming to recapture. Sadly, that initial sell-your-mother-to-get-it type of lust that characterises new relationships disappears all too quickly and sex gets relegated to a certain time-slot and place.

Sometimes this is not only sensible but necessary. If you've just started a new job, the last thing you're thinking about is whether the knickers you put on that morning are sexy enough for him to peel off that night. If he's struggling with family problems, chances are he's not going to surprise you with a sexy strip before the 6 o'clock news. But the rest of the time – when you're simply coping with the usual hiccups of routine, run-of-the-mill life – give sex the priority it deserves.

Memorise the next three sentences. Our most erogenous zone is the brain. The most erotic tool you have at your disposal is your imagination. The biggest turn-on of all is anticipation. Repeat them one more time. Learn how to combine the three and *wham!*, you've just raised your sex life from ho-hum to hellishly horny. Most of us think of foreplay as genital touching and oral sex. Wrong. Foreplay can start at 6 am in the morning, continue while you're both at work, be drawn out

'Paul and I have been together about 12 years but, I have to say, sex lately has been better than ever. We went out to dinner recently and ended up reliving the best sex we'd had. By the time we got in the cab we were both drunk and so excited, we completely ignored the driver and went for it in the back. I spread my legs really wide and Paul slid his fingers in and out. It was extremely obvious what we were doing and I got off on the fact that the cab driver could see exactly what was going on. When we got out, he refused payment, said he'd 'enjoyed the show'. I slithered out, pushed Paul against the wall outside the lift to his apartment and gave him the best head-job he'd ever had, right there, in the fully-lit foyer.'

Pamela, 36, armed forces

through dinner, then, when you're both *begging* to touch each other, the physical part starts.

Sceptical anyone actually *does* the things I'm suggesting? You're dead right. Few people do – that's why everyone's madly bonking everyone else behind each other's backs. It's easy to pick the couples who put effort into their sex lives. They're the two 60-year-olds next door who hold hands when they're out perusing the roses. That devilish gleam in their eyes isn't put there from bingo. Ditto the couple you've always envied because sexual sparks seem to *fly* between them yet they've been together five years. Here's how they do it . . .

- **Combine romance with eroticism.** You feel great when he sends you flowers, why not return the favour? If you think they aren't quite his style, then try sending a bottle of expensive vintage champagne, red wine or port. Now turn that loving gesture into a sexy one. Enclose a note explaining in great detail exactly what he did to deserve such luxurious spoils. (No, not washing your car – the to-die-for oral sex he gave you last week. Got it?) Your postscript details what you're aching for him to do to you that night!
- **Become a bookworm.** Invest £50 in your lovelife by walking into any good bookshop and walking out with an armful of sex books. You've already bought this one, now branch out into areas that particularly tickle your fancy: Tantric sex, fantasies, how to have a dozen orgasms an hour. You don't have to read them cover to cover, just dip inside once in a while to keep things fresh and imaginative. While you're there, splash out on a racy, erotic novel. Find the good bits and read them out to each other as a form of foreplay.

! ***The most popular places to have sex outside the bedroom? The car, the beach, in a swimming pool.***

- **For the confident.** Use your vaginal juices as perfume. Yup, I'm not kidding. Slip your finger inside, then touch it around your throat, your breasts, on your lips. He won't know what it is but he won't be able to keep his hands off you.
- **Have a bed picnic.** Set up chilled wine and an ice-bucket, foods you can eat with your fingers (fresh fruit, chocolates);

have an erotic movie playing in the background on the bedroom VCR.

- **Get snap happy.** Buy a Polaroid instant camera and take (flattering) shots of each other naked. (It's actually illegal for a processor to develop a pornographic film, not to mention the embarrassment of picking it up!) Destroy the pics after you've had fun if either of you feel uncomfortable about having them around. Personally, I wouldn't keep any of the explicit shots, no matter how much I loved and knew my partner.
- **Once isn't always enough.** There's a lot of hype about women having more than one orgasm but he likes double helpings too. Have sex in the morning on the weekend, then drag him back to bed an hour later.
- **Get wet.** Water does wonderful things: it makes us weightless and flexible and ensures every part of both of you tastes and smells wonderful. While I wouldn't recommend having intercourse in water (it dries up lubrication and forcing water up the vagina isn't recommended), the bath, a spa, a swimming pool or the sea are great places to start off.
- **Be her sex slave for a day.** An especially good idea if you're broke and her birthday is looming. All you need to do is offer to devote one entire day to pleasuring her. She gets to order you around unashamedly – and whether it's serving her an erotic breakfast in bed, feeding her grapes and strawberries Roman-style, or spending the day dressed only in your Calvins, you're not allowed to utter even a *word* of complaint.
- **Take a tip from *The Story of O*.** The character in the novel is taught not to give all of herself each time she makes love. Use the same philosophy and instead of each sex session running the gauntlet from kissing to intercourse, concentrate on one activity at a time: kissing and fondling-only sessions (no tongues, no penises, just fingers), oral sex without intercourse and intercourse without oral sex.

! ***Love hurts: 44 per cent of men and 41 per cent of women like getting love bites.***

- **Flirt with each other** – even if you've been together years! Experts say flirting sends natural amphetamines and endorphins surging through the body, stimulating an instant emotional 'high' not unlike orgasm. Pretend you've just met him and act as you did at the beginning. Dress sexily, look him dead in the eye when he's talking, twirl your hair around a finger. Be aware of your body when you move in front of him and chances are he'll sit up and take notice too.
- **Send sexy notes.** The written word is extremely powerful. Plant notes everywhere (preferably not just before her mother comes to visit). In the fridge stuck to the fruit juice, in her briefcase and make-up bag. Each one describes bits of her you find *so-o-o* sexy. The next time, make them 10 things you'd love to do to her right that second.
- **Tease.** You've got friends over for dinner? Smack him up against the fridge, cup his penis with your hand and give him a huge kiss while he's helping you in the kitchen. Chatter innocently away to your guests while he hides out there, waiting for his erection to go down.
- **Go out without knickers on.** This is one steamy idea even the least courageous of females can pull off. All you need to do is dress up for an evening out – and forget to put on your knickers. You can either tell him about it, or 'accidentally' show him by crossing your legs Sharon Stone-style.
- **Feeling a little bored at her next staff get-together?** Make things infinitely more interesting by feigning sickness,

> 'God knows what it was, but about three months ago, I went through a stage where all I could think about was sex. A lot of the time, I kept my mouth shut because we'd be over at Ian's mother's house or something. Then I started telling him about it and it built the sexual tension wonderfully. I rang him at work one day and told him I was masturbating and he cancelled a meeting, drove home and we had the best sex ever. It hasn't been this good since the beginning.'
>
> Helen, 32, mother

then take her with you to the bathroom. Emerge later feeling much better, thank you.

- **Be a voyeur.** Madonna's done it. So did Sabina in the erotic film *The Unbearable Lightness of Being*. We're talking mirrors and using them as sex props. Madonna and Sabina crawled and masturbated above mirrors laid flat on the floor. If yours is on the wardrobe door, it's pretty difficult to follow their lead. Instead, try making love in front of any available mirror in the house (angled so you can see her rather than vice versa if she's shy).
- **Be his mistress.** If he's going to have an affair, make sure it's with you. Arrange to meet him at lunchtime in the bar of a plain but presentable hotel. Book a room, buy a bottle of champagne and have forbidden, illicit, wild sex.
- **Get into the mood beforehand.** Masturbate several times during the day while you think about what the two of you will get up to that night – preferably telling her exactly what you're doing over the phone as you're doing it. Stop short of an orgasm, unless you're a premature ejaculator. If you are, masturbate an hour before you have sex – you'll last longer.
- **Remember kissing?** It's what you used to do when you first met. Many couples find that kissing stops once the relationship gets going or dwindles to a quick snog before getting down to business. A long, passionate kiss can do more to turn both of you on than putting your hands straight down the front of his trousers. It's more intimate than intercourse (which is why many prostitutes won't do it).
- **Have intercourse with your clothes on.** Feel each other through your clothing, put your leg in between her thighs and let her gyrate against it.
- **Be pushy.** Bearing down with your vaginal muscles during intercourse seems to trigger orgasm for many women.
- **Keep your eyes open.** Watch what's going on when you have sex, look into their face, watch your genitals moving in and out. Stimulate the sense of sight, not just touch.
- **Be unpredictable.** Let's face it – you're not going to widen his eyes with astonishment if you suggest having sex on a

Saturday night as you both climb into bed. But you will catch him unawares if you cuddle him from behind when he's washing the car, washing up or reading a book. Start fondling him, bring him to the brink of orgasm, then refuse to follow through until later.

- **Bare all.** For a truly original Valentine's Day gift, shave your pubic hair into the shape of a heart or shave it off completely. The sight of your totally exposed genitals will make him jump to attention!
- **Turn her on in the most inappropriate places.** This is a tricky one. Done at the right time, it works fantastically, but it does have a tendency to backfire. Many sex books advise you whisper suggestive somethings into her ear while you're out to dinner with her boss, for instance. Sounds fabulously erotic but, in practice her boss is likely to think you're horribly rude, or that they have got something stuck between their teeth and you're taking the mickey out of them. Ditto the ringing him at work bit. You want to get him hot and bothered but not so flustered he ends up blowing the deal of the century. By all means try it – just suss out the situation before you launch into your spiel.

> ***Great Timing . . .***
> ***When's the best time to have sex? In the morning. His testosterone levels peak around 9 am and if you've been together a while, your cycle probably echoes his. An orgasm? Midway through your menstrual cycle. You're twice as likely to orgasm because your nerve endings are at their most sensitive.***

- **Be anonymous.** Remember those silly masks you bought for the dress-up affair you both went to? Dig them out, put them on, laugh yourself stupid for five minutes, then have sex. Let your fantasies run wild and pretend you don't know each other.
- **Try Tantric.** It's the trendy thing to do. Basically, it's all about heightening and prolonging sexual arousal. To the newcomer, the most obvious thing about Tantric sex is that

things progress very slowly (you'll do nothing but stroke each other for hours); often, it ends with neither of you having an orgasm. Sounds ghastly? I'm with you but couples who fully explore Tantric or the Kama Sutra, swear the results are nothing short of spectacular.

- **Wake her up with the ultimate greeting** – licking her vagina. Do the same for him by licking his penis.
- **Make the move.** If your partner is always the one to initiate sex, the message you're sending is this: I do it to please you, not because I want to. This leaves both of you feeling cheated. The person who initiates sex feels sexier because they're taking control and giving themselves power. Surely you've watched enough movies by now to know that power's one of the biggest sexual turn-ons there is? Be the boss by suggesting sex and taking the lead role during lovemaking as well. Let them lie back while you do *all* the work.
- **Lie a little.** He's away on business? The next time he calls you late at night, skip the what-did-you-do-today stuff and tell him, in intimate detail, what you're wearing. No, not the truth – that Snoopy T-shirt and thick white socks are silky, black French knickers and a camisole. Move onto what you're going to do to him the minute you get your hands on him. The juicier and more explicit the better.

Q: What are most couples doing at 10.34 pm?
A: Making love. That's the average time researchers came up with when they asked 198 couples when they had sex.

- **Slide around on satin sheets.** So kitsch they're almost fashionable, you can't help but feel sensual with satin against bare skin. Great sex comes from indulging *all* the senses and satin sheets are one of a million ways to do it. Appeal to and vary one sense each time you make love and you'll never be bored again. Use music to stimulate his sense of hearing; talk to her while you're having sex, giving a blow-by-blow description of how she's making you feel. Ignite his sense of smell by burning oils, wearing perfume or letting him enjoy the naturally sweet scent your body emits when you're aroused. Touch is stimulated by different textures: use your hair, feathers and scarves as well as fingertips. Use food, champagne and all of your body parts to excite his taste buds.

- **Plan a dirty weekend.** More than one lack-lustre sex life has been saved by a spicy weekend bounding about on a king-size bed. Book the best hotel you can afford, pick her up from work on Friday night and disappear into the sunset for a weekend she won't forget in a hurry.
- **Dress for success.** He adores red lipstick, black stockings and high heels? You've got no excuse – any little black number suits this treatment. Make a night of it by playing the vamp, playing with your hair, playing with him under the table. She melts when you walk around the house in nothing but a pair of blue jeans, top button of the fly temptingly undone? Unless it's below freezing temperatures, indulge her on weekends.

'I've been married nine years but I could watch Sally undress for bed a million times and never be bored. She's always so distracted, she doesn't notice me watching but I love her breasts and the way she always fluffs her hair up and pouts in the mirror when she's naked . . . even if the only thing she's craving is sleep.'

Calvin, 43, architect

- **Make a pact to try one new thing each fortnight.** If you're too shy to launch into my other suggestions, start off simple. Have a bath together, give each other a foot massage, take off her top or his shirt without using your hands. Once you feel more comfortable, you can move into things like making love to them with their hands tied behind their back and (the real biggie) masturbating in front of each other. Get him to lick your fingers while you're masturbating yourself – you'll feel less embarrassed and both of you will find it a turn-on.
- **Turn undressing for bed into an art form.** It doesn't matter what you're wearing, it's how you take it off that counts. Unbutton tops slowly, stretch luxuriously as you pull

that sweater over your head, put one leg up on the bed as you roll down your pantihose. When you're naked, admire yourself for a minute in the mirror, running your hands over your breasts and hips. Not only will it keep him focused on your body and remove the familiarity of seeing you naked, it helps create a positive body image.

- **Suck each of his fingers as though it were a small penis.** Circle your tongue lazily around her palm to simulate oral sex.

> ***What do most women do straight after sex?***
> ***43 per cent have a shower***
> ***20 per cent clean their teeth***
> ***30 per cent roll over and go to sleep***
> ***7 per cent have a cigarette***

- **Learn to love oral.** Don't just do it to please him or her, revel in it. Crave it, concentrate, make noises to show you're enjoying it as much as they are. Switch from intercourse to oral and back again for sensational contrasts.
- **If you're excited, show it.** The biggest turn-on of all is seeing how much you're exciting your partner. If he's driving you wild, show him – better still, say so.

Enough already! In the midst of all this lust, it's worth pointing out that no-one can be a sexual dynamo all the time. If you don't feel like having sex, say so, and let him do the same. That way, it's guilt-free on both sides and it will save either of you putting on lukewarm performances.

SUGGESTIONS FROM THE SEXPERTS

Here, a sex therapist, relationships counsellor, sex worker, erotica expert and real people with really good sex lives share their secrets for keeping sex lusty long-term.

Dr Janet Hall

Sex therapist, relationships counsellor, author and public speaker on sexuality, Dr Janet Hall says:

- 'Put a magnet on the fridge which each of you move to show how horny you're feeling. If it's high it means "You're in luck"; if it's low, it means "Don't bother asking". This takes away the anxiety of "Does he/she want it or don't they?" Both of you have the right to move the magnet around – or have two!

- 'Use a dirty weekend as a reward for something – one of you gets a pay rise, you've finished doing up the house, etc. If a sexy weekend often follows a success or celebration, you'll condition yourself to enjoying them more because they're always associated with good times.
- 'Tape record your favourite fantasies and use the tapes as part of your sex warm-up. Have it playing as you sit down for dinner, slot one into her car tapedeck and press play as you kiss her goodbye for work.
- 'Make a list of your current, favourite sex things (position, toy, lubricant, fantasy) and stick them on the bedroom mirror. Both do it and constantly update for surprise and variety.
- 'Schedule kissing sessions once a week. Take in turns to be the leader and the follower.'

Amanda Dwyer

Owner/operator of Salon Kitty's in Sydney, which specialises in fulfilling fantasies and fetishes, Amanda says:

- 'You both have to be committed to the relationship. One-sided commitment isn't enough. You also have to trust each other. If you're suspicious, you'll always find something to doubt.
- 'Be honest about your sex life and never fake it. Tell the truth but use tact and sensitivity.
- 'Don't discuss former lovers in bed. If you must, do it some place else.
- 'Always practise safe sex until you're absolutely positive your lover is only involved with you.
- 'Look after your personal hygiene. Use deodorant, a mouthwash and shower regularly. Don't clutter the bedroom or other places you make love in with smelly old gym shoes and clothes thrown all over the floor.'

Jake Kubic

Jake is 26 and has been in a lusty, loving relationship for two years. He says:

- 'Keep each other on your toes and don't ever assume they'll never leave you. Recognise that you're both attractive to other people.
- 'Have common interests outside the bedroom. *Do* things together, not just shopping, going out to dinner, etc.
- 'Put some thought into your sex life. Think, "What can I do tonight to make it different?"
- 'Keep having sex even if you don't feel like it. It's a bit like exercise. Once you break the habit, it all becomes too hard.'

Grant Brecht

Psychologist and relationships expert, author and media personality, Grant Brecht of Corpsych says:

- 'There's no such thing as too tired for sex. Have it *before* you get too tired or turn yourself on mentally and have a lazy session. You don't always have to be swinging off chandeliers.
- 'Keep up the romance. In the beginning, couples are always planning picnics, dinners out, days in bed – keep them going *throughout* the relationship.
- 'Ask, continually, what turns your partner on and off. Communication is so important – it's commonsense to talk about sex but lots of people don't. Let your partner know you enjoy and value the lusty part of your intimacy. Don't just say, "I love you", say, "I think you're sexy."
- 'Look after the whole of the relationship. Make sure you've got a good balance in your life between work, play, time together, time alone.
- 'Switch on to the things you find sexy about your partner and use those thoughts and perceptions to turn yourself on when they're not around.'

Di Palmer

Manager of Club Femme (Sydney), the biggest chain of women's erotica stores in Australia, Di Palmer says:

- 'Think erotically. Sensuality is learnt. Constantly tell yourself, "I am sexually powerful and I love it, I am sensual and I love it." Don't give that power away to *anyone,* not even your partner. If your relationship isn't loving, caring and trusting, ask yourself, What the hell am I doing in it?
- 'Be open-minded. Be prepared to experiment: what was a turn-off with your last partner, might be a real turn-on with this one.
- 'Pull out all the stops and props when you really want to seduce each other. Light candles (they're flattering and great if you're body-conscious), wear lingerie or underwear that makes you *feel* as well as look sexy, experiment with body oils, try out some sex aids, play sexy music, put on an erotic video.
- 'Take him on a sex tour to find out what *really* turns men on. Go to a live peep show together, a strip show or a club that has tabletop-dancing. See how the female sex workers revel in their sexuality, unashamedly exposing their genitals. Learn from them. Men want to see your genitals spread: if you can reach that stage and be totally unembarrassed, he'll adore you.
- 'Wear duo-balls (balls you insert inside the vagina) while you're out to dinner. Tell him you've got them in; if the tablecloth's long enough for privacy, he can reach over and tug the string.'

Cheryl Nobel

Cheryl, 68, is retired and has enjoyed a happy sex life for 51 years with her husband. She says:

- 'Look after your health. You need energy to enjoy good sex.
- 'Keep the memories strong. Look at old photos together, reminisce about the great sex you had in the past. Pinpoint what made those times special and try to recreate them.
- 'Splash out on sexy night clothes. Whatever you wear to bed should be flattering.
- 'Stay young mentally. Be open to your partner's desires, find out what pleases them, then *do it*.

- 'Don't be unfaithful. If you find someone else attractive, weigh up what you'll lose and what you'll gain. As you get older, the devil you know is a safer bet than the devil you don't.
- 'Don't get upset if you're not having regular sex. If it's only once a fortnight, fine. Go for quality not quantity by making that one night really special. Have dinner outside, dress up, make a wonderful meal and make sex *outside* the dessert.'

GOOD VIBRATIONS: SEX TOYS TRIED AND TESTED

Will sex aids send you to heaven or the nearest hospital? Are they a waste of time and money or a wickedly easy way to electrify your sex life? If the question is 'Why use sex aids?' the answer has to be 'Why not?' After all, they've been around for the last 2500 years and show no signs of disappearing! The ancient Egyptians used dildos, the Romans made candles in the shape of (rather enormous) penises and the ancient Chinese invented the first 'cock ring' by binding the base of the penis with silk. According to the erotica shops I canvassed, sex aids, particularly *female* sex toys, are selling as fast as Big Mac's. While they'll never replace the 'real thing', say the managers, they put people in control of their own sexuality.

Today's toys are much more than playthings. The humble vibrator can be a lifeline for women who've had problems having an orgasm and many of the new aids are designed to improve vaginal muscle control. For every woman who squeals in horror at the mere mention of a sex toy, there's another who won't leave home without hers. Join the club. Don't just have a giggle at the hens' night, buy some of those strap-on dildos and balls that rattle noisily around inside. Men have more than a passing fascination with any type of sex toy and the thought of you being even remotely interested in trying one will get him *very* excited.

Rather than waste valuable pounds on an expensive aid, buy a few cheaper items to start with. A lot of the time, it's the novelty factor that appeals. If you enjoy these, then it's worth making a larger investment. Don't know where to start? Take a tip from the people who bravely volunteered (well, were bribed) to tell all about their trip to toyland . . .

Desensitising Spray

Cost: £10 – £25 (bought from a sex shop)
What is it?A spray-on potion designed to prolong his erection.
Tester: Peter, 32.
Satisfaction guaranteed? 'A friend recommended it, so I thought I'd give it a try. I put a bit on the end of my penis and massaged it in but it did nothing the first time. The second time, I slathered it on and felt a weird tingling sensation but that time it did work. I stayed harder for longer. No complaints.'

Fun Tongue

Cost: £35 (bought from a women's erotica shop)
What is it? A bizarre, cylindrical contraption with a tongue protruding from one end. It's designed to simulate oral sex and devotees swear it's as good as the real thing – if you can stop laughing for long enough to take it seriously. Insert lubricant into a special compartment and set the (washable) tongue on one of five settings. It licks up and down, side to side or moves in and out.
Tester: Susie, 40.
Satisfaction guaranteed? 'I saw it in the window of a sex aid shop and thought, "I've got to have it." I tried it on my hand and it felt sensational. The first time, I put on some crotchless knickers, dimmed the lights and watched in a mirror but it looked so ridiculous, I couldn't stop laughing. From then on, I closed my eyes. It's wild! It feels and licks like the real thing but it doesn't look the best. A friend of mine said he'd shoot it if he saw one lying on the side of the road.'

Push Pearl Vibrator

Cost: £55 (bought through mail order)
What is it? It's one of Australia's most popular vibrators with 'pearls' in the shaft that rotate in dizzy circles and a clitoral stimulator that also vibrates.
Tester: Marie, 31.
Satisfaction guaranteed? 'I saw a show on vibrators on TV and

thought the clitoral attachment thing would make me orgasm more often. I tried it inside and the rotating beads felt quite amazing but although the clitoral stimulator was buzzing madly, nothing happened. Then I used it outside, pressed it against my clitoris and *wow!* The only problem is it makes orgasm so easy, you forget how to have one any other way.'

Pink Pleasure Balls

Cost: £6.99 (bought from a sex shop)
What is it? Commonly known as duo balls, they're soft, prickly latex covered metal balls (the size of a golf ball), joined by a string. (Picture a kinky version of Click-Clacks that kids play with.) Inserted into the vagina they move around, supposedly making you feel sexy. Manufacturers also claim they help with muscle control.
Tester: Catherine, 23.
Satisfaction guaranteed? 'They were a present and I unwrapped them in front of my mother – I almost killed the friend who gave them to me, but thought, "Hey, give it a go." I slathered them with lubricant and inserted the first one, waited a bit, then put the second one in as well. A "tampon" string hangs down to get them out again. I felt full up, like I was walking around with a big penis inside. I couldn't walk naturally and took them out after about three minutes. Boring!'

Fur Play

Cost: £15 – £30 (bought from a women's erotica shop)
What is it? Designed for slaves to fashion as well as light bondage, the fur trimmed tie-me-up kit ensures you'll look trendy even when strapped to the bed starkers.
Testers: Simon, 24, and Linda, 29.
Her satisfaction guaranteed? 'Simon had been harping on for ages about tying me up so I bought him the kit for his birthday. Boy, was he impressed! It's really easy to use, feels soft and comfortable and we both found it a hell of a turn-on. It's our favourite (if only) sex toy.'
His satisfaction guaranteed? 'The best present I've ever had.'

Double dildos
Cost: £25 – £42 (bought from a sex shop)
What is it? It's a double 'dong' or dildo on a white leather harness. The wearer penetrates herself, then uses the other dildo to penetrate her boyfriend anally or, if she's a lesbian, her girlfriend either anally or vaginally.
Testers: Nathan, 36, and Rachel, 24.
Her satisfaction guaranteed? 'Nathan bought it – I hid around the corner. It didn't really appeal to me at all. He wanted to give it a go first and when he strapped it on I had to fight the urge to say "Ride 'em cowboy!" He used one dildo on me vaginally and it felt all rubbery and pinched a bit at first. But I got quite a kick out of penetrating myself and using it anally on him because I could experience what it's like to penetrate someone.'
His satisfaction guaranteed? 'Rachel wasn't into it that much and I was quite disappointed. But I think she got a kick out of playing "the man". Used with tonnes of lubricant, I quite enjoyed having it up my bum. Without lubricant, it hurts like hell.'

PORNOGRAPHY: WHY IT'S WORTH ANOTHER LOOK

Alex Comfort (in the infamous sex bible *The Joy of Sex*) says pornography is 'the name given to any sexual literature somebody is trying to suppress'. He goes on to say that 'most normal people enjoy looking at sex books and reading sex fantasies – which is why abnormal people have to spend so much time and money attempting to suppress them'. I'm inclined to agree with him. I strongly believe that your standard 'girlie' porn mag and video (those not involving torture, violence or children) should be available to the public. If *you* don't like them, don't buy or rent them. But you'd be surprised how many people, women included, who do.

After numerous bizarre tests, which involved wiring people's genitals to machines, scientists have officially declared that women get as turned on as men by reading or watching sexually explicit material. *Gosh*, we're amazed! The dispute has never really been that uninhibited, liberated women aren't turned on by watching or reading sexy things. It's just that we're not really into that hard-core stuff. X-rated films are often dull, repetitive and so unbelievable, we feel like laughing not bonking. Or they're so explicit, disturbing and in-your-face, we feel like throwing up. But even if you have suffered through one of his flicks and vowed never to watch one again, here's some good news. Switch off your preconceptions and switch on that VCR because pornography has finally given birth to erotica – a much subtler, softer style of erotic material, often targeted specifically at women.

If he wants to watch an X-rated video, say yes, but you pick it. Select one made by women for women (they promote it heavily on the back – try any of the Candida Royalle range) and you won't be forced to watch degrading scenes or silly performances by perfectly formed females who orgasm just by looking at an erect penis. If you really don't feel comfortable or have extreme moral objections even to this new range, at least give an R-rated a go. Pick up an old classic (like *The Postman Always Rings Twice*) or opt for a film like *Damage*, *The Unbearable Lightness of Being* or *9 1/2 Weeks* as a compromise. For those who *do* want to use erotica and pornography as an adjunct to sex, keep the following points in mind.

Do:

- Try a few before dismissing adult films, magazines or books totally. Take it in turns to pick one and approve the decision with your partner. If you fancy one and they don't, watch it alone.
- Have it playing in the background. Often, they're too boring to watch all the way through but looking up at the 'good bits' can be fun.
- Have a laugh and don't take them seriously. It's not real sex and there's lots of misinformation in them (like women don't need foreplay and enjoy penetration above all else).

Don't:

- Think it means your partner's not happy with you. It's a bit of fun, a way to spice things up, that's all.

- Feel guilty for feeling turned on. It doesn't mean you're perverted, dirty or sick; it means you're human.
- Force people to watch it if it does nothing for them or they're morally opposed. They're not a prude for not wanting to, and they're entitled to dislike it.
- Stop your partner indulging if you don't like pornography and they do. Just tell them you'd rather they watched/read it alone and kept it out of your sight. Unless it's extremely disturbing stuff (violent, a snuff film or involving children, for instance), it's his or her business, not yours.
- Rely on pornography to turn you on. If the VCR is on every time you have sex, you're getting lazy.

THE TOP FIVE QUALITIES MEN LOOK FOR IN A SEX PARTNER

1. Personality
2. Beauty
3. Brains
4. Humour
5. Good body

THE TOP FIVE QUALITIES WOMEN LOOK FOR IN A SEX PARTNER

1. Personality
2. Humour
3. Sensitivity
4. Brains
5. Good body

13

Dear Diary, I Had Great Sex Today

Six people kiss, copulate – and keep a record

'He was this big.'

'We had sex, non-stop, for 24 hours.'

'I had 12 orgasms in a row.'

Even if we are sceptical, claims like these make our own previously satisfying thrice-a-week-and-not-always-in-the-bedroom sex lives pale by comparison. It's unnerving to think everyone else has graduated to cyber-sex while we're still stuck with typewriter-sex, even if it is a sturdy, reliable old thing. Are they telling fibs or could it really be true? Am I missing out on something?

To find out exactly what great sex means to each of us, I asked three women and three men to keep a month-long sex diary. Each person was chosen to represent different ages, sex drives and stages in relationships. They were permitted to use false names but not allowed to alter or exaggerate any details and each diary is recorded in their own words. The result: a startlingly honest mish mash of appetites and activities ranging from one extreme to the other.

All the participants were shown the completed chapter, to see their reactions to what the rest of the team had recorded. There were snorts of disbelief ('She's lifted a page from a Jackie Collins novel!') and disgust ('Ughh! If he's one of your friends, I don't want to meet him'). But there was also envy ('I wish I could swap lives') and all-round fascination. Most thought everyone else's sex life sounded more interesting than theirs. Emma wanted to 'climax in one minute' like Maria could, Maria wanted Emma's freedom. David was desperately jealous of Robert's oral-sex-with-a-view encounter, Jane felt 'utterly, depressingly' out of her league. Which all points pretty obviously to one general conclusion: comparing and trying to measure up to other people's sexual standards will do little else but leave you constantly dissatisfied. Read this to satisfy your curiosity but please yourself, not your friends.

THE SEX FILES: AN INTIMATE GLIMPSE INTO REAL-LIFE SEX LIVES

Emma

Emma, 23, is single and living in Sydney. She works in the media and is bisexual, though doesn't classify herself as such. She says she's simply 'non-discriminatory' when it comes to choosing a sex partner. Emma has had many lovers and several long-term relationships.

Week one

Ryan came over on Friday night and we went out to dinner then stayed up late talking. When we finally got to bed, it was already past 2 am. Ryan's a great friend and a wonderful lover – sensual, erotic, experienced, funny, relaxed. I love that controlled intensity of his. We fuck and it's good, but I don't come the first time and he knows this so keeps touching me until I'm wet again. When he goes down on me, he knows exactly what he's doing and he enjoys doing it – an extra turn-on. He gets hard again and I put a condom on him using my mouth, which he finds very sexy. This time, when he makes love to me, I come and that makes him come too. It's amazing. He sleeps over and when he finally leaves, I ask if he's got everything (he likes to leave his mark). Of course, he 'forgets' a T-shirt that smells of his sweat and cologne and makes me horny, reminds me of him. I think about throwing it into the laundry with my stuff but end up sleeping with it under my pillow.

Later, I seduce myself, thinking about Ryan fucking me and going down on me with that great oral technique of his. Actually, I fantasise about other things too but I always like to imagine someone I know once I start to get aroused. It makes it more intimate. I wonder how he'd feel if he knew. He'd probably like to know I was thinking about him.

Week two

I'm in Melbourne on business and I meet Mark, a smart, sexy lawyer at a work function. There's an instant spark between us, one thing leads to another and I end up back at his apartment, in his bed. (Normally, I would have waited, but I'm flying back to Sydney tomorrow and I just can't resist!) Like most men, he's a little impatient and a tad heavy-handed at first, but I manage to convey my base-level requirements for enjoyable arousal and he does a pretty good job of fulfilling them. We fuck – using a condom that he provides – and it's sexy, athletic and abandoned. He goes down on me at one stage, quite expertly, and makes me extremely horny. Later, we do it 'doggie' and by the time he comes (loudly, which is great – I like his lack of inhibition and sense of theatrics), I'm so turned on that I only have to touch myself for 30 seconds or so and I also orgasm (not quite as loudly, which is probably just as well). We doze, cosily entwined, his hard body against my soft flesh. At seven, far too early, it's time to go. I leave him sleeping, again a stranger, creep into last night's clothes and steal away, leaving nothing but a hastily penned phone number and a kiss.

Today I miss Stephen, my ex, once the Love of My Life. Back in Sydney, I go to see a film by myself and it makes me nostalgic and miss him more. I want a love with intensity. I want to feel that strongly again, to fuck someone I would die for, someone I'd want to get pregnant to. Someone I'd miss. My friend Max calls and he's sweet and concerned but I don't feel passion for him. He's a darling though and it will be good to see him. I could use some steadying. I could use some more sex, too.

Week three

I'm at work and a big bouquet of tiny pink roses arrives from Mark. I call to thank him and we arrange to catch up next time I'm in town. He's great on the phone – he's got a really sexy English accent – but I shouldn't think this way when I'm in the office. I can't wait to go to Melbourne again.

I have spent the last 24 hours on a hot date at home. Max came over and we cooked Italian, drank a bottle of good red and watched a steamy video. It was quite good but I lost attention halfway through when Max took his shirt off. It was a shameless bid for my attention – and it worked. Great body. He used to have a hairy back and a white, pasty torso that reminded me of uncooked bread. But he waxes now, works out and goes to the solarium. He's too young but utterly charming and seductive, witty, quick, manually dextrous and great around the house. Kind of a nice package, don't you think? I was quite happy to go along with everything he suggested (again). I didn't like anal sex much before Max but he uses his fingers and tongue-fucks my anus and, for the first time, I actually contemplated having his penis inside my rectum. It's very addictive, what he does. Ryan called on my machine as Max was licking me and that was such a turn-on: hearing one guy on my machine saying how much he wanted me while another gives me the licking of my life. Max doesn't want me as his; we're just friends who fuck. He didn't put his shirt back on until 8.30 the *following* evening. Yum.

Ryan calls, just for a chat. We arrange to go out together next week and easily slip into friendship mode. He's the perfect escort – polite, sociable, good looking and he wears fantastic designer clothes. There's no guarantee we'll end up in bed together after our date and even if we do, we'll probably just cuddle and go to sleep. We're more friends than lovers really. Both of us know we're not soul mates but we're extremely fond of each other and I can imagine us being friends for life. If only more men were like him – most want to own you or run away.

Week four

I feel really horny tonight – it's that time of the month. I get out the trusty vibrator, read some porn to get off, go for quantity rather than quality. It's fun even though it's tacky. At least it stops me climbing the walls, gets the circulation going and I wake up satisfied. Guys – who needs them?

I've always slept with women and can't really imagine why anyone would write off half the population sexually just because they're the same sex. So when Natasha and I stay in, cooking dinner, dancing to the stereo, trying on clothes, it's natural that I start to feel horny. She comes up and starts stroking me and it feels sensual, comfortable and at the same time, very exciting. Girls having sex is still such a taboo it always gives me an illicit thrill. We kiss and her mouth is so soft, it couldn't possibly be a man. Both of us are horny but we take it slowly, like two sleepy cats. Going down on her is warm and erotic. As always, it makes me understand how guys feel – it isn't easy to give good head to a girl! I stop before she comes and she kisses me everywhere. We end up with our legs entwined and come that way. It's wild and wonderful and the best thing is, when it's over, we got back to being two girlfriends having a cosy evening. No pressure. No intimacy. I like girls, they have their own special charm, but I don't fall in love with them.

It's morning and I'm in Melbourne for the week. I'm at Mark's, trying to write this, and he's being very provocative. Later, maybe – or maybe really soon. He's shaping up rather nicely – lived up to the few phone calls we've had and we haven't stopped having sex since I got here. It's weird, the more sex I have, the more I need it and the less it seems to matter who it's with.

My sex life is . . . Exciting and satisfying – although I have my disappointments like everyone else. I know this diary makes me sound like I always have fantastic sex but I think you just caught me at a wild, wonderful time of my life. I guess you would say I'm promiscuous if you counted the number of lovers I've had but I don't think I sleep around at all. I pick my lovers very carefully because sex is extremely, extremely important to me. It's one of the most important things in my life and I put a great deal of energy into it. I'm definitely in tune with my body and my needs. Some of my friends say they envy my sex life but I think anyone can have great sex if they just learn to let go, relax and really listen to what their body is telling them. They seem so hung up on what their lovers will think if they do this or that. I say, forget the lovers, satisfy yourself first!

Jane

Jane, 32, has been seeing Brad, 27, for the past 10 months. Jane finds it difficult to trust men and has not had a relationship that's lasted more than three months since she was 18. Brad's clocked up four long-term lovers. They describe their relationship as 'shaky at best'.

Week one

I resigned from my job yesterday which was pretty nerve-racking because I'd been working there for five years. During the day, while I was waiting to see my boss, I made half a dozen phone calls to Brad so he could reassure me about what I was doing. He's very good at boosting my self-confidence. When I finally rang to tell him I'd done it, he told me he'd booked us into a five-star hotel for the night. We spent the night drinking champagne, eating room service food and making love. Brad's also very good at that. He's the only one who's ever been able to make me orgasm.

I don't know why, but I've always been uptight about sex. In my wild days, I used to hang around with a few girlfriends who I guess were quite promiscuous and I started to take a more recreational view of sex. It was probably quite good for me but I started having one-night-stands like they did and they hurt too much and put me off sex again. My friends were seriously in it for the sex but I only wanted the affection. I fell in love all the time.

Week two

My stress level's cranked up to maximum. I'm worried about whether I've done the right thing switching jobs, I've got work projects due and I'm paranoid about the weight I've put on since I gave up smoking. All of which means I don't feel particularly desirable or desiring of sex. Brad always says he doesn't want me to feel as though I have to make love but sometimes, like Thursday, I do even when I don't feel like it. It felt awful. I was so dry he can't have enjoyed it but I don't think he should pay just because I'm having a bad week.

Week three

This week was the worst on record. I start a new job then get the flu. Unfortunately, it's a bad week for Brad too. I want attention, he wants attention. So we both get it by arguing with each other – constantly. The end result is we haven't made love in eight days. Even though I'm not that fussed about sex, it makes me feel close to him. It's like the chicken and the egg thing: I can't feel close to him until we have sex but we can't because I don't feel close.
Figure that out.

Week four
All we've done is take turns at ending the relationship. One day we argue and I call it off. Then he back-pedals and it's on again. The next day, it's his turn to end it and I do the apologising. Last night, I told him I wanted him to sleep in the spare room. That's because I can deceive myself very easily when I'm asleep or half-asleep and pretend everything is okay. Ever since we started sharing a bed, we've been a very cuddly couple. In the middle of the night, I'll sometimes wake up and Brad is putting his arms around me and telling me he loves me. Even when we're fighting, I'll wake up to discover I'm wrapped around him and I forget about being angry. We did end up sleeping together in the end but that's all we did. I don't think we touched each other all night and then, this morning, he just got up and left. I'm scared. Where do we go now?

My sex life is . . . Sadly over for the moment! We're definitely off and I have no hope it will be on again. It's a shame because this was the best sex I'd ever had in terms of physical sensations. The touchy-feely side of the relationship was pretty good too. But we really are different personalities: he's laid-back and easygoing, I'm someone whose button is permanently stuck on fast-forward. I always wanted to move forward, he wanted to stop and smell the roses. Perhaps that's why he was so good in bed and I'm not.

Maria

Maria, 40, has been married to Ian, 39, for a year. She lives in Brisbane and works as a receptionist at a large community health centre. She is highly sexed and frustrated at her husband's lack of interest. She has just started having an affair with a married friend of theirs.

Week one
Had coffee with a girlfriend and we started talking about sex. I was going through one of my horny-as-hell times and trying to explain to her what it felt like. I told her I'm attracted to lots and lots of different kinds of men – often the main attraction is simply that they're new and I haven't conquered them yet. Unless a guy's really unattractive, I can usually find something about him that makes me

want him. He might look at me in a way that I know means he wants to sleep with me and that's enough to get the juices flowing. Sometimes, I'll look at his hands and imagine them dipping in and out of me. Once, I was at a barbeque and there was a guy there who was a complete jerk but he had the best body. At one stage, he took off his shirt to show us a scar and he had these fabulous back muscles and brown, gorgeous skin. I felt hot and flushed and if I could have, would have had him there and then. I think I've got more male hormones than female because men understand my feelings about sex totally. (Well, apart from my husband.) When I talk about sex to women they look at me like I'm crazy. But then, most of them don't like sex. I rarely act on my fantasies – though I would if I could get away with it.

Had another erotic dream last night about an old boyfriend. I often have dreams about guys I've dumped who want me back again. In my dreams, I'm sneaking around corners to see them, go back, then get bored again. I'm not that different in real life – once the game is over, I leave. I should never have got married because I miss the chase so much. When you're in the middle of someone pursuing you, you're so aware of your body, it feels like it's on fire. I'm like a dog on heat and if the person I'm lusting after comes near me, my body involuntarily arches toward them. That's what I miss about being married. I'm not supposed to have those thoughts anymore, I have to put a tight rein on my natural feelings.

It's funny how when Ian and I have had sex for a few nights running, it's assumed we won't do it for the next three. I looked over at him last night, all tucked in, peacefully asleep and I wondered if he really cared whether I was satisfied after sex or only interested in getting his own rocks off. Sex with Ian is fine, but that's the problem – it's just so totally, predictably, bloody okay.

Week two

It's now been five days since I last had sex. I've masturbated a billion times but feel like 'the real thing', not just me and a copy of Nancy Friday. Went to a party last night and flirted with Gary, this really old friend of ours. He's good-looking and always eyes me up and I think it's obvious we're both attracted to each other. Neither Ian or Gary's wife seem to notice, which is typical: if you're not in tune with sex, I guess you don't pick up vibes between other people either. I bet Gary would be more open to new things than Ian is. I heard a story once that he got caught fucking his secretary in the toilets at work. His wife was devastated but I was turned on. Anyone who screws someone in the toilets is into sex big time. Gary got married really young and his wife is now pregnant. I feel sorry for him. If I get that bored with Ian I can leave. He can't.

From my conversations with other people it seems to me that everyone is bored with their sex life. It's because we're all trying to be monogamous. The other day someone was saying how amazing it was that the boyfriend of this famous celebrity was caught playing around with another woman who wasn't half as attractive. I don't think it's amazing at all. Looks don't come into it: he just wanted someone new. Someone whose every move he didn't know off by heart.

I don't believe in PMT because I don't get it, but I do believe in bio-rhythms. Sometimes, I can imagine being faithful to Ian, other times it seems impossible. It's a Jekyll and Hyde thing. Reading what I've written so far now seems alien to me because I'm going through a happy-to-be-married period. Today I feel righteous and in love with Ian. We even talked about having kids. All I want to do is have slow, gentle sex with him. What a loony I am!

Week three

I'm still in my 'couldn't care less if I never got it again' mood. Had sex on Friday night but it was really frustrating because Ian was giving me oral and I was just about to come, then he did something and the delicious bit of the orgasm went and I was just left with the mechanics of it, the contractions minus the pleasure. I told Ian and he said male orgasms are always like that, that the intense, pleasurable bit lasts less than a second. Men are even more stupid than I thought. If their orgasm is so short, why are they in such a hurry to get to it? Why aren't they more into foreplay?

Ian was away on business for two days but the 'unsexy' period is coming to a close. I can feel the first stirrings of lust slowly uncoiling in my belly. It sounds dramatic but that's what it feels like. Sometimes I feel controlled by my body because desire takes over and I do things I regret later. It's like this big monster is about to take over my life again – the sheer force of my sexual urges frightens me. I really do love Ian but at those moments, I'd risk it all just to satisfy them.

Week four
I feel really nervous commiting this to paper. Remember Gary? The very-very-married-with-pregnant-wife guy I fancied? Well, I slept with him. Ian and I were round at their house on Sunday and we were all slipping into the champagne and swimming in their pool. Ian went off to the bottleshop to buy some booze and takeaways and the minute he left, Gary's wife said she wanted to pop over and see a friend who was sick. I mean, they asked for it! I felt quite embarrassed at first because it was just Gary and I in the pool. But we started chatting and flirting and next thing, he kissed me. A long, sexy, erotic French kiss. I think I knew it was coming but I was still startled. I laughingly tried to stop him but he kept kissing my neck and it was getting dark and I got so hot I didn't care anymore. He slipped his fingers inside my swimsuit and I was gone. Next minute we were frantically fucking on the side of the pool – and I mean *fucking* – and I climaxed in about one minute flat. I got up quickly afterward and was drying myself off when poor Ian came back, laden with booze, food and cigarettes. I felt guilty and sad. I've now betrayed him in reality, not just in my head.

Gary called me at work today and said he was sorry. I didn't want him to be sorry, I wanted more and I told him so. I still feel guilty but now I've thought about it, I've decided to see Gary again. Ian knows I need more from our sex life than he's giving me and yet he still doesn't make an effort. If he's not going to satisfy me, he can't expect me to be faithful. I feel bad about Gary's wife but she's never been a huge fan of mine anyway and I'm not taking him away from her permanently, just borrowing him for a few hours now and again.

My sex life is . . . Guilt-ridden. On one hand, sex gives me the very best moments of my life and I couldn't live without it; on the other, my urges get me in a lot of trouble – like the situation I'm in now. I do love Ian and would like to make it work but the 'bad girl' so often beats the 'good girl' side of me. I also feel resentful that we've slipped into 'married sex' even though we've only been married for a year. I have no idea what will happen now I'm having an affair but at least Gary's good in bed. Actually, it's not Gary, it's the forbidden part that appeals. In terms of technique, Ian's better.

Robert

Robert, 35, separated from his wife three years ago. He works as an account executive for a finance firm and describes his sex life as 'active but selective'.

Week one

I'm making love to Sarah but it's not really Sarah, it's Linda. Linda was a married woman I had an affair with over one year ago but she still haunts me. I met her through a mutual work friend at a function and we ended up getting drunk together and smooching on the balcony. Her husband was working. She was so beautiful and so unattainable, I thought that was it. But she called me soon after I met her and asked if she could drop in for coffee. So we started meeting and kissing and cuddling, then one day she came over and stripped right down to her underwear before snuggling up to me. I knew she wanted sex but I didn't want to push it. I mean, she was married and on this massive guilt-trip. We had intercourse but it felt like she wouldn't give herself fully although she had no trouble orgasming. I did – I was nervous as hell. For some reason, she didn't want much foreplay. It was like kissing, touching, then *bam!* she wanted penetration. I felt like I was starting halfway through. I'm not the sort of guy who can just drop my duds and get into it. She ended the affair soon after that so we only had intercourse three times. I knew the score. I knew she would end it but I've never forgotten her. I'd love to go out with someone as good-looking as her again and have other guys check out your girl. It's a huge ego-boost.

Sarah's probably a better fuck, if truth be told, and she gives a brilliant head job. She's the opposite to Linda: she wants a relationship and gives her all. The first time I slept with Sarah, we had sex with her six-month-old son asleep beside us. I thought it was a bit outrageous but the kid was fast asleep. It didn't turn me on at all – I actually felt quite uncomfortable and couldn't look at the child – but I admired Sarah for going for what she wanted. I'm the guilty one now. Sarah loves me and I love her but I make love to Linda whenever I touch her.

Week two

Sarah's gone away for a week with her folks so I meet some friends down at the local. There's a girl there who's exotic and very horny. We talk and I give her my phone number. She's called Cristina and is from South America. That was on Friday. On Tuesday, she called me at 11.30 pm, said she was lonely and would I like to come over. I was in bed but she said she was down, so off I went. Cristina lived in a penthouse apartment overlooking the city and her flatmates were out. She answered the door wearing a see-through lace teddy, led me to the couch, pushed me back and just went for it. Then she led me to the balcony and within five minutes of walking in the door, I was standing there, pants around my ankles, getting a head job while overlooking Sydney Harbour! She took me into her room and she had this mirror that she loved to watch herself in. She wanted it doggie style and kept on saying, 'Fuck me, fuck me like an animal.' I felt like I should write in to *Penthouse.* It was like one of those letters you read and never believe. I took her phone number but it was pretty obvious she only got off on someone new. I don't think I ever approach any sex session as just a fuck. I guess I hope they'll all lead to something. I told the guys at the pub what had happened. One of them said, 'Mate, that must have been the best sex of your life.' I guess it was because it was so unexpected but the best is always the last one you've had really. I thought my wife gave the best head job, then I thought Linda did, then Sarah. Now Cristina's in front.

Week three

Sarah's back. I expected her to be relaxed, tanned and keen for sex; instead, she's irritable and worn out because she had a shit time. Sex is awful because she's not responsive. I hate that more than anything. The worst sex I ever had was with a girl who led me from the lounge room to the bedroom by my penis. She instigated it all and I thought I was in for the ride of my life. But when I penetrated her, she lay there like a dead fish. I don't know if she was terribly pissed and it hit her then or what. She couldn't have been bored because we'd just started! Anyway, it goes down as the absolute worst sex of all and I think it's a worry that sex with Sarah reminded me of it. Sarah wants a commitment but I'm not sure I want to. I'm feeling incredibly pressured and also not sure I want to take on someone else's child. I've already got two of my own.

Week four

Cristina called and Sarah answered the phone. Neither was terribly impressed and even I wouldn't have believed the story I made up to try and get out of it. For some weird reason, Cristina was upset that I hadn't told her about Sarah. A bit much when she had her mouth wrapped around my penis before I'd even had a chance to speak! I feel guilty but pissed off for feeling like that. I've never promised Sarah a monogamous relationship – she just took it for granted – and Cristina was obviously just in it for the sex. My month ends where it started: with fantasies about Linda. Even though she was married, at least I knew where I stood.

My sex life is . . . A hell of a lot more interesting than it was when I was married. My wife was pretty conservative, and missionary was about it. I didn't have much experience before I got married so I'm making up for it now but aiming for quality, not quantity. I find women so much more liberated and in touch with their sexuality than the first time round. Sometimes it freaks me a little bit and I worry I'm not going to be able to satisfy them. I think that's why I'm so into foreplay; I feel more confident with my oral sex skills. Besides, intercourse is intercourse and most women's vaginas feel pretty much the same. There's only one girl who's stood out from the pack and she had a vice for a vagina. Her grip was incredible!

David

David, 21, admits he's 'as promiscuous as he possibly can be' and uninterested in a long-term monogamous relationship right now. He manages a gym.

Week one

Last night I was out at my usual club and made instant eye contact with a girl that oozed 'fuck me'. I got close to her and tried to pick up if the vibes were positive or negative, though even if they're negative, I'll still go for it. She started dancing so I danced with her and without speaking a word, we started kissing. I took her out to the back of my four-wheel drive and we had sex. Immediately it was over, I thought, 'Why did I bother?' I should have had a wank – it would have been much more pleasurable. The sluts never live up to expectations. There's no challenge. This girl left me, went back inside and I saw her leave to do the same thing with another guy within half an hour. When I say slut, I mean slut.

I went out with Diane tonight, a 'nice girl' I met through some friends. We had dinner and she's pretty, though pretty stupid as well. She came back to my place and it was obvious she expected sex which is weird. She comes from a well-to-do family and I thought she'd be different. I obliged but she freaked out because I couldn't come with a condom on. I never can. I have to almost get there, then pull out, take it off and finish myself off with my hand. Eighty per cent of girls don't mind but some react badly. They always think it's their fault. I can always get it up and going but ejaculating isn't the automatic process girls think it is. It goes back to when I was 17. I was with this girl and we had a wild weekend of sex and I came 21 times in three days. I don't know if it's psychological but since then, I've been pushing to come twice in a weekend. I remember feeling so drained and worn out afterward, I felt physically sick. It doesn't bother me though. Sex feels great even if I don't ejaculate.

Week two

Trish was at the club last night and I'm wondering if she's still a virgin. My best friend and I had a threesome with this girl a month ago. We met her at a party and had her outside, in full view of anyone who wanted to watch, but she'd only do oral. No penetration whatsoever. She said it was because she was a virgin and I was like, 'Yeah, right', but she loved sucking penises and she swallowed every drop. (It's a big thing swallowing. The only thing that's better is if she swallows most of it but some sperm's trickling out of her mouth. That is so hot!) I didn't for a minute believe Trish but her best friend swears it's true. She really is a virgin.

I've just had the worst sex experience of my life. I went to go down on this girl and I was hit by a cloud of odour that turned my stomach. I literally dry retched. The girl must have had a yeast infection because no-one could smell like that naturally. I still feel sick just thinking about it.

Week three

I watched a girl for two hours last night and she was something else. So beautiful and fresh. I didn't want to have sex with her; I knew I wanted a relationship just by looking at her. I blundered my way through a conversation but she's already got a boyfriend. Bummer. Despite what I sound like, I do think it's feasible to have sex with one person for the rest of your life. You'd have to love them incredibly and she'd have to be adventurous, open to new ideas and interested in doing the things I like, but it's possible. Every guy purves but I think you'd be surprised how many stay faithful when they really love their wives or girlfriends. In one sense, I'm relieved that girl had a boyfriend. I would have fallen for her for sure.

Week four

Writing this diary has made me think about my sex life. I counted up how many women I've slept with over the past year and didn't know whether to boast or be horrified. I go through periods where I'm picking up two to three girls a week for three to four months. Then I start feeling really dirty and think, 'Slow down. You're hurting people.' You bonk girls once and they want you to call them so I usually take them out one more time. But then, they want more and say 'Didn't that mean anything to you?' How do you tell them, 'No, the sex didn't and you didn't'? I don't mean to hurt them but I know I do.

My sex life is . . . Totally wild and depraved. I don't think I'll ever get sick of seeing a girl naked; I don't think men ever get over it even if they've been with the same woman for years. Single sex is better than the sex I had with a three-year live-in girlfriend. When she said no to sex, I used to feel very disheartened. I'd think, 'I'm losing it. She doesn't want me' and I'd never be sure if she was doing it to wield power over me, like 'I've got what you want but you can't have it'. I'd love to have sex several times a day – it doesn't matter that I couldn't ejaculate most of the time. My worst nightmare would be to fall in love with some girl who only wanted missionary-style sex. I hate it. I like doing it doggie-style because that's the only chance I have of coming.

Stephen

Stephen, 28, has been married for two years. He's a stockbroker and says he loves his wife more now than when they first got married.

Week one

I arrive home from a 14-hour work day and Jess is in a mad panic, running around with her underwear on because she's late meeting a girlfriend. I try to talk her into a quickie because she looks so sexy but no way. She won't even laugh with me. I get out a porn video (Jess hates them) and have a wank instead. When she comes home, she's tipsy and sits on my lap and gives me a deep kiss, using her tongue. Ironically, now it's me who can't be bothered. The day's caught up with me.

The next morning I wake up 'pee-proud' (my grandmother's term for a morning erection). I wake Jess by stroking and licking her back but she's hungover and not interested. I try really hard not to act pissed off but she knows I am and gets shitty herself. Somehow, this turns into a huge row and ruins the weekend.

Week two

The three-day war is over and Jess finally lets me have sex with her. She's really wet and I have to think about football to stop orgasming within a second. It's funny, even though she's really lubricated I get the feeling she's not really into it. Afterward, we watch the soaps and she's asleep within two minutes. I guess she was tired.

Jess's best friend has the best body I've ever seen in the flesh. She knows it and always wears the shortest skirts. Tanya was bending over at a lunch and she's got the most fabulous legs: no lumpy bits, just smooth flesh. Jess caught me watching, leant over and felt to see if I had an erection. It was certainly getting there. She was Not Impressed and announced to the whole table what had happened. I laughed it off but was totally pissed off. We had a huge row when we got home, so – no sex *again.*

Week three

Jess's sexual calendar is so predictable, I could literally circle the days when she'll feel like it and when she won't. The week before her period she turns into this intense nympho and screws really seriously, closes her eyes and concentrates like this is the last time ever. Jess also likes sex during her period and I have to pretend I do too. Actually, I hate it but Jess is a real feminist and if I dared to admit I'm turned off by menstrual blood I'd never hear the end of it.

My boss has just got a new secretary. She flirted with me today and asked me to go to lunch. I said fine, I like having women as friends, but made it very clear I was married and very happily so. Her behaviour changed after that – she wasn't interested in getting to know me as a person, just a potential Mr Right. Stupid woman. It really annoyed me.

Week four
I'm raring to go and so is Jess – a rare moment in our household. She pulls on this amazing two-piece underwear thing, all white and virginal, which she knows I love. She gives me a massage and I'm so tense and it feels so good, I almost lose the urge and just want to sleep. But then her tongue flicks over my penis and it responds, though not as quick as my brain does, so I move down on her. I love giving Jess oral. I love the smell of her. If I could bottle her vaginal juices I would. Sometimes, if she's really turned on and climaxes loudly, I'll almost come without any stimulation of my genitals at all. This session is so good, I feel really vulnerable afterward. I bury my nose in her hair and pray to God she'll never leave me.

My sex life is . . . Up and down but satisfying. I guess it reflects our relationship. We argue a lot which stops us having sex as often as I'd like but that's okay; I like Jess's spirit and married a passionate woman. I have no desire for sex with anyone else. Jess turns me on as much now as she did when I first met her and I don't see why her appeal will ever wear off. We're experimenting more now and she's not backward in coming forward about her desires. I think I scored lucky!

Appendix: A Sex Dictionary

'Those G-spot things sound great – where do you buy one?' Read this and you won't be the one who says it

abortion: Prematurely ending a pregnancy, usually through an operation called a termination.

AIDS (acquired immune deficiency syndrome): A condition caused by the human immunodeficiency virus (HIV) where the body loses its ability to defend itself against illness. The most feared sexually transmitted infection of all but avoided by using condoms and practising safer sex.

anal intercourse: When a man inserts his penis into his partner's anus. Some people's idea of heaven, others of hell.

aphrodisiac: Any substance believed to stimulate or enhance sexual desire. Everything from oysters and champagne to ground-up goat's toenails has been touted as one. Some work psychologically, few actually do anything.

areola: The pinky-brown bit surrounding the nipple.

arousal: Getting excited or turned on. The physiological and mental changes that happen to our body when someone we fancy touches us in all the right places.

A-spot: The 'anterior fornex erogenous', an extremely sensitive section of the front vaginal wall, about one-third of the way down from the cervix. The G-spot's neighbour.

bestiality: If your neighbour confesses to it, lock up your dog. It means they enjoy sex with animals.

bisexual: Being attracted to both John and Jane – and not really minding which one you end up with.

blow job: The everyday term for her giving him oral sex. The posh term is 'fellatio'.

bondage: Tying someone up before having your wicked way with them or vice versa.

breasts: Two, frequently ogled, mounds of flesh found at chest level on women. Breasts come in all different shapes and sizes and you can buy a new pair if you don't like your own.

buttocks: The fleshy, muscular cheeks of our bottoms that frequently dictate our jean size.

casual sex: Short-term affairs spent mostly in the bedroom.

CAT (coital alignment technique): A new way to have intercourse that involves rolling rather than thrusting.

celibacy: Voluntarily abstaining from sex for reasons the rest of us can't fathom.

cervix: The neck of the uterus which connects it to the vagina. Otherwise known as the bit that hurts when hit by an over-enthusiastic, long penis.

chemistry: The X-factor, the I-don't-know-why-I-like-him-I-just-do thing. Chemistry is God's way of ensuring we all don't fancy the same person since a healthy dose of it can make an ugly duckling seem like a swan to someone who's tuned into their vibes.

circumcision: Removal of the foreskin of the penis, usually done at birth for religious or 'hygienic' reasons. Now considered somewhat barbaric and unnecessary.

climax: Orgasm, coming, going off. The point during sex when someone could cut your big toe off and you wouldn't notice.

clitoris: A little, pea-sized organ at the top of a woman's vulva which becomes erect when stimulated. Plays a huge part in the process that leads to orgasm. Find hers, treat it with respect and she's yours forever.

come: Slang for the semen he ejaculates on orgasm. 'Coming' is slang for orgasm.

come out: A short form for 'coming out of the closet' or openly admitting you're gay – when you realise all that bending over with a low-cut top on was totally wasted on your best friend's flatmate.

compatibility: Sharing the same interest and outlook on life as your partner. *Dick and Dora are very compatible because they both like dressing up in latex.*

condom: A thin rubber sheath designed to stop sperm and nasty germs entering the vagina. Unfortunately, they don't work unless you take them out of the packet and place them over an erect penis before having intercourse.

contraception: Things you swallow, insert or put on to stop getting pregnant.

crotch: The genital area that both sexes emphasise with tight, body-hugging clothing if they think they've got something worth advertising.

cunnilingus: Giving her head, going down on her. The correct term for oral sex that no-one uses because they either can't pronounce it or think it's rude.

deep throat: A term inspired by the bottomless-mouthed porn queen, Linda Lovelace. She was able to take the entire length of the penis into her mouth and throat without gagging. The rest of us find our tonsils get in the way.

deviation: Any form of sexual activity considered to be abnormal by the majority of the population.

dildo: An artificial erect penis used for masturbation.

douche: A device for squirting water or other liquid into the vagina to cleanse it. Totally useless and quite harmful since the liquid often mucks up the natural pH level in the vagina.

ejaculation: Shooting your load, coming. The ejection of semen from the penis through a series of pleasurable, muscular contractions.

erection: Getting a hard-on, cracking a fat or a stiffy. The swelling and stiffening of the penis (or clitoris or nipples) during sexual stimulation.

erogenous zones: Parts of the body especially sensitive to sexual stimulation, differing dramatically from person to person and the situation. His forehead may turn into an erogenous zone if Pamela Anderson's the one touching it.

erotica: Something (usually a book, magazine, video or sex aid) that tastefully turns us on and makes us feel like having sex. (We call tasteless turn-ons pornography.)

erotic massage: Specific massage techniques that concentrate on the genitals.

ESO (extended sexual orgasms) technique: A long and involved (but worth trying) series of techniques designed to make your orgasms last longer.

exhibitionist: A sexual show-off. Someone who likes others watching them. Having sex on your dining table with the blinds open in full view of the neighbours innocently watching 'The Simpsons' is exhibitionistic behaviour.

Family Planning clinic: A special clinic that provides information and advice about contraception and all sex related matters.

fantasy: Imagining sexual situations or events involving real or imaginary people. The official term for those X-rated daydreams you amuse yourself with on the bus.

fellatio: Blow job, sucking him off. Using your tongue and mouth to excite his penis terribly.

fertile: Being able to fall pregnant or capable of making someone pregnant.

fetish: A sexual behaviour where the handling of a specific, often inanimate object (like rubber clothing or pre-worn panties) is necessary for sexual satisfaction. If he can only orgasm if you wear your high heels to bed, he's got a shoe fetish.

fidelity: Resisting going home with the best-looking guy at the party because you'd upset the one you already have. Staying faithful.

foreplay: Petting, feeling each other up, playing with each other. The stuff most people get up to before intercourse but should do during and after as well.

foreskin: The retractable fold of skin covering the tip of the penis on uncircumcised men that hurts if you yank it back too quickly.

frenulum: The string of particularly sensitive skin where the head of the penis meets the shaft. It's on the underside (the side closest to his testicles) and well worth introducing yourself to.

frigid: An outdated, Victorian term used to describe women who aren't interested in sex. Only used today by drunk men in pubs to explain why the woman they attempted to bonk wasn't interested.

gay: Homosexual, camp. This used to be a blanket term for all homosexuals but is now mainly used to describe men who are attracted to or have sexual relations with other men. Female homosexuals generally prefer being called 'lesbian'.

genitals: The external sex organs – a man's penis and testicles, a woman's labia, clitoris and vagina.

group sex: More than two people having sex with each other at the same time. Works a treat in fantasies, has a tendency to backfire in reality.

G-spot: A hot spot discovered by the German physician Dr Ernst Grafenberg. It's a small, slightly raised, sensitive area about 5 to 6 cm inside the vagina on the front wall.

hard on: *See* erection.

head (of the penis): The mushroom-shaped bit at the top of the penis that's softer than a baby's bottom.

heterosexual: People who are only being sexually attracted to the opposite sex. If you're female and can't have John, you wouldn't even consider Jane.

HIV (Human Immunodeficiency Virus): The virus that causes AIDS.

homophobes: People who are incredibly rude to and about homosexuals because they have psychological hang-ups about them.

homosexual: People who are attracted to people of the same sex.

hormone: A chemical substance produced by an endocrine gland which plays an important part in sexual and reproductive functions and alters moods. Why one day you feel like being Madame Lash, the next Mother Theresa.

hymen: A thin membrane that partly covers the entrance to the vagina before a woman first has intercourse. The hymen used to be considered proof a woman was a virgin. These days, tampons and physical exercise break it more often than penises do.

impotence: Not being able to get it up, the inability to achieve an erection. *Brewer's droop* is a term used to describe not being able to get an erection after one too many drinks.

inhibitions: Thoughts, morals or feelings that stop you letting loose and enjoying sex to the full.

Kama Sutra: Possibly the world's first sex manual and a literary classic. Written by Vatsyana in the fourth to fifth centuries AD.

Kegels: Exercises designed to strengthen the pubococcygeal muscle (PC) which controls the size and grip of the vagina. Men also have a PC muscle and should also exercise it.

kinky: Something sexual you do that others would love to but haven't the courage.

Kinsey (the Kinsey Institute): World respected American sexperts.

K-Y Jelly: The brand name of a popular water-based lubricant.

labia: The lips of the female genitals. The small ones are called the 'labia minora', the larger outer ones the 'labia majora'.

lesbian: A woman who has sexual relations with another woman.

libido: The desire or urge to have sex, your 'sex drive'.

love: A very strong feeling of attachment or desire to someone or something. Often confused with 'lust' (see below).

lubrication: Oils, creams or gels which are used to add moisture to the genital area to reduce friction and make sex more comfortable. Any couple who are serious about sex have some in their bathroom or bedside cabinet. K-Y Jelly is a lubricant.

lust: A strong desire to bonk someone. The havoc-wreaking emotion that makes us go for the hunk on the Harley over the sensible accountant our mother wants us to date.

making love: Having sex with someone you're happy to wake up with in the morning as opposed to simply having sex.

masochist: Someone who gets pleasure from pain.

Masters and Johnson: Pioneer sex researchers.

masturbation: Playing with yourself, frigging (means 'to rub' in Latin). Stimulating your own genitals to achieve orgasm. Mutual masturbation is when you and your partner stimulate each other's genitals.

ménage à trois: The French term for a threesome.

menstruation: Period. The monthly discharge of blood that takes place if no eggs are fertilised.

missionary: The most famous, most used position for intercourse. He lies on top of her.

monogamy: Only having sex with one person over a specific period of time.

mons pubis or mound of Venus: The soft, mound-shaped pad of fat, covered in hair, that cushions the woman's pubic bone so it doesn't hurt when he's on top.

Morning After Pill (MAP): A pill containing a high dose of oestrogen that can prevent pregnancy if taken up to 72 hours after unprotected intercourse.

necrophiliacs: Seriously weird people who want to have sex with dead bodies.

nipple: The tip of the breast that becomes erect if sexually stimulated (or it's bloody freezing).

Nonoxynol-9: A chemical present in most spermicides. It kills the HIV virus in laboratories, but unfortunately doesn't appear to be as successful in real life.

normal: Like everyone else, average, not different. The most commonly asked sex question in relation to any behaviour is 'Am I normal?' Somehow, being 'normal' makes people feel better. Strange, when normal often equates to boring.

nymphomaniac: A woman who wants lots of sex or sex with more than one man. Commonly used by men to describe a girlfriend who wants it more than they feel like providing.

oral sex: Using the mouth to stimulate the genitals. *See also* cunnilingus, fellatio.

orgasm: Climax, coming. The peak of sexual excitement usually accompanied by muscular contractions.

orgy: A wild, abandoned group sex experience usually involving excessive drinking and drugs. A favourite in Roman times and Joan Collins films. Good luck finding one outside California.

ovaries: The two female sex glands on either side of the uterus.

ovulation: The monthly release of an ovum (egg) from an ovary.

Pap test: A smear test used to screen against cancer, particularly cancer of the cervix. If you're over 16, sexually active and female, you should be having them regularly.

PC muscle: *See* Kegels.

penetration: Putting something inside something, him 'entering' you. Usually used to describe the insertion of his penis into a vagina or anus.

penis: The erectile male sex organ. The long, hard thing that prods you in the back while you're trying to sleep.

perineum: In women, the area between the vagina and the anus; in men, the area between the scrotum and the anus. In both, a highly charged sexual area.

period: *See* menstruation.

pervert: Anyone who gets sexual satisfaction from doing something unusual. Definitions of 'perverted' behaviour vary depending on who's using the word. To a 96-year-old virgin, tongue-kissing may be seen as perverted. To a 21-year-old male, smearing chocolate sauce all over his girlfriend's body and licking it off while she's tied to the fridge isn't.

petting: Feeling each other up. *See also* foreplay.

pheromones: Substances secreted by the body, with an often undetectable odour, that stimulate sexual desire in others. Perfumes attempt to simulate the effect of natural pheromones; some are more successful than others.

Pill, the: A tiny tablet that turned a set of sexual mores upside down. Taken daily and correctly, it's an oral contraceptive that stops women getting pregnant.

platonic relationship: A close relationship between two people that doesn't involve sex. Liking but not lusting after someone.

pornography: Material designed to stimulate sexual excitement that's rarely left on people's coffee tables. Hard core porn is explicit, nothing-left-to-the-imagination stuff. Soft-core porn doesn't require any imagination either but you don't get to see any pink bits.

pre-come or pre-ejaculatory fluid: The stuff that comes out of his penis before the real whoosh. Mother Nature thoughtfully provided it so the penis slips easily into the vagina.

pregnant: Knocked up, having a bun in the oven, about to have a baby. A time of great joy or desperation depending on the woman it happens to and what's happening in her life.

premarital sex: Sex between two people who aren't married. What just about everyone under the age of 25 is doing. Extramarital sex is sex between two people when one, or both, are already married to someone else. What lots of people over the age of 25 are doing.

premature ejaculation: When he ejaculates before his partner or he are finished with his erect penis. This could be before he's even penetrated, three thrusts in or an hour later – it all depends on what the couple's definition of 'too early' is.
promiscuity: Sleeping with lots of people on a casual basis. Promiscuous to one person might mean three partners a year, another might define it as more than three a week.
prostate gland: The male gland that surrounds the neck of the bladder and the urethra. The male G-spot (found in his rectum).
prostitute: Someone who gets paid for having sex. Women or men who marry purely for money aren't called prostitutes but they technically fit the definition.

quickie: Sex in a hurry, usually when both of you are so hot you don't need foreplay and want penetration NOW!

rape or sexual abuse: To force someone, either with violence or verbal threats, to have any type of sexual contact against their will.
rear entry: Him penetrating her from behind.
rubber: Slang for condom.

sadism: When a person gains pleasure from inflicting pain or 'disciplining' another. S and M is short for 'sadism and masochism', getting turned on by inflicting and/or receiving pain.
safe period: The stage in a woman's menstrual cycle when she's least likely to get pregnant.
safe sex: Sex that carries a relatively low risk of contracting STIs or HIV, like kissing, mutual masturbation or using a condom during other activities.
scrotum: The pouch of loose, wrinkled skin that contains a man's testicles.
semen: The mixture of sperm and seminal fluid ejaculated from a man's penis during orgasm. We usually say sperm but the correct term is semen.

sex aid or toy: Any object used to generate or enhance sexual arousal and/or orgasm. If a jar of Vegemite puts a twinkle in your eye when used in a certain way, it's a sex aid.

sex drive: *See* libido.

sex therapist: A psychologist who is specially trained to solve your sexual problems. A good one is worth their weight in gold.

shaft: The length of the penis.

69er: Two people simultaneously giving each other oral sex. The position they adopt – head to toe – resembles the number 69 when viewed from certain angles.

sleeping with someone: A euphemism usually meaning you did everything but.

smegma: A smelly, cheese-like substance that accumulates under the foreskin of an uncircumcised male or under the hood of a woman's clitoris because of poor hygiene. Capable of putting either sex off oral sex for good.

sodomy: Anal intercourse.

sperm: The male reproductive cell. Millions of sperm are produced in the testicles and mixed with seminal fluid before being ejaculated from the penis.

spermicide: A substance placed in the vagina or used with condoms or diaphragms to kill the hardy little buggers.

squeeze technique: A method of curing premature ejaculation where a man or his partner squeezes the head of the penis before he reaches the point where ejaculation is inevitable.

STD: *See* STI. STD is the old term for STI. They dropped 'disease' and replaced it with 'infection' because it sounds less off-putting.

STI (sexually transmitted infection): Infections that are passed from one person to another during some form of sex. Not high on anyone's wish list.

straight: *See* heterosexual.

stripping: Removing your clothes provocatively rather than yanking them off willy-nilly and leaving them in a heap at the end of the bed.

swinging: Partner swapping with other singles or couples. Dangerous stuff.

testicles: Balls, nuts, testes. The two male sex glands carried in the scrotum that manufacture sperm and produce sex hormones. Extremely sensitive, they produce a pain quite unlike any other if knocked or kicked.

testosterone: The primary male sex hormone responsible for the male sex drive. Women also produce it and it's responsible for our sex drive as well.

thrusting: The act of him pushing his penis in and out of a vagina or anus.

transsexual: A man or woman who feels they are really a member of the opposite sex trapped in the wrong body. Many undergo sex change operations.

transvestite: A man (sometimes a woman) who has a compulsion to cross-dress (i.e., dress in the clothes of the opposite sex). Him popping on your dressing-gown to get you both a cup of tea on a cold winter morning doesn't make him a transvestite.

uncut: An uncut penis is one which is uncircumcised.

unprotected sex: Sex without a condom which puts you at risk of pregnancy and STIs.

urethra: The tube through which urine is passed from the bladder. In men, it's also the tube through which semen is ejaculated.

uterus: The womb. A tranquil place where the baby lives until it's ready to face the world. Not surprisingly, most refuse to budge and have to be pushed out.

vagina: The soft, short passage that leads from a woman's vulva to her cervix. Also the bit where he puts his bit during intercourse.

vas deferens: Either of the two tubes that carry sperm from the testicles.

vasectomy: A male sterilisation procedure that cuts or seals the vas deferens so sperm can't pass into the semen.

VD (venereal disease): An old-fashioned term for STIs.

vibrator: Battery or electrically powered device, often penis-shaped, that's used to stimulate the genitals. Guaranteed to fall out of a cupboard when your mother-in-law visits.

virgin: Any person who has not had sexual intercourse.

voyeur: Peeping Tom. Someone who enjoys watching others have sex (often more than doing it themselves).

vulva: The external sex organs of a woman. Everything you can see.

water sports: Playing polo or volleyball in water, skiing on top of it – or having sex that somehow involves urination.

wet dreams: Previously used to describe a nocturnal experience which made men involuntarily ejaculate in their sleep and stick the sheets together. Now, sexperts believe women have wet dreams too (though they're a lot less messy). Any dream where either sex is so turned on, they have an orgasm in their sleep or wake during the throes of one.

withdrawal method: A somewhat risky method of contraception where he agrees to remove his penis from the vagina just when he's enjoying being in there the most.

Xmas: The time of the year when no-one has sex very much because they're either (a) too drunk, (b) too full, or (c) too broke to go out and get some.

Index